Yauf friedrich
Reckmir

QL1211890025.7

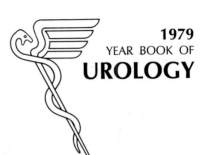

1979
YEAR BOOK OF
UROLOGY

THE 1979 YEAR BOOKS

The YEAR BOOK series provides in condensed form the essence of the best of the recent international medical literature. The material is selected by distinguished editors who critically review more than 500,000 journal articles each year.

Anesthesia: *Drs. Eckenhoff, Bart, Brunner, Holley and Linde.*

Cancer: *Drs. Clark, Cumley and Hickey.*

Cardiology: *Drs. Harvey, Kirkendall, Kirklin, Nadas, Paul and Sonnenblick.*

Dentistry: *Drs. Hale, Hazen, Moyers, Redig, Robinson and Silverman.*

Dermatology: *Dr. Dobson.*

Diagnostic Radiology: *Drs. Whitehouse, Bookstein, Gabrielsen, Holt, Martel, Silver and Thornbury.*

Drug Therapy: *Drs. Azarnoff, Hollister and Shand.*

Endocrinology: *Drs. Schwartz and Ryan.*

Family Practice: *Dr. Rakel.*

Medicine: *Drs. Rogers, Des Prez, Cline, Braunwald, Greenberger, Bondy and Epstein.*

Neurology and Neurosurgery: *Drs. DeJong and Sugar.*

Nuclear Medicine: *Drs. Quinn and Spies.*

Obstetrics and Gynecology: *Drs. Pitkin and Zlatnik.*

Ophthalmology: *Dr. Hughes.*

Orthopedics and Traumatic Surgery: *Dr. Coventry.*

Otolaryngology: *Drs. Strong and Paparella.*

Pathology and Clinical Pathology: *Drs. Carone and Conn.*

Pediatrics: *Drs. Oski and Stockman.*

Plastic and Reconstructive Surgery: *Drs. McCoy, Brauer, Dingman, Hanna, Haynes and Hoehn.*

Psychiatry and Applied Mental Health: *Drs. Romano, Freedman, Friedhoff, Kolb, Lourie and Nemiah.*

Sports Medicine: *Drs. Quigley, Anderson, Krakauer, Marshall and Mr. George.*

Surgery: *Drs. Schwartz, Najarian, Peacock, Shires, Silen and Spencer.*

Urology: *Drs. Gillenwater and Howards.*

The YEAR BOOK of

Urology

1979

Edited by
JAY Y. GILLENWATER, M.D.
*Professor and Chairman, Department of Urology, University of
Virginia School of Medicine*

and

STUART S. HOWARDS, M.D.
*Professor, Department of Urology, University of Virginia School
of Medicine*

YEAR BOOK MEDICAL PUBLISHERS, INC.
CHICAGO • LONDON

Printed in U.S.A.

Library of Congress Catalog Card Number: CD38-103

International Standard Book Number: 0-8151-3469-X

Introduction

The YEAR BOOK of UROLOGY has become one of the most widely read books in the field under the editorships of W. W. Scott and John T. Grayhack. More than 3,000 articles were reviewed and approximately 10% were abstracted for the 1979 YEAR BOOK. It is a challenge for us to continue the high standards set by Doctors Scott and Grayhack. Their comments on the articles were excellent and were enjoyed and valued by the readers. We elected to continue this feature and asked eight consultants to assist us: Drs. Roscoe R. Robinson, Robert A. Gutman, Calvin M. Kunin, Patrick C. Walsh, E. Darracott Vaughan, Jr., Donald C. Martin, Carl A. Olsson and William E. Bradley. We extend to them our warmest appreciation.

Jay Y. Gillenwater, M.D.
Stuart S. Howards, M.D.

Table of Contents

The material covered in this volume represents literature reviewed up to February, 1979.

General Considerations

Studies of Introital Colonization in Women with Recurrent Urinary Infections: X. Adhesive Properties of *Escherichia coli* and *Proteus mirabilis*—Lack of Correlation with Urinary Pathogenicity. The ability of a bacterial strain to adhere to the vaginal and urinary mucosa seems to be important in the pathogenesis of urinary infection. Jackson E. Fowler, Jr. and Thomas A. Stamey[1] (Stanford Univ.) examined the adhesive properties of various strains of *Escherichia coli* and *Proteus mirabilis* of known clinical virulence to evaluate the importance of this factor in determining ability of a bacterial strain to colonize the urinary tract. Bacterial adherence to vaginal epithelial cells was measured in vitro for 37 strains of *E. coli* and 18 strains of *P. mirabilis* isolated from the anus, bladder and renal pelvis. *Escherichia coli* strains were from women with frequent lower urinary tract infections and *P. mirabilis* strains were from patients having nephrolithotomy for renal pelvic stones. Vaginal epithelial cells were collected from normal women.

No correlation was evident between the adhesive properties of the bacterial strains and their clinical pathogenicity (Fig 1). The difference in adhesive properties between the *E. coli* and *P. mirabilis* strains was only weakly significant. The in vitro measure of bacterial adherence was found to be quite reproducible.

These findings suggest that host factors determining bacterial adherence are more important than bacterial adhesive factors in determining susceptibility to urinary infections. Different strains of *E. coli* adhere to vaginal cells with varying affinity and the capacity of different *P. mirabilis* strains to adhere to vaginal cells is markedly vari-

---

(1) J. Urol. 120:315–318, September, 1978.

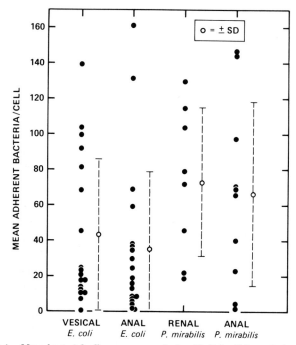

Fig 1.—Mean bacterial adherence per vaginal epithelial cell for vesical and anal *E. coli* and renal and anal *P. mirabilis*. (Courtesy of Fowler, J. E., Jr., and Stamey, T. A.: J. Urol. 120:315–318, September, 1978.)

able. Such host factors as the presence of vaginal antibody specific for anal bacteria and perhaps unrecognized virulence factors of fecal bacteria may help determine the ability of bacterial strains to colonize the vaginal introitus and urinary tract.

▶ [This study provides evidence against the notion that certain bacteria have "uropathic" properties which permit them to colonize the periurethral region and invade the urinary tract. Stamey and his group have marshalled considerable evidence that local host factors are more important.—Calvin M. Kunin] ◀

Immunologic Basis of Recurrent Bacteriuria: Role of Cervicovaginal Antibody in Enterobacterial Colonization of Introital Mucosa. Carriage of *Enterobacteriaceae* in the vaginal vestibule precedes bacteriuric episodes. Thomas A. Stamey, Nancy Wehner, Gladys Mihara and Mercy Condy[2] (Stanford Univ.) used indirect immuno-fluorescence with antiserums to human immunoglobulins to determine whether introital carriage in susceptible women is related to absence of specific cervicovaginal antibody (CVA) and whether absence of introital carriage in resistant women is related to the presence of CVA against their predominant fecal *Escherichia coli* organisms. Studies were done in 51 premenopausal, 1 postmenopausal and 11 hysterectomized women with recurrent bacteriuria. Controls included 10 premenopausal and 3 hysterectomized women who had never had urinary tract infections. Antibody coating of bacteria was assessed in cervicovaginal fluid (CVF) by the indirect immunofluorescence technique of measuring serum antibody titer.

In controls, the predominant fecal *E. coli* was coated with CVA 78% of the time after exposure to CVF. Among 23 patients with enterobacterial introital carriage who were not bacteriuric, antibody coating occurred in only 27% of 37 collections. Coating with CVA was twice as frequent in bacteriuric patients without introital colonization as in those whose bacteriuric organisms persisted on the introitus. The most common immunoglobulin coating bacteria was IgA, but IgG was nearly as prominent. Neither lactobacilli nor *Staphylococcus epidermidis* ever demonstrated fluorescent antibody. Immunoglobulin concentrations were comparable in patients and controls.

The findings strongly suggest that introital colonization with *Enterobacteriaceae* in susceptible women, a prerequisite for reinfections of the urinary tract, is associated with an absence of CVA. Specific vaginal antibody to *Enterobacteriaceae* was found in the absence of the cervix and uterus in this study, indicating that local vaginal antibodies occur in vaginal fluid despite the presence of only a stratified squamous epithelium. The immunologic implications of this finding and the common occurrence of IgM in cervicovaginal secretions deserve further study.

▶ [Dr. Stamey and his colleagues have exhaustively studied each of the potential factors that may lead to periurethral colonization with *E. coli* and subsequent occurrence of recurrent urinary tract infections. Having ruled out many other local factors, they now present evidence that women with recurrent infection may not effectively produce local vaginal antibodies, mostly of

(2) Medicine (Baltimore) 57:47–56, January, 1978.

the IgA variety. This is an exciting observation. It will be of great interest to see how he relates the current findings with his other recent observation that bacterial adherence to vaginal epithelial cells is also altered in women with recurrent urinary infections.–Calvin M. Kunin] ◄

Urine Bacterial Counts after Sexual Intercourse. The association of sexual intercourse with subsequent acute symptomatic urinary tract infection in women is well known. It has been explained by trauma to the urethra, allowing bacteria colonizing the introitus to ascend to the bladder. R. Michael Buckley, Jr., Maryanne McGuckin and Rob Roy MacGregor[3] (Univ. of Pennsylvania) studied the effect of intercourse on bladder bacterial counts in women. Twenty couples aged 21–40 years participated in the study. Three women had never had a symptomatic urinary tract infection, and 14 had had only one or two infections in recent years. None had had symptomatic bacteriuria in the 6 months before the study or had taken antibiotics. Clean-catch midstream urine specimens were collected within 4 hours before intercourse and within an hour and 8–10 hours after intercourse. A total of 76 intercourse episodes was available for study.

Less than a 1 log increase in bacterial counts was found after intercourse in 53 of the 76 intercourse episodes. Twenty-three episodes with an increase of over 1 log in counts occurred in 11 women. Four had such an increase after every intercourse studied. Counts of over 10^5 colony-forming units per ml developed after 7 episodes, 6 involving the urinary pathogens *Escherichia coli* and *Enterococcus*. Eleven of 16 episodes with lower counts involved organisms of lower pathogenic potential. All specimens contained fewer than 10 white blood cells per high-power field. No episode was symptomatic. One patient with symptoms of cystitis had over 10^5 colony-forming units of E. *coli* per ml in a preintercourse specimen. The rise in bacterial counts after intercourse was transient. Durations of the increase were similar in early- and late-voiding subjects. Urine bacterial counts were not obviously related to the types of birth control measures used.

Sexual intercourse resulted in increases in bacterial colony counts of over 1 log in nearly a third of intercourse

(3) N. Engl. J. Med. 298:321–324, Feb. 9, 1978.

episodes studied. The increases were asymptomatic and transient. Early voiding after intercourse did not prevent these increases. Failure to prove the protectiveness of early voiding, however, may not apply to a more susceptible population.

▶ [Urinary tract infections appear to be more common in sexually active women. Sexual intercourse, however, does not explain the high frequency of significant bacteriuria in young girls or the very high rates of colonization in elderly women. This study demonstrates transient, higher bacterial counts in urine of women following intercourse. This may be due to mechanical introduction of bacteria into the urethra. The urinary stream appears to effectively wash away the organisms. We are still left without a clear notion as to how the bacteria gain entrance into the bladder and produce persistent colonization.—Calvin M. Kunin] ◀

Advances in the Diagnosis of Renal Candidiasis. Urinary tract candidiasis usually is discovered at autopsy. The number of *Candida* in the urine that is to be considered significant is uncertain. P. J. Kozinn, C. L. Taschdjian, P. K. Goldberg, G. J. Wise, E. F. Toni and M. S. Seelig[4] conducted a retrospective study of 64 patients with findings suggestive of renal candidiasis to develop guidelines for the laboratory diagnosis of this condition. Eighteen of the 64 had positive renal pathology at autopsy. One other case was proved by biopsy and 1 at surgery for a candidal ball. *Candida* colony counts were done on 30 subsequently autopsied patients, 16 with indwelling Foley catheters. Prospective studies were done on urine from 165 randomly selected hospital patients. *Candida* colony counts were made on midstream and catheter urine specimens.

Candiduria was present in all 20 patients with confirmed renal candidiasis and in 10 of 44 without renal pathology. Five of the latter patients had indwelling catheters. Colony counts in catheterized urine averaged 19,000 in patients with renal candidiasis and 3,500 in those without. Respective average counts in clean-catch specimens were 23,500 and 20,300/ml. Seven randomly selected patients had *Candida* colony counts above 10,000/ml in midstream urine, with negative bacteriologic study results; 4 of the 7 had pyuria. Fifteen other subjects had significant bacteriologic counts. The agar gel diffusion precipitin test for *Candida*

---

(4) J. Urol. 119:184–187, February, 1978.

antibodies gave a positive result in 15 of 18 proved cases. False positive results were obtained in 5 cases. The sensitivity of the test was 83%, and its specificity was 89%.

The most consistent diagnostic findings of renal candidiasis in this study were candiduria and a positive serum *Candida* precipitin test result. A colony count below 10,000 /ml in a midstream specimen can only militate against the diagnosis of renal candidiasis. A high colony count must be confirmed in a catheter specimen.

Candida pyelonephritis is most often due to hematogenous spread. In the presence of an anatomical abnormality, it may be caused by ascending infection.

▶ [Differentiation is often difficult between renal candidiasis and simple colonization of the urine with *Candida.* There may be, however, some useful clinical clues such as presence of a contaminated intravenous catheter, a positive blood culture or colonization of the urine in a patient who is receiving immunosuppressive agents. Serologic tests for antibodies to *Candida,* as indicated in this report, may also be helpful. Unfortunately, antibody responses take time and may only be helpful in retrospect. The test, however, should become more sensitive and specific as knowledge is gained concerning which antigen(s) gives the best serologic response and as more sensitive serologic methods are developed.—Calvin M. Kunin] ◀

Xanthogranulomatous Pyelonephritis: Critical Analysis of 26 Cases and of the Literature. Xanthogranulomatous pyelonephritis is an atypical form of severe chronic renal parenchymal infection that may mimic neoplastic and other inflammatory parenchymal diseases. Reza S. Malek and Jack S. Elder[5] (Mayo Clinic and Found.) reviewed data on 26 patients treated in 1918–75. The 15 females and 11 males had a mean age of 50 years. Most had multiple symptoms and physical findings. Urolithiasis was a factor in 9 cases, prostatic obstruction in 4, diabetes in 4 and primary hyperparathyroidism in 2. Ten patients had had urologic procedures. All patients had pyuria and 17 were anemic. Fourteen patients exhibited urosepsis, and cultures of renal tissue were positive in 22 cases. All 13 patients studied exhibited hepatic dysfunction. The urographic findings included a renal mass with stippled calcification (Fig 2), caliceal deformity, nephrolithiasis, a functionless (Fig 3) or poorly functioning kidney and hy-

(5) J. Urol. 119:589–593, May, 1978.

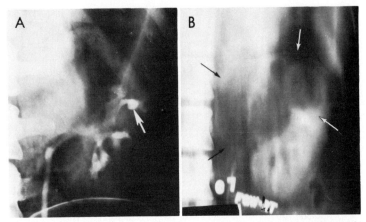

Fig 2.—Xanthogranulomatous pyelonephritis appearing as mass in kidney with stone. **A,** intravenous pyelogram reveals mass involving upper half of left kidney and causing caliceal deformity. Arrow points to small, dense caliceal stone. **B,** nephrotomogram shows solid-appearing mass with thick capsule *(arrows)*. (Courtesy of Malek, R. S., and Elder, J. S.: J. Urol. 119:589-593, May, 1978.)

dronephrosis. Only 1 case was diagnosed preoperatively. Malignancy was considered in 11 cases.

Two patients had biopsy only, and 2 had conservative renal operations. One had biopsy with pyelolithotomy and ureterolithotomy. Nephrectomy was done in 21 patients. The process was confined to the kidney in 5 patients. Seventeen of the 25 patients followed are living after a mean of 4.4 years; 8 died of unrelated causes after a mean of 13.4 years. Hypertension was observed in 11 patients. Urosepsis has recurred in 5 of 9 survivors who presented initially with chronic urinary tract infection.

The correct diagnosis was missed in all but 1 of 26 patients in this series. Localized disease may be amenable to partial nephrectomy, particularly in children. More often, previously unrecognized disease is diffuse and advanced, necessitating removal of the diseased kidney and perirenal fat. Fistulization of adjacent bowel may result, as it did in 1 of these patients. Xanthogranulomatous pyelonephritis does not seem to recur, and the prognosis in patients with otherwise normal urinary tracts is excellent. Some conditions associated with the disease, such as bacteriuria and

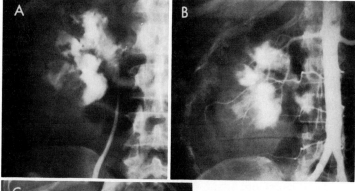

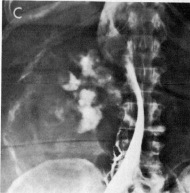

Fig 3.—Xanthogranulomatous pyelonephritis in functionless kidney. **A,** retrograde ureteropyelogram reveals caliceal deformity, irregularity and filling defects in right kidney. **B,** selective renal arteriogram shows bizarre distribution of contrast medium, thought to represent puddling in necrotic hypernephroma. Note laterally displaced ascending colon. **C,** inferior venacavogram shows displacement deformity of inferior vena cava. Note laterally displaced ascending colon. (Courtesy of Malek, R. S., and Elder, J. S.: J. Urol. 119:589-593, May, 1978.)

hypertension, however, may continue to be a problem in certain patients.

▶ [Xanthogranulomatous pyelonephritis is a severe form of chronic pyelonephritis in which histiocytes appear to be heavily laden with foreign material, probably bacterial products. It usually occurs in individuals with chronic complicated infections. This article provides considerable useful descriptive clinical information concerning this entity. A case presentation of this disease might prove useful in testing candidates for boards in urology (and medicine).—Calvin M. Kunin] ◀

Unusual Renal Manifestations of Wegener's Granulomatosis: Report of Two Cases. Wegener's granulomatosis is characterized by necrotizing granulomatous lesions in the upper and lower respiratory tract, glomerulonephritis and a generalized vasculitis involving both arteries and veins. Hypertension is unusual. Stuart B. Baker and

Dwight R. Robinson[6] (Boston) recently encountered 2 patients with features previously ascribed only to polyarteritis nodosa. One patient, who presented with typical necrotizing granulomatous sinus disease and cavitary lung lesions, had multiple bilateral renal arterial aneurysms, one of which ruptured, leading to a massive perinephric hematoma (Fig 4). Gelfoam embolization obviated the need for nephrectomy. The other patient presented with glomerulonephritis and mononeuritis multiplex 2 years before classic necrotizing granulomatous disease of the sinuses and nose and pulmonary nodules developed. A ureteral obstruction resulted from necrotizing vasculitis of the periureteral vessels (Fig 5). Both the patients responded dramatically to cyclophosphamide therapy.

The diagnosis of Wegener's granulomatosis should be considered in patients presenting with multiple renal aneurysms, spontaneous perinephric hematoma, necrotizing glomerulitis or ureteral obstruction due to vasculitis, even if typical granulomatous respiratory tract involve-

Fig 4.—Angiogram of right kidney of man aged 24 years. **A,** note compression of the lateral aspect of the right kidney. Multiple aneurysms of varying size *(arrows)* are seen throughout the parenchyma. **B,** note extravasation of dye from a ruptured aneurysm in the upper pole *(a)* tracking into a massive perinephric hematoma *(h)*. (Courtesy of Baker, S. B., and Robinson, D. R.: Am. J. Med. 64:883–889, May, 1978.)

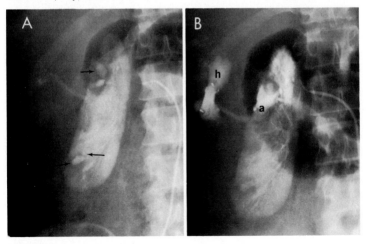

(6) Am. J. Med. 64:883–889, May, 1978.

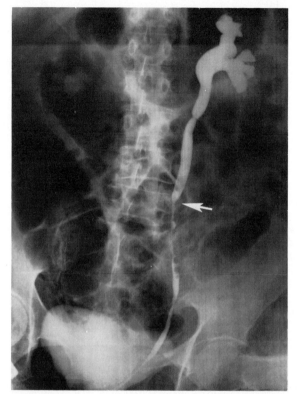

Fig 5.—Left retrograde pyelogram of a woman aged 60 years. There is hydrone-phrosis, with an upper ureteral partial obstruction. In addition, there is a 6-cm irregular, nodular narrowing in the lower ureter, beginning at the level of the L5 *(arrow)*. (Courtesy of Baker, S. B., and Robinson, D. R.: Am. J. Med. 64:883–889, May, 1978.)

ment is absent. The differential diagnosis between Wege-ner's granulomatosis and polyarteritis nodosa is of more than academic interest because of the dramatic efficacy of cytotoxic immunosuppressive therapy in Wegener's gran-ulomatosis.

▶ [Wegener's granulomatosis is a generalized vasculitis with an alarmingly virulent course. Renal involvement is a major complication as pointed out in this interesting clinical study. The disease is more than a medical curiosity now that effective therapy is available. It is essential that this disease be considered in the differential diagnosis of unexplained hematuria.–Calvin M. Kunin] ◀

Papillary Plasma Flow in Experimental Pyelone-phritis in Rats: Effect of Antibiotic Therapy and Indomethacin. A defect in maximum renal concentrating ability (U_{max}) is the earliest functional abnormality in human and experimental pyelonephritis. Inhibitors of renal prostaglandin synthesis rapidly reverse the defect in experimental pyelonephritis. Medullary prostaglandin synthesis may increase papillary plasma flow and result in a defect in U_{max}. Sandra P. Levison and Matthew E. Levison[7] (Med. College of Pennsylvania), with the technical assistance of Peter Pitsakis, determined papillary plasma flow in normal rats and rats with early bilateral enterococcal pyelonephritis, with and without antibiotic or indomethacin administration. Papillary plasma flow was determined by measuring accumulation of ^{125}I-albumin in the renal papilla. Antibiotic therapy was with sodium ampicillin. Indomethacin was infused in a dose of 10 mg/kg in 4-day-infected rats.

The U_{max} was significantly less in 4-day-infected than in normal rats. Papillary plasma flow was significantly lower in infected rats. Blood pressures did not differ significantly. Mean papillary water content was similar in the two groups of rats. Ampicillin-treated rats with significantly reduced renal enterococcal titers had significantly higher U_{max} and papillary plasma flow values. Urine osmolality rose to peak values an hour after indomethacin administration and then fell steadily, with erratic changes in papillary plasma flow (table).

The findings suggest that the defect in U_{max} in pyelonephritis may not be caused by abnormal papillary plasma

U_{max} AND PAPILLARY PLASMA FLOW 1 HR AFTER INDOMETHACIN IN 4-DAY-INFECTED RATS

	No. of rats	Umax (mOsm/kg H₂O)[*]		Papillary plasma flow (ml/min/100 gm)[*]
		Pretreatment	Posttreatment	
Indomethacin-treated	8	1,158 ± 55	2,518 ± 54	24.3 ± 1.0
Diluent-treated	8	1,161 ± 45	1,082 ± 31	25.9 ± 1.7

[*]Mean ± S.E.M.

(7) J. Lab. Clin. Med. 92:570–576, October, 1978.

flow, and that different mechanisms may be responsible for the defects in U_{max} and papillary plasma flow in pyelonephritis. The reversibility of the defect in papillary plasma flow after antibiotic therapy suggests a transient cause, rather than profound structural damage.

▶ [This is an elegant study demonstrating that the reversible renal concentrating defect in acute pyelonephritis is related to production of renal prostaglandins. This provides more detail concerning the early biochemical effects of inflammation on renal function. It is too early to extrapolate these findings to the renal defense against infection, but they may turn out to be valuable clues.–Calvin M. Kunin] ◀

Sequelae of Covert Bacteriuria in Schoolgirls: A Four-Year Follow-up Study is reported by the Cardiff-Oxford Bacteriuria Study Group.[8] Renal growth and renal scarring were investigated in schoolgirls with asymptomatic bacteria who were followed, with or without treatment, for 4 years, and the findings were related to the amount of bacteriuria observed during this period. The study consisted of 208 girls, aged 5–12 years, who had bacteriuria on screening during 1971–72. Ninety-eight were observed for 4 years without treatment, and 110 were treated, usually with cotrimoxazole. Initially, 1- or 2-week courses were given, but 3–12-month courses of low-dose maintenance therapy were sometimes administered to girls with recurrent bacteriuria. At the beginning of the study, the treated and control groups had respective mean ages of 8.7 and 8.6 years.

Eight control girls had infection during follow-up and were treated. No significant differences in blood pressure or in blood urea and serum creatinine levels (Table 1) were noted at follow-up. At the end of the study, 15% of treated girls and 45% of untreated girls had bacteriuria. No treated girl had persistent bacteriuria, but 30% of control subjects did. Renal growth is shown in Table 2. Nine girls with unscarred kidneys, 6 in the control group, showed impaired kidney growth. No new scars were found in girls whose kidneys were normal at initial radiologic study. Treatment failed to prevent the progression of kidney damage.

New renal scars did not develop in girls in this study whose kidneys were normal at the outset. Treatment did

---

(8) Lancet 1:889–893, Apr. 29, 1978.

TABLE 1.—BLOOD UREA AND SERUM CREATININE
CONCENTRATIONS IN TREATED AND CONTROL GROUPS

Test		Treated	Controls
Blood-urea (mmol/l)	Initial	4·0±0·8 (98)	4·0±0·9 (87)
	Final	4·0±1·0 (105)	4·0±0·9 (89)
Serum-creatinine (μmol/l)	Initial	63±12 (97)	60±9 (90)
	Final	66±10 (103)	67±11 (89)

Results given in mean ±SD.
Numbers in parentheses refer to number of girls.

not influence renal growth. Screening of schoolgirls for covert bacteriuria cannot be recommended, since treatment that markedly reduces the duration of bacteriuria has no significant beneficial effects. Further attempts to prevent the renal scarring associated with infection and its possible late sequelae should focus on children less than age 5 years and should aim at identification of high-risk factors, the most important of which appears to be vesicoureteral reflux.

▶ [Uncomplicated urinary tract infections in schoolgirls rarely lead to

TABLE 2.—MEANS (±SD) OF RENAL GROWTH RATES (MM/YEAR)

Radiological findings	Side	Treated group	Control group
Normal	Right	3·8±1·4 (78)	3·6±1·6 (70)
	Left	3·8±1·5 (84)	3·5±1·4 (66)
v.-u. reflux	Right	3·8±1·2 (12)	3·5±2·0 (14)
	Left	3·6±1·6 (12)	4·3±1·7 (20)
Kidney scarring	Right	3·5±1·7 (8)	2·1±1·3 (5)
	Left	2·6±0·9 (6)	4·2±1·5 (4)
Kidney scarring and v.-u. reflux	Right	1·8±1·8 (12)	2·7±1·1 (7)
	Left	1·1±1·2 (8)	3·0±2·0 (7)

Numbers in parentheses refer to number of girls.

end-stage renal failure. This study is somewhat confusing because of the variety of therapies used in the treated group and the controls. Nevertheless it is a useful contribution to our understanding of the natural history of uncomplicated urinary infections.–Calvin M. Kunin] ◄

Urinary Tract Infection Localization in Women. The site of urinary tract infection is an important determinant of successful therapy. Fairley et al. found that the bladder-washout (BW) method compared favorably with the Stamey procedure using serial ureteric specimens. Thomas et al. found an excellent correlation between the presence of antibody-coated bacteria (ACB), detected by direct immunofluorescence, and renal infection. Godfrey K. M. Harding, Thomas J. Marrie, Allan R. Ronald, Shirley Hoban and Patricia Muir[9] (Winnipeg, Man., Canada) correlated the results of the ACB and BW tests with symptoms in 51 adult women, most of whom had experienced recurrent urinary tract infections. Nineteen patients had upper tract symptoms and signs and 8 had lower tract symptoms only at the time of BW localization. Seven specimens were used in the BW tests. The ACB test included two controls, a positive one and a negative one.

Pyelograms were abnormal in 11 of 33 patients. All 31 women whose infecting bacteria were coated with antibody were proved on BW testing to have an upper tract infection. None had lower tract infection. Fourteen of 20 other women had a lower tract infection, and 6 had upper tract infection on BW study. Three of the latter patients had had upper tract symptoms and signs, 1 had lower tract symptoms and 2 were asymptomatic. Two of the patients had abnormal pyelograms. The presence of ACB was significantly associated with proved upper tract infection on BW study. All 11 patients with abnormal pyelograms had upper tract infection only. Nine had their infecting bacteria coated with antibody. Three of 19 patients with upper tract symptoms and signs had lower tract infection. Three of 8 with lower tract symptoms only had upper tract infections. Both gram-negative and gram-positive organisms were coated with antibody.

The presence of ACB in the urine sediment of women with reported urinary tract infections indicates upper tract

(9) J.A.M.A. 240:1147–1150, Sept. 8, 1978.

infection. Some women with antibody-coated organisms and upper tract infection have organisms emanating from their ureters at BW study that are not coated with antibody. Caution is needed in interpreting ACB-negative results. The presence of upper tract symptoms and signs is a better predictor of localization of infection than are lower tract symptoms.

▶ [The antibody-coated bacteria phenomenon is an interesting laboratory test to help localize infection to tissues as opposed to simple bladder urine colonization. It should be considered at present as a research tool. In my view, underlying anatomic or neurologic abnormalities and response to therapy are far more important prognostic indicators than localization of the site of infection.—Calvin M. Kunin] ◀

Evaluation of a Dip-Slide in a University Outpatient Service. Use of the conventional calibrated loop method of culturing urine requires transport of specimens to the laboratory, causing delay in culture and the possibility of increased bacterial counts during transportation. Mary Jane Martin and Maryanne B. McGuckin[1] (Univ. of Pennsylvania) evaluated the feasibility of using the agar-coated dip-slide in a hospital walk-in clinic. Studies were done in 31 women aged 17–40 years who had been treated for urinary tract infection and in 85 women with no definite predisposition to urinary tract infection. The clinic staff inoculated dip-slides in the former group, and laboratory personnel in the latter. Specimens were collected in clean-catch midstream urine containers. Dip-slides were inoculated just after specimens were voided, while conventional cultures were delayed 1–2 hours by transport to the laboratory.

Overall agreement between the dip-slide and conventional culture methods was 51.7%. Qualitative disagreement for bacterial type was noted in 37% of cases and disagreement on counts in 11.2%. The two methods agreed in 42% of patients with past infection and in 55% of the nonpredisposed group. The respective rates of quantitative disagreement were 6.5% and 13%. The dip-slide method gave quantitatively false results in 16.3% of 110 cases. Ten of these were falsely positive, and 8 were falsely negative.

The dip-slide was not feasible for this clinic population. It seems better suited to a situation in which cultures will

(1) J. Urol. 120:193–195, August, 1978.

be 70–80% negative or less than 10^4 organisms/ml will be present. Laboratory personnel were needed to keep contamination during inoculation to a minimum. They also were needed for more accurate reading of the dip-slide. Dip-slide results should be evaluated carefully along with clinical impressions in complicated cases of urinary tract infection.

▶ [This study documents the failure of a hospital clinic to use dip-slides effectively. I had previously thought that dip-slides were highly reliable. As with any test unless the staff understands the method and applies it conscientiously the results will be poor.—Calvin M. Kunin] ◀

Etiology of Nonspecific Urethritis in Active Duty Marines. John W. Klousia, David L. Madden, David A. Fucillo, Renee G. Traub, Janet M. Mattson and Aurella G. Krezlewicz[2] (Marine Corps Training Command, Quantico, Va.) reviewed the findings in 187 patients seen at a marine dispensary in an 18-month period with urethral discharge, dysuria, frequency or urgency. Elimination of patients with gonorrhea, clinical prostatitis, concomitant genitourinary problems, pyuria only or a history of antibiotic therapy in the preceding 6 weeks left 64 patients acceptable for study. Control subjects had nongenitourinary, noninfectious conditions, mostly orthopedic in nature.

Positive cultures were obtained in 87% of patients with nonspecific urethritis and in 92% of controls. Only one positive viral culture was obtained, herpesvirus simplex type II. The recovery of mycoplasma and ureaplasma is shown in the table. The frequency of mycoplasma was not related to race, but those of higher rank had a higher frequency, and a positive correlation with the number of sexual partners was noted. About a third of study and control patients

INCIDENCE OF UREAPLASMA AND CLASSIC MYCOPLASMA ISOLATED FROM
PATIENTS AND CONTROLS

	Non-Specific Urethritis	Controls
	No. Pts.* (%)	No. Pts.* (%)
Ureaplasma	25/64 (39)	25/47 (52)
Classical	13/64 (20)	13/47 (27)

*Number of marines with positive isolation/total number studied.

(2) J. Urol. 120:67–70, July, 1978.

with two or more sex partners had positive cultures. Circumcision did not appear to influence the isolation rate.

These findings support the absence of significant differences between men with nonspecific urethritis and controls matched for sexual activity. The increased incidence of positive cultures of ureaplasma found in higher socioeconomic group subjects may reflect a difference in the partner population.

▶ [Ureaplasma, a subgroup of the mycoplasma family, is an organism in search of a disease. It appears to be spread in part by sexual contact. It is too frequently found in asymptomatic individuals, however, to be considered as a major cause of the urethritis syndrome.–Calvin M. Kunin] ◀

Recognition and Management of Genital Chlamydial Infection. Shirley J. Richmond and J. D. Oriel[3] observe that *Chlamydia trachomatis* is a widely prevalent obligate intracellular bacterial parasite with distinct genital and ocular strains. "Nonspecific" genital infection is now a major health problem in Western society, and genital chlamydiae have been implicated as an important cause of such infection. Genital chlamydiae are commonly found in the genital tract in promiscuous populations. Epidemiologic evidence for their sexual transmission has been obtained. Chlamydiae probably cause up to half of unselected cases of nongonococcal urethritis in men attending venereal disease clinics. Chlamydiae can be isolated from 20–30% of unselected women attending such clinics. Ocular infection by genital chlamydiae in Western society is sporadic. A definitive diagnosis can be made only by isolation of the organism from the genital tract, usually the urethra in men and the cervix in women.

Tetracyclines are used to treat men presenting with gonococcal urethritis, whether or not they have *Chlamydia* organisms. True relapse of urethral chlamydial infection in men is rare. The proper management of infected women is unclear. Attention should be focused on women with cervical discontinuity and a purulent cervical discharge and isolation attempted if facilities are available. If not, a trial of tetracyclines is probably justified in women with the syndrome. Chlamydial ophthalmia should be considered in all infants who develop mucopurulent conjunctivitis 4 or

(3) Br. Med. J. 2:480–483, Aug. 12, 1978.

more days after birth. Chlortetracycline eye ointment and oral erythromycin therapy are used if the diagnosis is made or strongly suspected. Gonococcal infection may act as a potent chlamydial reactivator, and vigorous measures to control gonorrhea may be one of the most effective means of controlling chlamydial infections in the community.

▶ [It is now clear that chlamydiae are major etiologic agents in nongonococcal urethritis. This provides an explanation for the efficacy of tetracycline in management. It is also becoming more clear that chlamydial infections account for serious neonatal infection as well. Rapid inexpensive diagnostic tests are needed to detect infection in females who may have unrecognized infection.—Calvin M. Kunin] ◀

Chlamydia Trachomatis as a Cause of Acute "Idiopathic" Epididymitis. Fifty-five to 100% of cases of acute epididymitis seen in recent series have been idiopathic. Nongonococcal urethritis is often present in men with acute idiopathic epididymitis, and *C. trachomatis* has been isolated from the urethras of these patients. Richard E. Berger, E. Russell Alexander, George D. Monda, Julian Ansell, Gerald McCormick and King K. Holmes[4] (Seattle) found evidence in a study of 23 men with acute epididymitis that *C. trachomatis* is the major cause of "idiopathic" epididymitis and that coliforms are the major cause of epididymitis in older men. Twenty-three consecutive men seen during 1976–77 with unilateral pain and swelling of the epididymis for less than 2 months were studied. None had received antibiotics in the previous month. Epididymal aspirates, anterior urethral specimens, prostatic massage specimens and urine were obtained for bacteriologic study. Serum microimmunofluorescence antibody to *C. trachomatis* was determined.

Coliforms were isolated from midstream urine in 8 of 10 men more than age 35 years and none of 13 younger men. *Chlamydia trachomatis* infection was documented in 11 of the 13 younger men and in no older patients (table). *Neisseria gonorrhoeae* was not isolated from any patient in this series. *Chlamydia trachomatis* was isolated from epididymal aspirates from 5 of 6 younger men. Coliforms were isolated in 5 of 10 older patients. Two of the 5 younger patients had urethral cultures negative for *C. trachomatis*.

(4) N. Engl. J. Med. 298:301–304, Feb. 9, 1978.

ISOLATION OF PATHOGENIC AGENTS FROM 23 PATIENTS WITH ACUTE
EPIDIDYMITIS ACCORDING TO SOURCE OF ISOLATE AND AGE OF PATIENT

PATHOGEN	MEN <35 YR OF AGE		MEN >35 YR OF AGE	
	ANY SOURCE	EPIDIDYMAL ASPIRATE	ANY SOURCE	EPIDIDYMAL ASPIRATE
N gonorrhoeae	0/13	0/6	0/10	0/10
Coliform organisms*	0/13	0/6	8/10	5/10
C trachomatis†	10/13	5/6	0/10	0/10

*Coliform species isolated in concentration ≥10^5/ml of midstream urine included *Escherichia coli* only (6), *E. coli* plus *Proteus mirabilis* (1) and *P. mirabilis* alone (1).

†An eleventh patient was culture negative but had a fourfold rise in microimmunofluorescent antibody to *C. trachomatis*.

All 10 patients with positive urethral or epididymal cultures for *C. trachomatis* had serum antibody to the organism. Both patients with negative urethral cultures showed seroconversion. *Ureaplasma urealyticum* was isolated from the urine of 7 of 11 men with *C. trachomatis* infection, none of 8 with coliform infection and 2 of the 4 others. Midstream pyuria was most prominent in men with coliform infection. Inguinal pain was largely confined to those with *C. trachomatis* infection. Scrotal edema and erythema were more marked in men with coliform infection.

Epididymitis can be added to the list of diseases caused by *C. trachomatis*. Morbidity caused by *C. trachomatis* now parallels and rivals that caused by *N. gonorrhoeae*.

▶ [This is a beautifully conducted study that provides extremely useful information concerning the etiology of acute epididymitis. Holmes and his group have provided convincing evidence of the key role of chlamydiae in epididymitis occurring in young men. This study pretty well eliminates the sterile urine reflux theory and provides a rational basis for antimicrobial therapy.—Calvin M. Kunin] ◀

Efficacy of Single-Dose and Conventional Amoxicillin Therapy in Urinary Tract Infection Localized by Antibody-Coated Bacteria Technique. The rate of recurrence of acute, uncomplicated urinary tract infection in women after treatment with a wide variety of antimicrobial agents is unacceptably high. The great majority of treatment failures and recurrent infections with the original infecting organism occur in patients with renal infection. Leslie S. T. Fang, Nina E. Tolkoff-Rubin and Robert

H. Rubin[5] (Boston) evaluated the usefulness of the anti-body-coated bacteria assay and of single-dose amoxicillin therapy in 61 women with symptoms of cystitis who were infected with amoxicillin-sensitive organisms. Patients with positive assays received conventional therapy. Those with negative assays received either 250 mg amoxicillin orally 4 times daily for 10 days or a single 3-gm oral dose.

Forty-three patients had negative assays for antibody-coated bacteria, and 22 of them received single-dose therapy. All 22 were free from symptoms 24–48 hours after treatment. One was reinfected after 1 week, and 3 had negligible numbers of the same urinary pathogen but were asymptomatic. All 21 assay-negative patients who received conventional therapy did well. Two were reinfected at 4 weeks. Nine of the 18 patients with positive assays had relapses with the same pathogen at 1 week. Three continued to relapse despite retreatment with sulfisoxazole or ampicillin for 2 or 3 weeks. Pyelograms were normal in these patients. One other patient was reinfected at the 1-week follow-up. Three patients on single-dose therapy had mild gastrointestinal disturbances, and in 1 patient a rash of mononucleosis became worse. Eight patients given conventional therapy had mild gastrointestinal symptoms, and 9 had symptomatic monilial vulvovaginitis.

Single-dose therapy is convenient and less expensive than conventional therapy. Patient compliance is greater and side effects are reduced. The response to single-dose therapy could become a useful guide to future management. Single dose therapy fails in a sizable minority of patients with asymptomatic renal involvement. These patients become candidates for radiologic assessment of the urinary tract and more intensive antimicrobial therapy.

▶ [This is a well-documented study of the efficacy of a single large dose of amoxicillin in treatment of urinary tract infections localized to the bladder urine by the antibody-coated bacteria method. I suspect that the cost of the test and the delay in receiving a report from the laboratory will be greater than that of a 7–10 day course of therapy.—Calvin M. Kunin] ◀

Treatment of Urinary Tract Infection with a Single Dose of Trimethoprim-Sulfamethoxazole. Antimicrobial therapy is commonly prescribed for 5–21 days in treat-

(5) N. Engl. J. Med. 298:413–416, Feb. 23, 1978.

ment of urinary tract infection, but there is no convincing evidence that a short course of therapy is less successful. Ross R. Bailey and George D. Abbott[6] (Christchurch, New Zealand) compared a single oral dose and a conventional course of trimethoprim-sulfamethoxazole (TMP-SMX) in 40 women with asymptomatic bacteriuria, cystitis or acute pyelonephritis and in 20 children who were asymptomatic or had cystitis. Only patients with a urinary tract pathogen sensitive to TMP-SMX were included. The women were given either a single 2.88-gm dose (0.48 gm TMP and 2.4 gm SMX) or 0.96 gm (0.16 gm TMP and 0.8 gm SMX) every 12 hours for 5 days. Children were given a single dose or a 7-day course of age-related dosages.

In both groups of women, 85% were cured. A new organism appeared in the urine within a week of treatment in all 3 women in whom single-dose therapy failed. Only 2 women had impaired renal function. Two of 3 women with acute pyelonephritis who received a 5-day course of therapy were cured. Two women given a 5-day course had mild skin reactions. Seven of the 10 children who received a single dose of TMP-SMX and 8 of the 10 given a 7-day course were cured. Diarrhea developed in 1 child given a 7-day course and a mild urticarial skin rash in another.

Single-dose treatment with TMP-SMX for uncomplicated urinary tract infections is simple, effective and economical. It is well accepted and well tolerated by patients.

▶ [This is one of several excellent studies that indicate that most of the effect of antimicrobial therapy in uncomplicated urinary tract infections is gained in the first day or two of treatment. More prolonged therapy adds little except perhaps to prevent early recurrence. Since recurrence is the major problem in managing urinary tract infections in females, periodic follow-up cultures are still needed to guide effective long-term management.—Calvin M. Kunin] ◀

Controlled Trial of Prophylactic Treatment in Childhood Urinary Tract Infection. Few controlled trials of long-term, low-dosage prophylaxis in prevention of recurrent symptomatic urinary tract infection in children have been carried out. J. M. Smellie, G. Katz and R. N. Grüneberg[7] report a randomized comparison of low-dosage prophylaxis with cotrimoxazole and nitrofur-

(6) Can. Med. Assoc. J. 118:551–552, Mar. 4, 1978.
(7) Lancet 2:175–178, July 22, 1978.

antoin and no prophylaxis in 53 children aged 2–12 years with bacteriologically proved, symptomatic urinary tract infection and normal urograms and cystograms. Five boys and 40 girls completed the trial. After initial treatment with cotrimoxazole for 7–10 days, one fourth of the group received prophylactic nitrofurantoin in a dosage of 1 to 2 mg/kg daily, one-fourth received low-dosage cotrimoxazole (10 mg sulfamethoxazole and 2 mg trimethoprim per kg daily) for 6–12 months and half received no further treatment. The groups were similar in age and social class, but more of those on prophylaxis had a history of symptomatic infection.

No child on prophylaxis (for an average of 10 months) had a recurrence of infection, but 11 of 22 controls had further infections. After completing prophylaxis, 32% of children had an infection within 1 year, compared with 59% of children not on prophylaxis. All children with previous infection who were not on prophylaxis had further infection during the year of follow-up, compared with 44% of 18 who received prophylaxis. Predisposing factors were identified in nearly all children who had further infections. Antibiotic sensitivity of the organisms did not differ significantly before and after treatment. No trimethoprim-resistant organisms emerged in either the urine or the bowel flora during the study.

Long-term, low-dosage prophylaxis prevents further infection of the unobstructed urinary tract while it is being given. The main cause of recurrent infection in the absence of outflow obstruction appears to be breakdown of the host defenses, allowing colonization of the susceptible bladder by bowel commensals ascending the urethra.

The principal uses of low-dosage antibacterial prophylaxis at present are control of recurrent symptomatic infections and prevention of infection in infants and children with vesicoureteral reflux.

▶ [This study reinforces the evidence that low doses of nitrofurantoin or tri-methoprim-sulfamethoxazole are highly effective agents in prophylaxis of highly recurrent urinary tract infections. The study also suggests that prophylaxis may be effective in diminishing the rate of recurrences even after treatment is stopped. It should be emphasized that long-term prophylaxis is not needed when recurrences are spaced widely apart.–Calvin M. Kunin] ◀

Serum Antibody Titers in Treatment with Trimethoprim-Sulfamethoxazole for Chronic Prostatitis. Tri-

methoprim-sulfamethoxazole (TMP-SMX) has been found to be useful in treating chronic bacterial prostatitis due to various pathogens. Edwin M. Meares, Jr.[8] (Univ. of California, San Francisco) compared the clinical, bacteriologic and serologic responses of 22 men given TMP-SMX therapy for chronic prostatitis due to various strains of *Escherichia coli*. All the patients, aged 29–64, were in good general health and had no evidence of obstructive uropathy. All had at least two positive diagnostic bacteriologic localization cultures for prostatic infection due to *E. coli*. Nine men received 2 tablets of TMP-SMX (80 and 400 mg) twice daily for 2 weeks and 13 received 2 tablets twice daily for 12 weeks. Antibody was measured by a direct bacterial agglutination method.

Before treatment 18 patients (82%) had serum antibody titers of 1:320 or above against somatic O antigen of the *E. coli* pathogen. Seven patients were cured, 5 after treatment for 12 weeks; 6 of them had elevated serum antibody titers which fell to normal after treatment. Ten patients were improved, 5 after short-term treatment; 7 had elevated antibody titers that were essentially unchanged during and after treatment. All 5 patients who were unchanged had elevated serum titers that were unchanged during and after treatment. All pathogens were sensitive in vitro to TMP-SMX. No change in sensitivity patterns was noted in patients who were not cured. No significant adverse drug reactions were observed.

Treatment with TMP-SMX can cure some men who have chronic prostatitis due to sensitive strains of *E. coli*.

▶ [The initial observations that trimethoprim penetrated into prostatic secretions indicated that this drug would be effective in the management of bacterial prostatitis. Meares now provides evidence that this promise is only partially fulfilled. Cure is accompanied by a fall in antibody titers to the invading bacteria. Unfortunately, persistent infection is still frequent and is accompanied by continued high levels of antibody in the blood. Serologic studies should therefore provide a useful marker of continued infection and serve as a helpful guide to evaluate new agents.—Calvin M. Kunin] ◀

Antibiotic Irrigation and Catheter-Associated Urinary Tract Infections. Both closed drainage systems and antimicrobial irrigation have been used to prevent urinary tract infections in catheterized patients. John W.

(8)   Urology 11:142–146, February, 1978.

Warren, Richard Platt, Robert J. Thomas, Bernard Rosner and Edward H. Kass[9] (Boston) conducted a prospective randomized trial of neomycin-polymyxin irrigation in a closed catheter system. Irrigation consisted of vials containing 40 mg neomycin sulfate and 20 mg polymyxin B sulfate. Each vial was mixed into a 1 L bag of physiologic saline for irrigation. Ninety-eight patients were catheterized with a double-lumen, nonirrigated system and 89 with a triple-lumen, antibiotic-irrigated system. The groups were similar in age, sex and renal function. The mean duration of catheterization was 3.5 days in the group without, and 3.3 days in that with, irrigation.

The prevalence of urinary tract infection is shown in Figure 6. Infection occurred in 18% of the group without, and 16% of the group with, irrigation. At low volumes of daily urine output, infection was more frequent in the group with no irrigation, but the collection junction was disconnected on more low-output days in this group. Only one of sixteen organisms isolated from irrigated patients was sensitive to neomycin, compared with 58% of twenty-four or-

Fig 6.—Prevalence of indwelling catheters and cumulative prevalence of urinary tract infections during the first 12 days of catheterization. Three of the 18 patients without irrigation who became infected did so after the 12th day of catheterization and do not appear in the figure. (Courtesy of Warren, J. W., et al.: N. Engl. J. Med. 299:570–573, Sept. 14, 1978.)

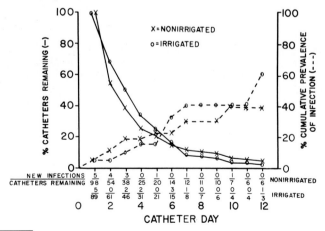

ganisms isolated from the other group. The two junctions present in the triple-lumen irrigated catheters provided twice the opportunity for disconnection as occurred in the other group. Disconnections had a strong influence on the acquisition of urinary tract infections. No bacteremia was observed in 12 patients having blood cultures.

This irrigation method had no ultimate effect on the rate of acquisition of urinary tract infections and selected a more antibiotic-resistant population as infecting agents. The extra junction of the irrigating catheter provides an increased opportunity for breaks in the integrity of the closed catheter apparatus. Irrigation as now used cannot be recommended, but more stringent catheter care, a different irrigant, increased irrigant volumes or changes in irrigation technique might substantially lower infection rates in patients receiving irrigation.

▶ [The important message in this article is that no system of aseptic or prophylactic urinary catheter care will be effective without meticulous attention to care of the equipment. If, as shown here, the major break in the system was due to opening of the junction between catheter and collection tubing, the lesson seems to be to seal them to foil meddling hands.–Calvin M. Kunin] ◀

CALCULI

Calcium-Containing Renal Stones are discussed by Lynwood H. Smith[1] (Mayo Clinic and Found.). Most stones that form within the urinary tract contain calcium. Various crystalline forms of calcium oxalate and calcium phosphate are the most common types of stones. A major problem in evaluation of patients with calcium urolithiasis relates to the metabolic activity of the stone formation. Irrespective of the underlying cause, stone formation varies among patients with the same disorder. Type I renal tubular acidosis (RTA) is characterized by inability of the distal nephron to generate or maintain steep luminal-peritubular hydrogen ion gradients. Type II RTA is associated with a proximal renal tubular defect in bicarbonate reabsorption. Urolithiasis and nephrocalcinosis have occurred with type I RTA but not to date with type II. Patients with type I are managed by correction of their

(1) Kidney Int. 13:383-389, May, 1978.

metabolic abnormalities. Hypercalciuria usually accompanies hypercalcemia and has been considered to be important in the formation of urinary tract stones. Neoplastic disease is the most common cause of hypercalcemia, but stone formation is rare.

The syndrome of idiopathic urolithiasis includes various metabolic disorders, and is the most common cause of calcium urolithiasis in industrialized countries. The diagnosis currently is applied to perhaps 80% of patients who have formed stones in the urinary tract. It is a diagnosis of exclusion. Typically the serum calcium concentration is normal, the serum phosphorus concentration is low-normal or low and hypercalciuria is present. Calcium oxalate, calcium phosphate and uric acid can all be present. Abnormal calcium absorption from the gut has been demonstrated, as has renal hypercalciuria. Some patients with idiopathic urolithiasis and hypercalciuria may prove to have primary hyperparathyroidism. Others may exhibit primary defects of crystal growth and aggregation inhibitors, increased urinary oxalate excretion, increased urine alkalinity or abnormal uric acid metabolism. Treatment of idiopathic urolithiasis is directed toward correction of these various abnormalities. Stone formation often is variable between patients and within the same patient.

▶ [This article does not lend itself to abstracting and should be read by the urologist.–J.Y.G.] ◀

Physicochemical Aspects of Urolithiasis are reviewed by Birdwell Finlayson[2] (Univ. of Florida). Supersaturation of urine with the salts that stones consist of gives rise to the thermodynamic driving force for stone formation. Stone-formers' urine is supersaturated with the salt of the stones that they are growing, but some non-stone-formers' urine at times seems to be just as supersaturated. Nucleation is the initial event in stone salt precipitation. Classic heterogeneous nucleation occurs when a foreign surface reduces the metastable limit by catalyzing nucleation. Nonclassic nucleation may operate through spinodal decomposition with spherulitic growth, or secondary nucleation. The detailed growth history of urinary stones is unknown. Investigatively, perhaps the most informative

(2) Kidney Int. 13:344-360, May, 1978.

studies have been on the rate of particle growth of precipi-
tates in urine.

There is no doubt that crystal growth and aggregation
inhibitors are present in urine, but their role in the pathogenesis of stone disease is unclear. Differences in urinary
inhibitor concentration between stone-formers and normal
subjects may result from solution depletion by adsorption
on crystalluria particles. Accordingly, inhibitor concentration becomes a correction on the estimate of supersaturation. This could explain the apparent success of the saturation inhibition index, as well as the more obvious
hypothesis of urinary inhibitors directly reducing crystallization activity in stone disease. A valid understanding of
the supersaturation and inhibitor concentration profile
along the nephron will make it possible to start development of a comprehensive kinetic picture of what can hap-
pen in urine as it moves through the urinary passages.

▶ [It is good to see urologists involved in the scientific study of urolithiasis.—
J.Y.G.] ◀

Inhibitors and Promoters of Stone Formation. Herbert Fleisch[3] (Univ. of Berne) observes that the main mechanisms thought to be important in urinary stone formation
are the relation between the concentration of precipitating
substances in urine and the solubility of the mineral phase
formed; promoters of crystallization and aggregation; and
inhibitors of crystal formation and aggregation. An epitac-
tic mechanism of precipitation could explain why most
stones are formed not just by one salt, but by a mixture of
different salts. The role played by various compounds in
the total inhibitory activity against calcium phosphate formation is unclear. Many types of crystal aggregate in
urine, and substances that disaggregate crystals have
been identified. The diphosphonates probably are the most
potent inhibitors of calcium oxalate precipitation known.

Many patients who form stones exhibit a defect in urinary inhibitors. A decrease in inhibitory activity of calcium phosphate precipitation has been demonstrated in
stone-formers by use of the rat cartilage system. Only a
few ways to increase urinary inhibitors are known. One is
oral administration of orthophosphate, which increases py-

(3) Kidney Int. 13:361–371, May, 1978.

rophosphate excretion. Diphosphonates given orally have reduced formation of induced bladder stones experimentally and have decreased calcium oxalate crystal aggregates and the growth of brushite in human urine. Urolithiasis is probably a multifactorial disease, in which several predisposing factors can play roles. Not all are likely to be present in the same patient, and treatment probably has to be individualized.

▶ [One of the more interesting developments reported by Howard (Johns Hopkins Med. J. 139: 239, 1976) is that a complex, citrophosphate, enables the soft shell crab to store calcium in an amorphous form in the liver. Before discarding its shell the crab mobilizes the calcium to the liver and uses it to form a new shell hours later. This compound may be the low molecular weight inhibitor of calcium phosphate stones. Studies are underway to identify a high molecular weight inhibitor (possibly similar to heparin) of calcium oxalate stones. Hopefully in the future we can measure inhibitor activity in the patient's urine and thereby develop an appropriate therapeutic program.– J.Y.G.] ◀

Use of Phosphates in Patients with Calcareous Renal Calculi is reviewed by William C. Thomas, Jr.[4] (Univ. of Florida). Considerable success has been achieved in recent years by use of various phosphatic compounds to prevent growth or recurrence of calcareous calculi. Oral administration of Calgon, a polyphosphate water conditioner, or similar amounts of phosphate as orthophosphate salts is effective in causing calculous patients to excrete urine that will not mineralize rachitic cartilage in vitro. Diphosphonates, which inhibit crystal formation, have also been suggested to prevent stone formation. A daily dosage of 1,500 mg phosphorus appears to be the minimal effective amount in men, whereas 1,250 mg has been adequate in most women. Patients who form multiple stones may require up to 2,250 mg phosphorus daily to prevent formation of new calculi. Orthophosphates markedly reduced or prevented stone formation in 90% of 270 patients, most of them treated for 1–12 years. Diarrhea is the most troublesome side effect. At present, oral diphosphonate therapy holds little promise in treatment of calcareous calculi. Calcium excretion in urine can be reduced by limitation of dietary calcium and administration of compounds that interfere with its intestinal absorption. Sodium phy-

(4) Kidney Int. 13:390–396, May, 1978.

tate and cellulose phosphate have been evaluated for this purpose.

Cost, palatability and absence of ill effects on long-term treatment must be considered in selection of an agent to use in patients with renal stones. Regardless of the treatment chosen, continuous supervision of patients is necessary.

▶ [Our experience with using phosphates to prevent calcium stones has also been good. Thiazides and phosphates should not be given together since they are reported to cause renal damage. Phosphates and magnesium therapy should not be used together since they are reported to cause newberryite stones.–J.Y.G.] ◀

Prevention of Calcium Stones with Thiazides. Edmund R. Yendt and Moussa Cohanim[5] (Queen's Univ., Kingston, Ont.) observe that the mechanism by which thiazides reduce urinary calcium excretion is still not entirely clear. There is fairly good evidence that intestinal calcium absorption may decrease during long-term thiazide administration. There is some confusion regarding the effects of thiazides on serum calcium concentration. Other effects of thiazides include an increase in urinary magnesium excretion, a marked rise in urinary zinc excretion and a decrease in urinary oxalate excretion.

A standard dosage of 50 mg hydrochlorothiazide twice daily has been used. A lower dosage is used at first to minimize side effects. The authors have initiated thiazide therapy in 346 patients with renal calculi and have observed progression of stone disease in 16 patients complying well with a full dosage of hydrochlorothiazide. No new stone formation was seen in 28 normocalciuric patients with calcium stones during 103 patient-years of observation. Stone progression has ceased in 30 hypercalciuric patients with tubular ectasia who received thiazides. Side effects have occurred in about 30–35% of thiazide-treated patients. They have tended to be most severe during the initial phase of treatment and have often disappeared in time. Metastatic calcification has not been observed during long-term thiazide therapy.

Stone progression ceases in at least 90% of patients who take hydrochlorothiazide regularly. A dosage of only 25 mg twice daily appears to be effective in a significant propor-

(5) Kidney Int. 13:397–409, May, 1978.

tion of patients. Thiazides are effective in normocalciuric and in hypercalciuric patients and in most patients with tubular ectasia (medullary sponge kidney). Side effects have necessitated discontinuance of thiazide therapy in about 7% of cases. The therapeutic efficacy of thiazides in stone prevention cannot be accurately predicted by the degree of the hypocalciuric response. Thiazides also reduce urinary oxalate excretion and increase urinary zinc and probably magnesium excretion, and these effects probably contribute to the efficacy of thiazides in prevention of stone disease.

▶ [More patients with recurrent calcium stones should be on such a medical program.–J.Y.G.] ◀

Calcium-Uric Acid Nephrolithiasis. A small fraction of patients with nephrolithiasis form mixed calcium-uric acid stones or pass both types of stone. Fredric L. Coe[6] (Michael Reese Hosp.) reviewed 23 cases, found among 539 renal stone patients. The patients constituted 4.7% of patients for whom the stone type was known. At least 1 mixed stone was documented in 17 patients. Patients with idiopathic hypercalciuria were treated with 2 mg trichlormethiazide twice daily and those with hyperuricosuria with 100 mg allopurinol twice daily or a low-purine diet. Patients without metabolic disorder were treated with allopurinol or a low-purine diet. A thiazide derivative was also used in 2 patients to control high blood pressure.

Stone disease was unusually active in this group; the patients formed 67.8 stones per 100 patients per year, nearly twice the rate for calcium stone formers in general. In 3 patients primary hyperparathyroidism was documented by excision of an adenoma. Two patients had gout. Hyperuricosuria was found in 11 patients, always in association with hypercalciuria, which was idiopathic in 9. Two patients had hypercalciuria alone. Only 1 patient had a low 24-hour urine pH. Ten patients had no detectable urine chemistry abnormality of calcium or uric acid. Four patients had continuing stone disease on treatment with allopurinol and alkali, but the new stones frequently were composed only of calcium salts. Treatment appeared to reduce stone formation. When 4 patients who formed only 1

(6)   Arch. Intern. Med. 138:1090–1093, July, 1978.

stone were excluded, new stones were 13.7% of those predicted on the basis of the pretreatment recurrence production rate.

Combined idiopathic hypercalciuria and hyperuricosuria was found in about 40% of patients with calcium-uric acid nephrolithiasis in this series. The natural history was reminiscent of that in hyperuricosuric calcium stone formers, with high recurrence rates. The pathogenesis of mixed stones is not obvious, but treatment directed against both calcium and uric acid crystallization seems to be effective in prevention of new stones.

▶ [Stone analysis and metabolic studies are obviously needed to diagnose and treat these patients.−J.Y.G.] ◀

Hyperuricosuric Calcium Oxalate Nephrolithiasis. Fredric L. Coe[7] (Michael Reese Hosp.) points out that hyperuricosuria is frequent in patients with calcium oxalate nephrolithiasis. Excessive dietary purine intake is a major factor in hyperuricosuria. Uric acid overproduction from endogenous purine metabolism contributes in some patients. A tubular defect of urate reabsorption is unlikely in view of the absence of hypouricemia. Idiopathic hypercalciuria was found alone in 32.2% of calcium stone-formers and with hyperuricosuria in 11.7%, whereas 14.6% had only hyperuricosuria and 20.2% had no discernible metabolic defect. Hyperuricosuric patients formed most of their stones at a slightly greater average age than other types of patients. Robertson obtained evidence that sodium acid urate may promote calcium oxalate stone disease by forming a gel phase in urine, which adsorbs or interferes with naturally occurring urine inhibitors of calcium oxalate crystal growth. The inhibitors may be acid mucopolysaccharides.

Perhaps the most dramatic evidence linking hyperuricosuria to calcium oxalate stones is the apparent ability of allopurinol to reduce new stone formation to far below pretreatment rates. Stone production was reduced greatly by allopurinol therapy in 48 patients with recurrent calcium stones who had hyperuricosuria as the sole metabolic disorder and who were treated for at least a year. A group of 34 patients without detectable metabolic disorder, who received no specific treatment, formed less than two thirds

(7) Kidney Int. 13:418–426, May, 1978.

of the stones expected during follow-up, suggesting that nonspecific factors related to follow-up probably foster a moderate decline in stone formation, but one that is far less impressive than that which occurs with allopurinol therapy. Dietary measures have not been evaluated as a treatment approach. They may be as effective as allopurinol and offer the advantages of simplicity and avoidance of a drug.

Acetohydroxamic Acid: Clinical Studies of a Urease Inhibitor in Patients with Staghorn Renal Calculi. The hydroxamic acids are inhibitors of urease. Acetohydroxamic acid is relatively nontoxic and is noncarcinogenic, although high doses may be teratogenic. It inhibits alkalization of urine and crystallization of struvite and apatite in vitro, despite the growth of *Proteus,* and prevents the formation of struvite bladder stones in rats with chronic *Proteus* urinary infection. Donald P. Griffith, J. R. Gibson, C. W. Clinton and Daniel M. Musher[8] (Baylor Univ.) examined the pharmacokinetics of acetohydroxamic acid and its effects on urine pH and ammonia in patients with staghorn renal calculi and chronic urinary infection due to urease-producing bacteria. The agent was given orally in gelatin capsules. The first 8 patients received single weekly doses of 500–2,000 mg and then multiple daily doses of the same amount. Twenty-three patients have been treated continuously with 500 mg twice daily for 2–12 months.

Major side effects have been infrequent. A reversible hemolytic anemia occurred in 2 patients taking 1.5–2 gm daily and in 1 with azotemia who took 1 gm daily for 2 months. No significant biochemical changes have been observed. The drug is absorbed rapidly from the gut and excreted in the urine. Excretion was significantly lower in patients with reduced renal function. Urinary alkalinity and ammoniuria were reduced in all patients. Reductions were incomplete in patients with urinary appliances, who generally had much higher urinary ammonia concentrations and greater urinary alkalinity. Long-term sterilization of the urine with antibiotics had failed before administration of acetohydroxamic acid. Two patients had sterile urine while receiving acetohydroxamic acid and culture-

(8) J. Urol. 119:9–15, January, 1978.

specific antibiotics, with little or no change in the radiographic size of the renal stones.

Acetohydroxamic acid therapy should significantly reduce the incrustation of catheters and the formation of bladder stones in patients requiring long-term catheter drainage. Urease inhibition may facilitate the dissolution of infection-induced urinary stones and reduce the urinary virulence of urea-splitting bacteria. Acetohydroxamic acid is well tolerated clinically. It potentiates the effect of a number of antimicrobial agents against several bacterial species in vitro; the exact nature of this synergy is unknown.

Pharmacokinetics of Acetohydroxamic Acid: Preliminary Investigations. Acetohydroxamic acid (AHA), a bacterial urease inhibitor, is being studied as an agent for use in treatment of infection-induced urinary stones and as a potentiating agent for antimicrobials. It effectively inhibits bacterial urease in urine and is well tolerated clinically. Stuart Feldman, Lakshmi Putcha and Donald P. Griffith[9] (Houston) examined the pharmacokinetics of AHA in normal volunteers and in male Sprague-Dawley rats. Two healthy subjects received 250, 500 and 1,000 mg AHA in aqueous solution and a third received a 1,000-mg dose. Patients with staghorn renal calculi and chronic urinary tract infection due to urease-producing bacteria received 250-mg capsules of AHA after overnight fast. Fasted rats were dosed orally and intravenously. The oral doses were 50 and 100 mg/kg and the intravenous doses were 10, 50 and 100 mg/kg.

In rats the biologic half-life of AHA increased with dose after oral and intravenous administration. Bioavailability was less with oral than with intravenous administration. In normal subjects the apparent biologic half-life of AHA also increased with increasing doses. The drug was distributed throughout the total body water. Patients showed an increased AHA half-life with a decreasing creatinine clearance and a decrease in the percentage of the dose recovered in the urine as intact AHA.

Acetohydroxamic acid is subject to nonlinear pharmacokinetics. The data indicate saturation of the metabolic con-

(9) Invest. Urol. 15:498–501, May, 1978.

version of AHA to its metabolites. Acetohydroxamic acid is absorbed rapidly from the gastrointestinal tract after oral administration to human subjects. It has a biologic half-life of about 5–10 hours in subjects with normal renal function and may be dose dependent in its disposition. Pharmacokinetic studies of patients given repetitive daily doses of AHA are in progress.

▶ [AHA is shown in patients to block the urease enzyme and thereby prevent further struvite formation. Its role in clinical medicine is not defined. Bacteriuria can be suppressed in some patients with proteus infections and struvite stones by chronic antibiotic administration. The hematologic complications with long-term AHA administration must be defined. The acid is not available for use because it is not patentable and no drug company will undergo the expense of testing in patients. Vernon Smith is studying the effect of hydroxyurea, another urease inhibitor, in patients with struvite stones. The persistence of Don Griffith and his group is to be congratulated and encouraged.–J.Y.G.] ◀

Struvite Stones are discussed by Donald P. Griffith[1] (Baylor Univ.). Stones of struvite, or crystalline magnesium ammonium phosphate, have been termed infection stones and triple phosphate stones. Human struvite stones are a mixture of struvite and carbonate-apatite. Numerous reports attest to the association of urea-splitting bacteria, struvite and carbonate (apatite) stones. Experimental studies indicate that urease-producing bacteria are the primary, if not the sole, bacteria involved in infection-induced stones. Ureolysis by urease leads to chemical changes in the urine that bring about urine supersaturation by struvite and carbonate-apatite, and crystal formation. An associated increase in urinary proteins may also play a role in calculogenesis. Elimination of infection or inhibition of urease or both may reverse the pathologic process. Infection stones account for 15–20% of all urinary stones. Staghorn renal calculi are commonly infection induced. Bladder stones of struvite and carbonate-apatite occur often in association with long-term urethral catheterization.

Treatment is directed toward removal of all stones and correction of anatomical abnormalities; eradication or suppression of urinary tract infection or both; and treatment of any underlying metabolic disorder. Surgical re-

(1) Kidney Int. 13:372–382, May, 1978.

moval of infected renal calculi, with or without removal of focal areas of pyelonephritis, is usually practical and successful. Antibiotics are given before and after operation. Long-term, low-dosage, culture-specific antibiotics are probably indicated. Restriction of dietary phosphorus with Basaljel supplementation is of some use in prevention of recurrence or growth or both, of infection stones. Specific antimicrobial therapy should significantly reduce the calcium phosphate saturation of urine. Treatment with acetohydroxamic acid (AHA) reduces urine alkalinity and ammonia excretion. Combined AHA and specific antibiotic therapy has sterilized the urine in previously resistant cases. Side effects of AHA have been minimal. Significant stone dissolution has not been observed in patients given AHA. Of the hydroxamates studied biologically, AHA appears to have the greatest pharmacologic potential.

▶ [In our experience the Shorr program (10W phosphate diet plus Basaljel) and sterilization of bacteriuria have usually prevented recurrences. The diet, however, is difficult to adhere to. The successful use of the Shorr program at New York Hospital is reported in the Journal of Urology (108: 368, 1972).–J.Y.G.] ◄

Oxalic Acid and the Hyperoxaluric Syndromes are discussed by Hibbard E. Williams[2] (Univ. of California, San Francisco). Calcium oxalate stones are the most common type of renal calculus found in the United States. Oxalate absorption from the gut is normally small, and most urinary oxalate is derived from endogenous sources. Hyperoxaluria may be due to increased endogenous production, primarily from the major precursor glyoxylate, or to increased oxalate excretion, secondary to increased intake or gastrointestinal oxalate absorption. Increased oxalate production has been attributed to intake of a metabolic precursor of oxalate, pyridoxine deficiency and primary hyperoxaluria associated with a genetic defect in oxalate synthesis. Both types of primary hyperoxaluria are inherited as autosomal recessive traits. Enteric hyperoxaluria recently has been recognized in patients with a variety of malabsorptive states in which gastrointestinal absorption of oxalate is increased. This is because calcium is bound to fat, leaving the oxalate free to be absorbed.

In patients with hyperoxaluria secondary to increased

(2) Kidney Int. 13:410–417, May, 1978.

ingestion of oxalate or a precursor, the offending agent is removed and acute renal failure is treated. Acute hemodialysis may be of use in reducing the serum oxalate concentration. Vitamin replacement is indicated in the rare patient with pyridoxine deficiency. Attempts to reduce oxalate production in primary hyperoxaluria have generally been unsuccessful. Large doses of pyridoxine may be helpful in these cases. Maintenance of large urine volumes is important. Calcium restriction probably is not indicated. A low-oxalate diet may be of some help. Treatment becomes more difficult once chronic renal failure develops. Enteric hyperoxaluria is managed with a low-oxalate diet, control of fat malabsorption and careful calcium supplementation. Cholestyramine may be helpful in patients in whom calcium therapy causes an increase in urinary calcium that offsets the reduction in urinary oxalate.

▶ [The role of urinary oxalate excretion in calcium stones has not received the attention it deserves since oxalate increases have 10 to 20 times the effect of calcium increases on stone formation. A drug analogous to allopurinol needs to be developed for such patients.–J.Y.G.] ◀

Urolithiasis in Patients with a Jejunoileal Bypass. Ralph V. Clayman, Henry Buchwald, Richard L. Varco, William C. DeWolf and Richard D. Williams[3] (Univ. of Minnesota) studied 517 patients (426 women and 91 men) for up to 11 years after jejunoileal bypass surgery for obesity. The proximal 40 cm of jejunum was joined to the distal 4 cm of the ileum in an end-to-end manner. The distal limb of the defunctionalized segment was attached end-to-side to the cecum and its proximal limb oversewn. Patients received KCl, Lomotil, diphenoxylate and atropine after discharge, as well as calcium carbonate in a dose of 0.84 gm 3 times daily. Monthly injections of vitamin B_{12} were also given.

Symptomatic urolithiasis was recorded in 34 of the 365 patients contacted (9%). It occurred in 7% of women and 19% of men. Urolithiasis was verified by pyelography or the recovery of stones in all but 3 patients. About one third of the patients passed more than one stone. Stones were recovered from 47% of the patients and analyzed in 32%. All but 1 patient passed calcium oxalate stones. Open sur-

(3) Surg. Gynecol. Obstet. 147:225–230, August, 1978.

gery was necessary in 21% of affected patients. The average interval to symptomatic stone disease in 27 patients was 22 months. Stone formation could not be related to diet, family history, fluid intake, medications, renal disease, age or postoperative weight loss. No stone disease was recorded in 91 patients operated on more recently. These patients drank less coffee than the earlier ones, and more of them continued to use calcium carbonate. These patients were younger than the study group and had lost less weight when evaluated.

Recent findings support the hyperoxaluria theory of colonic hyperabsorption. The simplest and often the most effective approach to reducing oxalate absorption has been to attempt to eliminate the substrate. The present findings indicate that calcium supplementation may help prevent urolithiasis in patients who undergo jejunoileal bypass operation. Both metabolic and roentgenographic studies are necessary before and at regular intervals after operation to identify "silent" stone formers.

▶ [This is an excellent example of a situation in which correction of one problem (obesity) creates another medical problem (urolithiasis). Oxalate stone formation has stimulated much research into oxalate metabolism in these patients. In addition to the theory of increased oxalate absorption secondary to calcium binding by fat, others have suggested a toxic effect from the increased bile salts and oxalate which causes increased oxalate absorption.– J.Y.G.] ◀

Nephrolithiasis during Pregnancy. Previous studies of women with renal stones have focused on pregnancies complicated by stone passage. Fredric L. Coe, Joan H. Parks and Marshall D. Lindheimer[4] (Univ. of Chicago) analyzed the obstetric histories of 78 women with established nephrolithiasis, in whom stones had no adverse effects on pregnancy other than an increase in number of urinary tract infections. Pregnancy did not alter the activity or severity of stone disease. The women, aged 45 and under, had a total of 148 pregnancies, 90 before and 58 after diagnosis of overt nephrolithiasis. Forty had no further pregnancies after stone disease was diagnosed. Eleven women were pregnant both before and after their disease became evident, and 27 became pregnant at the time they began forming stones or afterward. Calcium oxalate or calcium

(4) N. Engl. J. Med. 298:324–326, Feb. 9, 1978.

phosphate stones were present in all but 12. Ten patients had struvite stones and 2 had cystine stones. Idiopathic hypercalciuria was found in 42% of the women, hyperuricosuria in 13%, primary hyperparathyroidism in 10%, infection stone in 13% and cystinuria in 3%.

Stones were passed during 20 pregnancies of 15 patients. Six calculi were discovered during evaluation for pain or urinary tract bleeding. Most patients were hospitalized, but bladder catheterization, cystoscopy and surgery were not performed. The rate of stone passage did not appear to be increased during pregnancy. Six pregnancies ended in abortion. Symptomatic urinary tract infection complicated 11 of 58 pregnancies that occurred after the onset of stone disease and 6 of 90 pregnancies that occurred before onset of stones, a significant difference. Other complications were no more frequent in pregnancies complicated by stones than during stone-free or prestone pregnancies.

Stone disease has no prejudicial effect on pregnancy other than an increased frequency of urinary tract infection. Pregnancy appeared to exert no influence on stone disease in this series. Seven of 8 women with hyperparathyroidism had relatively uncomplicated gestations.

▶ [Little is written on this subject since, as the authors confirm, stone disease does not affect pregnancy except by increasing the frequency of urinary tract infections.–J.Y.G.] ◀

Evaluation of Calcium Urolithiasis in Ambulatory Patients: Comparison of Results with Those of Inpatient Evaluation. Charles Y. C. Pak, Christopher Fetner, Judith Townsend, Linda Brinkley, Cheryl Northcutt, Donald E. Barilla, Melvin Kadesky and Paul Peters[5] (Univ. of Texas Health Science Center, Dallas) evaluated a protocol for evaluation of ambulatory patients for various causes of calcium urolithiasis. It consists of collection of two 24-hour urine samples with subjects ingesting a random diet, and another when subjects are adhering to a diet restricted in calcium and sodium. A test of "fast" and "oral calcium load" follows. The results were compared with those of inpatient evaluation in 24 patients with calcium urolithiasis of various causes, 19 men and 5 women with a mean age of 42 years. Twelve normal subjects were also evaluated.

(5) Am. J. Med. 64:979–987, June, 1978.

The match in defining abnormalities between outpatient and inpatient evaluations was virtually complete with respect to urinary calcium during fasting and after an oral calcium load, urinary oxalate excretion and urinary cyclic adenosine monophosphate and serum calcium and parathyroid hormone concentrations. Six patients with normocalciuria as inpatients on a low-calcium diet had hypercalciuria on the restricted outpatient diet. Serum phosphate and renal threshold phosphate values were generally lower in the outpatient setting. Urinary uric acid values were significantly higher in outpatients. The two evaluations gave the same diagnoses in 18 patients, including 7 with absorptive hypercalciuria during both low and high calcium intakes. One patient was found to have hyperuricosuric calcium oxalate nephrolithiasis only on outpatient study. Hyperuricosuria coexisted with other causes of calcium stones in 14 patients during outpatient evaluation and was present in 3 patients during inpatient study. The ambulatory evaluation confused absorptive hypercalciuria type II (only with a high calcium intake) with type I in 4 patients. Hypophosphatemic absorptive hypercalciuria was erroneously diagnosed in 1 patient.

The ambulatory protocol may have the distinct advantage over inpatient study in detection of hyperuricosuria. The only serious deficiency concerned the 1 erroneous diagnosis of hypophosphatemic absorptive hypercalciuria.

▶ [In an era in which everyone is trying to cut medical costs, this article shows that the cheaper ambulatory evaluation of stone patients is as reliable as evaluation conducted during hospitalization.–J.Y.G.] ◀

Simultaneous Measurement of Vitamin D Metabolites in Plasma: Studies in Healthy Adults and in Patients with Calcium Nephrolithiasis. Angela E. Caldas, Richard W. Gray and Jacob Lemann, Jr.[6] (Med. College of Wisconsin, Milwaukee) measured the three major circulating metabolites of vitamin D simultaneously to determine whether alterations in vitamin D metabolism other than elevated plasma 1,25-$(OH)_2$-D levels may result in changes in plasma 24,25-$(OH)_2$-D levels in calcium stone formers. Studies were done in 36 healthy adults, aged 20–46 years, and in 23 patients, aged 18–75 years, with a history of

(6) J. Lab. Clin. Med. 91:840–849, May, 1978.

calcium oxalate and/or apatite nephrolithiasis. All but 3 of the patients were men. None had primary hyperparathyroidism or urinary infection. All subjects were on a normal diet that included one daily serving of dairy products.

Plasma 25-OH-D concentrations averaged 48 nmol/L in healthy adults. The average plasma 24,25-$(OH)_2$-D concentration was 4.3 nmol/L, and the average plasma 1,25-$(OH)_2$-D concentration was 82 pmol/L. The plasma levels of 24,25-$(OH)_2$-D and 25-OH-D were significantly positively correlated. The patients with calcium nephrolithiasis had an average plasma 25-OH-D concentration of 45 nmol/L and an average plasma 24,25-$(OH)_2$-D concentration of 3.7 nmol/L, not significantly different from the means for normal subjects. A positive correlation between plasma 24,25-$(OH)_2$-D and 25-OH-D levels, similar to those observed in normal subjects, was also evident in the stone formers. The plasma 1,25-$(OH)_2$-D concentrations were significantly elevated in the patient group, averaging 132 pmol/L. This metabolite was not correlated with the others in either group.

These findings suggest that the synthesis of 24,25-$(OH)_2$-D is, to a large extent, dependent on the availability of precursor 25-OH-D in healthy adults and in calcium stone formers. Hypophosphatemia may be responsible for the high plasma 1,25-$(OH)_2$-D concentrations in calcium stone formers, either as a result of a primary defect in phosphate metabolism or as a result of secondary hyperparathyroidism. The elevation appears to be specifically dependent on disturbances of regulation of the renal mitochondrial 1α-hydroxylase system that determines synthesis of the hormone.

▶ [Vitamin D metabolism is being studied to understand the etiology of calcium nephrolithiasis. One difficulty in such studies is the development of an accurate and sensitive assay for vitamin D_3. 7-Dehydrocholesterol is converted by ultraviolet light to vitamin D_3. This is converted in the liver to 25-hydroxyvitamin D_3, then in the kidney to 24,25-dihydroxyvitamin D_3, and finally to its most active form, 1,25-dihydroxy-vitamin D_3, which is synthesized only in the kidney under the stimulus of low serum phosphate. Caldas et al. postulate that one mechanism of the disordered calcium metabolism in stone formers is an elevated vitamin D_3 stimulated by hypophosphatemia. Physiologic functions of vitamin D_3 are to increase intestinal calcium absorption, mobilize calcium from bone, which requires the presence of both vitamin D and parathyroid hormones and, possibly, increase renal tubular reabsorption of calcium.–J.Y.G.] ◀

Relative Deficiency of Plasma Calcitonin in Normal Women. Calcitonin appears to protect the skeleton, as well as maintain plasma calcium homeostasis, and its relative deficiency in women may be a factor in the etiology of postmenopausal osteoporosis. C. J. Hillyard, J. C. Stevenson and I. MacIntyre[7] (Royal Postgrad. Med. School, London) used a new radioimmunoassay for plasma calcitonin to study 19 normal men and 30 normal women aged 17–35 years; 18 women taking oral contraception; and 13 women in the 3d trimester of pregnancy. No drugs other than contraceptives were being used. The estrogens included mestranol and ethinyl estradiol and the progestagens were norethisterone, norethisterone acetate, *d*-norgestrel, *dl*-norgestrel and lynestrenol.

The findings are shown in Figure 7. The plasma calcitonin concentration was at least 4 times higher in men

Fig 7.—Plasma calcitonin concentrations in four groups. Group means are shown. Mean plasma calcitonin concentration was significantly lower in normal women than in the other three groups (P < 0.001). (Courtesy of Hillyard, C. J., et al.: Lancet 1:961–962, May 6, 1978.)

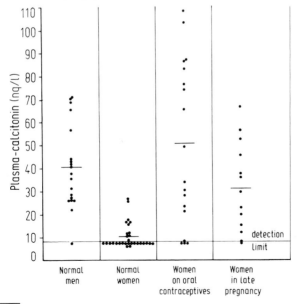

(7) Lancet 1:961–962, May 6, 1978.

than in women, but both pregnancy and oral contraception increased the concentrations in women to those found in men.

It is tempting to suggest that testosterone, estrogen and perhaps progesterone are responsible for the sex difference, but that testosterone is by far the most potent stimulator of calcitonin secretion. The findings are compatible with the view that calcitonin acts to protect the skeleton during times of calcium stress such as pregnancy and perhaps during growth and lactation. If so, calcitonin may have a role in the etiology of postmenopausal osteoporosis. Plasma calcitonin is heterogeneous, and it is conceivable, though unlikely, that the differences observed reflect changes in biologically inactive but immunologically reactive species.

▶ [These authors report one of the first measurements of plasma calcitonin in normal subjects, possibly because of a new radioimmunoassay technique. The hypothesis that a deficiency of calcitonin may be involved in the etiology of postmenopausal osteoporosis remains to be proven.–J.Y.G.] ◀

Divalent Cation Metabolism: Familial Hypocalciuric Hypercalcemia versus Typical Primary Hyperparathyroidism. Although it has been suggested that metabolism differs in primary hyperparathyroidism and familial hypocalciuric hypercalemia, analyses of parathyroid gland histologic findings and plasma parathyroid hormone concentrations have not clearly differentiated these groups. S. J. Marx, A. M. Spiegel, E. M. Brown, J. O. Koehler, D. G. Gardner, M. F. Brennan and G. D. Aurbach[8] (Natl. Inst. of Health) investigated 23 members of three families with familial hypocalciuric hypercalcemia and 64 subjects with hyperparathyroidism.

Serum concentrations of sodium, potassium, chloride, bicarbonate and phosphate were similar in the two groups; hypophosphatemia and mild hyperchloremic acidosis were present in both. Serum magnesium concentrations were significantly higher in the familial group, even when controlled for age, sex and renal function. Serum calcium and magnesium concentrations were inversely related in the group with primary hyperparathyroidism and positively related in the familial group. The severity of hypercal-

(8)   Am. J. Med. 65:235-242, August, 1978.

cemia was similar in the two groups, but creatinine clearance was higher in the familial group and no different from the age-adjusted and sex-adjusted normal mean. Urinary calcium excretion was strikingly lower in the group with familial hypocalciuric hypercalcemia. Serum protein concentrations were similar in the two groups. Plasma ionized and ultrafilterable calcium concentrations were increased in both groups in similar direct proportion to the increase in plasma total calcium concentration. The plasma ultrafilterable magnesium concentration showed a similar proportional relation to the plasma total magnesium concentration in all patients.

Increased serum concentrations of the physiologically active forms of both calcium and magnesium are present in familial hypocalciuric hypercalcemia. The renal handling of the filtered load of these divalent cations differs from that in primary hyperparathyroidism.

▶ [Patients with hypocalciuric hypercalcemia rarely have nephrolithiasis and need to be differentiated from those with hyperparathyroidism. The mechanism of hypocalciuria despite hypercalcemia is unknown.–J.Y.G.] ◀

Radionuclide Kidney Function Evaluation in the Management of Urolithiasis. Renal and ureteral stones may cause asymmetric renal damage that is not assessed accurately by serum creatinine and blood urea nitrogen measurements, urography, nephrotomography and arteriography. Anton J. Bueschen, L. Keith Lloyd, Eva V. Dubovsky and W. Newlon Tauxe[9] (Univ. of Alabama) performed renal scintillation camera studies in 77 patients seen in 1975–76 with renal or ureteral lithiasis. Renal calculi were present in 53 patients and ureteral calculi in 24. The 64 men and 13 women had a median age of 55 years. A total of 114 studies was performed. The adult dose of ^{131}I-orthoiodohippurate was 300 μCi in patients with 2 kidneys and 150 μCi in those with a solitary kidney. Upper abdominal radioactivity was recorded after nuclide injection, and a blood sample was obtained 44 minutes after injection to calculate effective renal plasma flow (ERPF). The mean normal ERPF in a study of 67 kidney donors was 514 ± 46 ml/minute.

The ERPF was more sensitive than the serum creatinine

(9)   J. Urol. 120:16–20, July, 1978.

level as an indicator of total renal function. It was as low as 300 ml/minute in some patients with normal serum creatinine values. The ERPF to individual kidneys often was unequal in the presence of a normal serum creatinine level. In differential studies, the ERPF often was equal in the presence of abnormal total ERPF and often unequal in the presence of normal total ERPF. The time of peak activity often was delayed with equal and unequal differential ERPF. Serial studies gave very reproducible results or demonstrated easily explained changes. No patient except those with small nonobstructing stones had a normal camera study with an abnormal pyelogram (IVP). The IVP failed to quantitate the degree of decreased unilateral renal function.

The comprehensive renal function study is helpful in evaluating patients with urolithiasis by providing an accurate measure of total and differential renal function. It is a noninvasive procedure, requires no patient preparation and produces low radiation exposure. No allergic reactions occur.

▶ [Radionuclide measurement of kidney function is a noninvasive procedure that allows the accurate measurement of differential renal function. Experimental studies in our laboratory have shown that the ^{131}I-orthoiodohippurate scan could reliably predict whether a hydronephrotic kidney would recover function after release of obstruction. Our few clinical studies have also shown the scan's ability to determine the amount of renal function in the kidney damaged from ureteropelvic junction obstruction or reflux.–J.Y.G.] ◀

Homocystinuria in New South Wales. Bridget Wilcken and Gillian Turner[1] (Sydney, Australia) reviewed the findings in 27 patients (17 male and 10 female subjects) with homocystinuria from fifteen families in New South Wales. All 27 patients had biochemical findings consistent with cystathionine synthetase deficiency. The condition in 1 patient was found on newborn screening, but the condition in the others was detected because of symptoms. For patients born during 1960–69, the ascertainment rate for the total population was 1 in 58,000. When the diagnosis was confirmed, patients received 200–500 mg pyridoxine daily in divided doses, and the plasma amino acids and serum and red blood cell folate levels were determined.

Five patients were referred with poor vision and 1 with

(1) Arch. Dis. Child. 53:242–245, March, 1978.

apparent traumatic lens dislocations. Two others were aphakic after operation. Seven other patients with dislocated lenses were investigated for other reasons. Fourteen patients were overtly mentally retarded, with IQs less than 70. Many others were considered slower than their unaffected siblings, even before homocystinuria was diagnosed. Seven patients had thrombotic episodes, which in 4 patients were severe. All six deaths were probably related to thrombosis. A marfanoid habitus was noted at diagnosis in 6 patients. Thirteen patients responded to pyridoxine therapy. One required folic acid as well. Temporary biochemical improvement was observed in two of the families not responsive to pyridoxine. All but 1 of the 9 patients considered to be very mildly affected were in the pyridoxine-responsive group. One of these sibships included 2 subjects of superior intelligence.

One third of patients in this series were very mildly affected by homocystinuria. There is clearly a group of patients who remain relatively asymptomatic until adult life. Physicians must consider the possibility of homocystinuria in adults who present with thromboses. The diagnosis also must be considered in otherwise normal girls presenting with tallness at the time of puberty. It is not clear whether cases requiring folic acid therapy as well as pyridoxine represent a different enzyme activity response or a variant of "classic" homocystinuria.

▶ [The urologist must be aware of the clinical syndrome of homocystinuria: dislocation of the ocular lens, marfanoid habitus, osteoporosis, arterial and venous thromboses, and mental retardation in moderately to severely affected cases. No renal stones were described in these patients.–J.Y.G.] ◀

X-RAY AND DIAGNOSIS

Enhanced Detection of Asymptomatic Renal Masses with Routine Tomography during Excretory Urography. L. Keith Lloyd, David M. Witten, Anton J. Bueschen and William W. Daniel[2] (Univ. of Alabama) found in a prospective study of a diagnostic scheme for evaluating renal masses that a significant number would have gone undetected without routine tomography. A scout film of the ab-

(2) Urology 11:523–528, May, 1978.

domen and a single tomographic cut through the renal area are first obtained. An injection of 50 or 100 cc of contrast material is then given, with external ureteral compression, and tomographic cuts are made at three or four levels through the renal area 1–3 minutes after contrast material injection. Further films are obtained after compression is released.

Of 109 patients having this evaluation during 1974–75, 32 (29%) had renal masses that did not deform the collecting system and were detected only on tomographic films. Only 23 patients had symptoms that could have been referable to the renal masses detected, including 6 patients in the tomography-detected mass group. The diagnosis in all the latter patients was benign renal cyst. The diagnoses are given in the table. Benign renal cyst was the most frequent diagnosis, followed by renal cell carcinoma. Virtually all masses in the tomography-detected mass group were benign renal cysts, but two highly significant findings were an asymptomatic renal cell carcinoma and a papillary cystadenoma.

Routine tomography permits detection of a large number of asymptomatic renal masses and defines the renal anatomy sufficiently for standard nephrotomography or renal gamma camera studies to rarely be needed. The diagnostic enhancement of routine tomography and its ease of appli-

DISTRIBUTION OF DIAGNOSES

Diagnosis	Total Group	Tomography-Detected Mass Group
Benign renal cyst	88	29
Renal cell carcinoma	8	1
Papillary cystadenoma	1	1
Adrenal adenoma	1	—
Hamartoma	1	—
Perinephric abscess	2	—
Polycystic disease	2	—
Pancreatic pseudocyst	1	—
Atrophic pyelonephritis	4	1
No mass	1	—
TOTALS	109	32

cation should make it a standard feature of excretory urography.

▶ [Our experience is similar. The incidence of asymptomatic renal masses detected by tomography is reported by Lang to be as high as 4% in the general hospital population and as high as 15% in patients with benign prostatic hypertrophy (Radiology, 109:257, 1973). Certainly more masses will be detected with routine tomography and even more with the CT scan. The paucity of hard data about false positives or negatives with ultrasound, CT scanning, arteriography or mass puncture prevents the development of a definite protocol. However, institutions seem to be moving in a more conservative direction, i.e., using renal exploration less to decide whether a cystic-appearing lesion is malignant.—J.Y.G.] ◀

Radioimmunoassay for Urinary Renal Tubular Antigen: Potential Marker of Tubular Injury. Richard A. Zager and Charles B. Carpenter[3] report development of a radioimmunoassay capable of quantitating a single human renal tubular epithelial antigen (HRTE-1) in unconcentrated urine and serum. Antiserum was produced in rabbits by use of renal tubular epithelial fractions, and immunofluorescence staining was carried out. Human RTE antigens were identified by immunodiffusion in agarose and by immunoelectrophoresis in agarose. The competitive protein-binding assay was based on antigen purified from a crude tubular preparation by salt fractionation, DEAE anion exchange chromatography and Sephadex G-200 gel filtration. The antigen was labeled with ^{125}I for use in the assay.

The HRTE-1 antigen was demonstrated in serum and urine and in extracts of a variety of organs. All but 1 of 24 patients with chronic nephropathy or prerenal azotemia had normal urinary antigen concentrations, despite wide differences in urine flow rate, degree of renal function and amount of proteinuria. Ten of 12 patients with acute tubular necrosis had significantly abnormal HRTE-1 levels. Eight had high levels, whereas in 2 HRTE-1 was not detectable.

The findings suggest that HRTE-1 antigen can be detected in both normal and pathologic urines, and that altered antigen concentration can be documented in at least one renal disorder, acute tubular necrosis. Quantitation of HRTE-1 in urine may have clinical value as a marker of

(3) Kidney Int. 13:505–512, June, 1978.

acute tubular injury. The present assay can detect antigen over a range of 6 ng/ml to 50 μg/ml. The degree of reproducibility is high. A large, blind, prospective study is needed to determine the ultimate clinical utility of the assay.

▶ [This technique is exciting in that the amount of renal tubular antigen in urine does seem to correlate with loss of brush border elements in acute tubular injury. Since this antigen is not entirely kidney-specific, more studies are needed to accurately define its role in clinical medicine.–J.Y.G.] ◀

Urologic Applications of Computerized Axial Tomography: Preliminary Report. Bruce H. Stewart, Robert James, John Haaga and Ralph J. Alfidi[4] (Cleveland Clin. Found.) reviewed experience with computerized tomographic (CT) scanning in 190 urologic patients with proved disorders of the genitourinary system and retroperitoneum. At present the Delta-50 Fast Scanner is used. A bolus of 50 ml 60% sodium and meglumine diatrizoate was injected after the preliminary scan when additional contrast was needed.

All but one of 34 cysts were diagnosed correctly by CT scanning. In many cases, patients with cysts in central sites suspected on pyelography were found on CT scanning to have additional cysts in other locations. Guidance by CT in cyst aspiration and injection was useful. Fifteen patients with renal neoplasia were studied. Study by CT can differentiate angiomyolipomas from renal cell carcinoma, and local extension of disease into pararenal structures and regional nodes often can be demonstrated. Fetal lobulation and renal fibrolipomatosis were shown by CT scanning in several cases, obviating the need for angiography and/or renal exploration. Small renal pelves associated with relatively acute obstruction were identified and aspirated under CT guidance. Percutaneous nephrostomy was facilitated in several instances. The CT scan is also helpful in demonstrating larger retroperitoneal lesions and their relation to other organs and in evaluating adrenal disease. Demonstration of genitourinary pathology in the pelvis by CT scanning has been somewhat limited to date. In localizing foreign bodies, CT scanning is of great value. The study has also been helpful in defining the location and extent of abscesses in some instances.

---

(4) J. Urol. 120:198–204, August, 1978.

Initial experience has shown that CT scanning is of value in helping determine the etiology, site and extent of various diseases of the kidneys, adrenals, retroperitoneum and pelvic organs. In most cases it will probably augment rather than replace conventional diagnostic procedures, although it undoubtedly will eliminate the need for potentially hazardous procedures in some cases. The procedure also makes possible the accurate placement of needles for aspiration, biopsy, antegrade pyelography and temporary percutaneous nephrostomy. It is noninvasive and carries a low risk of radiation exposure.

▶ [In our experience both computerized axial tomography and ultrasonography have been very accurate diagnostic tools. It is difficult, however, to keep abreast of these new fields. The urologist and radiologist *must* define the accuracy of these methods (false positives and negatives) and not stamp on the patient's chart that the renal mass is a "cyst" without knowing the chances of error. It is worrisome to see a patient admitted for a problem, undergo an ultrasound or CT scanning procedure, and *then* be referred to the urologist for an intravenous pyelogram. According to William R. Fair, of 35 cases at Barnes Hospital called "cyst" on CT scanning, 2 were false positive and 1 false negative as shown by surgery, autopsy and other methods.–J.Y.G.] ◀

Comparative Diagnostic Accuracy of 105 mm versus Conventional and Magnification Radiographic Techniques in Arteriographic Diagnosis of Renal and Perirenal Masses. David Wixson, Harold A. Baltaxe, Stephen Balter and Lawrence N. Rothenberg[5] (New York Hosp.-Cornell Univ. Med. Center, New York) evaluated the diagnostic accuracy of 105 mm photofluorography (23 cm mode) versus magnification and/or conventional radiography in the arteriographic study of renal or perirenal masses. The results obtained in 106 selective renal arteriograms in which the 105 mm technique and at least one other radiologic technique had been used were reviewed. The findings in 88 patients were evaluated. Photofluorography and magnification radiography were compared in 82 patients for diagnostic accuracy. Photofluorography and conventional radiography were performed and compared in 33 patients.

There were no interobserver differences in the diagnosis of the presence or absence of a mass. The findings determined by the different methods are compared in Figure 8. In three instances, the pathology was not apparent on the

(5) Invest. Radiol. 12:527–533, Nov.-Dec., 1977.

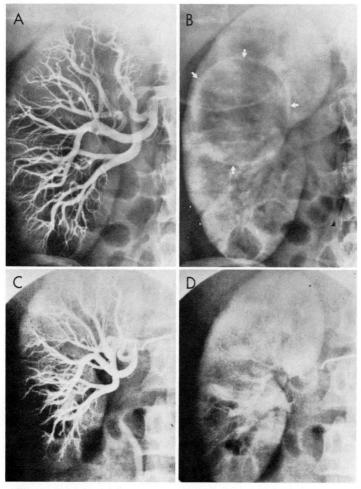

Fig 8.—**A** and **B,** an avascular right renal mass *(arrows)* is seen with the magnification radiographic technique but not with 105-mm photofluorographic technique (**C** and **D**). Ultrasonography confirmed the presence of 8-cm right renal cyst. (Courtesy of Wixson, D., et al.: Invest. Radiol. 12:527–533, Nov.-Dec., 1977.)

105-mm photofluorographs but was evident on magnification radiographs. The limited field size was a frequent disadvantage with 105 mm photofluorography and to a lesser extent with magnification radiography. Part of the kidney or pathology was excluded from the field in 49 of 100 patients with single renal arteries examined by 105 mm photofluorography and in 12 of 77 having magnification radiography. Severe exclusions were present in 24 and 6 patients, respectively. The kidney and pathology were included in the field in all 33 selective renal arteriograms done by conventional technique.

Photofluorography is not presently suitable for use as a sole radiographic technique in the arteriographic evaluation of renal pathology. Conventional radiography offers a compromise between the advantages and disadvantages of the magnification and photofluorographic techniques. A larger photofluorographic mode is needed for routine renal arteriography to provide adequate field size and decrease the frequent need for repeat examinations; however, the field size must not be increased at the cost of further reduced resolution.

A Rapid Method for Diagnosis of Acute Uric Acid Nephropathy. Acute uric acid nephropathy is an oliguric state that is rapidly reversible with appropriate therapy. It is thought to be due to deposition of uric acid crystals in the collecting tubules. About 50 cases have been reported. The disorder may become more prevalent as neoplastic diseases are treated more aggressively. John Kelton, William N. Kelley and Edward W. Holmes[6] postulated that the ratio of the concentration of uric acid to that of creatinine in a random urine specimen might differentiate acute uric acid nephropathy from acute renal failure of other causes. Five patients with acute uric acid nephropathy and 27 with acute renal failure from other causes were studied. No patient was receiving allopurinol therapy.

The mean serum urate concentration tended to be higher in patients with acute uric acid nephropathy, but there was considerable overlap between the two groups. The ratio of the mean urinary uric acid concentration to creatinine concentration differed significantly in the two groups. The highest uric acid to creatinine ratio obtained in any patient with acute renal failure was 0.90, whereas the lowest obtained in any patient with acute uric acid nephropathy was 1.0. In 7 previously reported cases, the

(6)   Arch. Intern. Med. 138:612–615, April, 1978.

serum urate related to the blood urea nitrogen did not distinguish the patients from those with other types of acute renal failure.

The ratio of uric acid to creatinine in urine distinguishes individual patients with acute uric acid nephropathy from those with acute renal failure of other causes. A uric acid to creatinine ratio more than 1.0 in a random urine specimen may be a useful adjunct in supporting the clinical diagnosis of acute uric acid nephropathy.

▶ [Treatment of acute uric acid nephropathy with diuresis by mannitol and Lasix, alkalinization with Diamox and sodium bicarbonate, and reduction of the uric acid load with allopurinol has been successful in our hands.–J.Y.G.] ◀

Ultrasonic Evaluation of the Prostatic Nodule. Physical examination alone does not distinguish benign from malignant prostatic lesions, and many clinicians perform biopsy whenever a hard nodule is palpated. Martin I. Resnick, James W. Willard and William H. Boyce[7] (Bowman Gray School of Medicine) used transrectal prostatic ultrasonography as an adjunct in evaluating patients who had prostatic nodules on rectal examination. A rotatable transrectal ultrasonic probe was passed into the rectum, and serial sonograms of the prostate and surrounding structures were obtained. Perineal needle biopsy was done where prostatic calcification was absent or if the site of nodules did not correspond to that of prostatic calculi on radiography and ultrasonography.

Malignant nodules are seen as focally dense, asymmetric areas that do not fade with increased instrument attenuation. Often sound waves are not transmitted through the tumor. Larger tumors distort the capsule, and seminal vesicle invasion may be detected. Areas of chronic prostatitis may be difficult to distinguish from malignancy. Prostatic calculi do not distort the prostatic capsule, and their position can be confirmed radiographically.

Fifty patients with a mean age of 70.2 years who had undiagnosed prostatic nodules were studied. In 5 with prostatic calcifications, the ultrasonic and radiographic position corresponded to the site of the palpable nodule. All 21 patients with ultrasonic findings suggesting malignancy had biopsy evidence of adenocarcinoma. Biopsy specimens

(7) J. Urol. 120:86–89, July, 1978.

in 20 patients with ultrasonic findings of benign tissue all showed benign hyperplasia. Biopsy of a suspicious area in the palpably normal opposite lobe in 1 case showed adenocarcinoma. Prostatitis was predicted in 2 of 4 cases from the ultrasonic findings. Ultrasonography clearly showed the degree of tumor involvement in patients with malignancy. The operative findings corresponded closely to the ultrasonic findings in 8 patients who were suitable candidates for radical prostatectomy.

Transrectal ultrasonography appears to be a useful adjunct in evaluating patients with prostatic nodules. It is helpful in differentiating malignant and benign lesions and in selecting patients for further evaluation. It also is a useful noninvasive staging technique.

▶ [This is the only experience I am aware of in using ultrasound to evaluate prostatic nodules. Its role is yet to be determined. I do not think it will replace the rectal exam and most clinicians will still want a needle biopsy or cytologic exam from a thin needle. Our experience using the thin needle has been that we can get an accurate diagnosis within minutes.–J.Y.G.] ◀

Urinary Tract after Abdominoperineal Resection. Radiographic changes in the urinary tract after abdominoperineal resection may make it difficult to recognize recurrent neoplastic disease. Zoran L. Barbaric, Daniel E. Wolfe and Arthur J. Segal[8] reviewed the findings in 33 patients (22 men and 11 women, with a mean age of 59 years) who had uroradiologic examinations after abdominoperineal resection. All patients were operated on for rectal carcinoma.

All patients showed medial deviation of the ureters; this was much more marked in the men. The right ureter could cross the midline in the region of the pelvic brim or sacral hollow (Fig. 9). This positional change could be explained by the removal of supporting structures and the occurrence of postoperative fibrosis. Hydronephrosis was noted in 11 patients, 7 of whom were asymptomatic. Unilateral obstruction always occurred on the left. Benign stricture could not be distinguished radiographically from ureteral invasion by recurrent tumor. All patients had some form of bladder deformity. This was much more marked in the men. Recurrent tumor deforming the bladder usually occurred at the inferior aspect of the bladder on the left (Fig. 10). Six patients had bladder outflow obstruction. Five men

(8) Radiology 128:345–348, August, 1978.

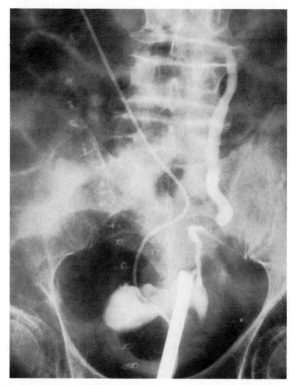

Fig 9.—Retrograde pyeloureterogram. Both ureters are positioned medially. Right ureter is crossing the midline; 1-cm long left ureteral narrowing proved to be due to recurrent rectal carcinoma. The bladder is deformed. (Courtesy of Barbaric, Z. L., et al.: Radiology 128:345–348, August, 1978.)

had a retrovesical abscess. One patient had a ureterocutaneous fistula complicating inadvertent ureteral ligation. One man had a urethroperineal fistula. Urinary tract infection was a common complication. Reflux, abscess formation, ureteral obstruction and fistulas could all be detected radiographically. Emphysematous cystitis and pericystitis were also observed. Osteitis pubis was noted in 1 patient. In 3 patients, phleboliths were displaced after operation.

The most difficult diagnostic radiologic problem is the differentiation of ureteral stricture from recurring invasive

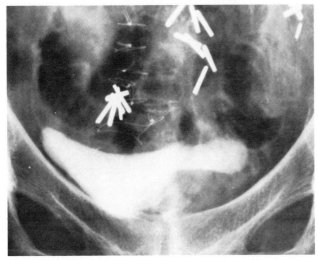

Fig 10.—Recurrent rectal carcinoma deforming left bladder floor several months after operation. In 3 patients with recurring neoplasm affecting the bladder, the displacement or deformity was always present on the left. (Courtesy of Barbaric, Z. L., et al.: Radiology 128:345–348, August, 1978.)

neoplasm. This can be effectively solved by thin-needle aspiration biopsy of the area in question. Cystography and voiding or retrograde urethrography are useful in evaluating retrovesical abscesses. This study suggests the necessity for a baseline postoperative excretory urogram in all patients undergoing abdominoperineal resection.

▶ [In our experience medial deviation of the ureters at the sacral promontory is common and is assumed to be due to reapproximation of the edges of the posterior peritoneum during closure. Since urologists are unable to perform adequate pelvic examinations in these male patients, it is difficult to determine if symptoms are due to urologic pathology (i. e., the prostate), recurrent tumor or abscess formation. In some of these patients with perineal pain in whom I suspect recurrent rectal carcinoma, I have done "blind" biopsies through the perineum and obtained a histologic confirmation of recurrent cancer.–J.Y.G.] ◀

Urine Cytology Findings in Analgesic Nephropathy. B. Jackson, J. A. Kirkland, J. R. Lawrence, A. S. Narayan, H. E. Brown and L. R. Mills[9] (Univ. of Adelaide) found 3 urothelial carcinomas and 1 case of severe urothe-

(9) J. Urol. 120:145–147, August, 1978.

lial dysplasia by urine cytology screening in 98 patients with analgesic-induced papillary necrosis. Eighteen other patients had changes suggesting that they were at risk of malignancy in the near future. Freshly voided urine was processed by filtration through a Millipore filter, and the cellular elements were stained with Papanicolaou, hematoxylin, orange-green 6 and Ehrlich's acid 50 reagents. The diagnosis of analgesic nephropathy was based on a definite history of analgesic abuse of over 3 powders or tablets daily for at least 5 years and radiographic or histologic demonstration of papillary necrosis.

A mean of 4.2 cytologic studies per patient was performed, with an average cytologic follow-up of 17 months. Twenty-two patients (22.4%) had changes suggestive of malignancy. Two of the 19 who were adequately investigated had bladder carcinoma, and 1 had a presumed renal pelvic carcinoma. A 4th patient had advanced dysplastic changes. The degree of cytologic abnormality was not related to the amount of analgesic consumed, but the more severe changes tended to occur in more severe renal failure. More marked changes tended to occur in males. A preparation of aspirin, phenacetin and caffeine, "Bex," was used in 84% of cases. About half the patients abstained from analgesics during the survey, and in a few cases the cytologic changes tended to improve slowly over a period of 1–2 years. However, class C and D cells were found in several patients who had stopped abuse up to 8 years previously.

Routine urine cytology is recommended in all cases of analgesic nephropathy. It appears reasonable to avoid phenacetin and its derivatives when analgesics must be used over the long term and to change the analgesic compound at intervals.

▶ [Analgesic abusers have been reported to have an increased incidence of uroepithelial tumors (Leistenschneider: Schweiz. Med. Wochenschr. 103:433, 1973 and Bengtsson: Scand. J. Urol. Nephrol. 2:145, 1968). In Jackson's study, 3 of 19 patients with positive cytology had malignancies and 1 had advanced dysplastic changes. Whether the remaining have "false positive" cytologies or will develop tumors is unknown.–J.Y.G.] ◀

Cytologic Changes Due to Urinary Calculi: Consideration of Relationship between Calculi and Development of Urothelial Carcinoma. M. E. Beyer-Boon, L. H.

R. I. Cuypers, H. J. de Voogt and J. A. M. Brussee[1] examined the cytologic changes induced by calculi in 62 patients with urinary tract lithiasis and the relationship between calculi and urothelial carcinoma in 92 patients with proved cancer of the renal pelvis or ureter. Most cytologic studies were done on fresh, spontaneously voided specimens. Smears of sediments were stained by the Papanicolaou method and by the May Gruenwald Giemsa (MGG) method. Most specimens were examined by phase contrast microscopy. Calculi from 45 patients were analyzed chemically.

The cytology report was positive for cancer in 10 patients, suspicious in 1, atypical in 7 and negative in 44. In 9 patients, the cytologic picture was thought to be compatible with grade 2 carcinoma. The cytologic picture became normal after the calculi were removed and remained normal for periods of 1–5 years in all of the 9 patients. In 1 of these, the cytologic pattern remained abnormal after pyelolithotomy but returned to normal after litholapaxy. Both nuclear changes and multinucleated urothelial cells were noted in abnormal sediments. The proportion of multinucleated cells increased during an attack of renal colic. Similar types of stones were found in patients with normal and abnormal cytologic findings. No patient has manifested urothelial carcinoma to date. In 9 of 11 patients with "false positive" lithiasis, the cytologic picture was less polymorphic than in most patients with carcinoma in situ. Fewer abnormal cells were present in the lithiasis patients, and an inflammatory background was frequently present. The mean proportion of multinucleated, morphologically malignant cells was 12.3%. Morphologically benign multinucleated urothelial cells were often found in the lithiasis patients in contrast with patients with carcinoma in situ.

Severe cellular changes may be found in the urothelium adjacent to a calculus, and a review of the findings in 92 patients with urothelial carcinoma showed a possible relation between a long history of lithiasis and the development of upper tract cancer. It is conceivable that the atypia

(1) Br. J. Urol. 50:81–89, April, 1978.

associated with lithiasis may prove to have clinical importance comparable with the drug-induced atypia that was thought to "mimic" cancer. Patients who have stones and shed abnormal cells must be followed closely.

▶ [In our experience squamous cell carcinoma of the renal pelvis is frequently associated with long-term calculi. Perhaps the changes in urine cytology will prove to be the precursor of malignant changes. Longer follow-up of these patients is certainly needed.–J.Y.G.] ◀

Urinary Cytology as a Screening Study to Detect Urinary Malignancies. Nelson A. Moffat[2] (Marshfield Clin., Marshfield, Wis.) performed cytologic examination of voided urine in a population of 1,337 persons aged 50–65 years in the Greater Marshfield Community Health Plan, a prepaid health-care program in central Wisconsin with an enrollment of about 40,000 persons, to look for malignant cells arising from the urinary tract. Contact with patients was made by mail. Of 5,342 notified of the study, 1,337 (25%) responded. Thirteen specimens contained abnormal cells, and two contained markedly atypical cells strongly suggesting carcinoma. One patient had flank pain and was found on pyelography to have a ureteral tumor; a cervical lymph node was positive for transitional cell carcinoma. The other 12 patients had negative pyelograms and cystoscopic studies. Some patients also underwent bladder biopsy. All had repeated cytologic studies which were negative.

The cost of this study was about $1,000, not including the cost of follow-up studies on "abnormal" subjects. The response rate was low and a relatively small number of lesions were detected. However, the method was an inexpensive one for screening a population. The possibility of false negative results requires further investigation.

▶ [In our experience, the reliability of urine cytology is dependent on the skill of the person reading the data and varies tremendously from institution to institution. The yield will also vary with the populations screened since uroepithelial tumors are relatively uncommon (20 per 100,000).

The largest experience of controlled cytologic screening I am aware of is at the Mayo Clinic. Drs. Charles Rife and David Utz in 2 years (1975–77) did 10,323 paired procedures (cystoscopy and cytology) on 8,140 patients. Of these patients, 2,800 were known to have had previous uroepithelial tumors. Cytology picked up 67% of the 1,310 bladder cancers, and cystoscopy missed 12.2% (of which most were in situ or sessile). Cytology most fre-

(2) Wis. Med. J. 77:S37–S38, April, 1978.

quently missed the low grade papillary lesions. The false positive rate was 4%, most of which later turned out to have cancer. The false negative rate was 3–4%.–J.Y.G.] ◀

Infusion Intravenous Pyelography and Renal Function: Effects in Patients with Chronic Renal Insufficiency. Tahir Shafi, Shyan-Yih Chou, Jerome G. Porush and Warren B. Shapiro[3] (Brookdale Hosp. Med. Center, Brooklyn) prospectively studied a group of patients with renal insufficiency undergoing infusion pyelography to evaluate factors that might play a role in the nephrotoxic effects contrast mediums. Forty patients with various degrees of renal insufficiency who underwent pyelography in 1975 and 1976 were studied. Patients received fluids intravenously from the night before examination; about 1.5 L was given in 15 hours. Each patient received 300 ml of 30% sodium diatrizoate by intravenous drip in 10–15 minutes, after bisacodyl administration and overnight fast.

Twenty-eight patients had a 25% or greater rise in serum creatinine concentration or decrease in creatinine clearance or both after pyelography. Prestudy serum creatinine concentrations were similar in these patients and those without nephrotoxicity. Fractional excretion of sodium increased in nephrotoxic patients. Eleven of 12 diabetics had further deterioration in renal function after pyelography. Seventeen nephrotoxic patients were nondiabetic. Four nephrotoxic patients and 1 nontoxic patient became oliguric after pyelography. The serum creatinine concentration usually peaked on the 3d day after pyelography and generally returned to the baseline level after 7–10 days. No patient required dialysis.

Infusion pyelography entails a risk of producing acute renal failure in patients with chronic renal failure, with and without diabetes. The procedure should be ordered only for patients in whom the potential benefits outweigh the potential risk. Renal function should be monitored daily for several days after the procedure. Preexistent vascular disease in the kidney, possibly associated with the known vasoconstrictive effects of contrast mediums, may be important in the production of acute renal failure after infusion pyelography.

(3) Arch. Intern. Med. 138:1218–1221, August, 1978.

Renal Injury Associated with Intravenous Pyelography in Nondiabetic and Diabetic Patients. Currently used radiographic contrast agents may be nephrotoxic for diabetic patients. Bruce E. VanZee, Wendy E. Hoy, Thomas E. Talley and John R. Jaenike[4] (Univ. of Rochester) reviewed experience with 23 patients in whom renal function deteriorated after intravenous pyelography; 16 were nondiabetic. The patients had an abrupt rise in serum creatinine concentration of over 1 mg/dl, with or without oliguria, after pyelography; no other nephrotoxic factors were apparent. In 6 patients preexistent deterioration of renal function was accelerated or oliguria occurred abruptly after pyelography. Pyelography was done with 300 ml Reno-M-Dip (30% diatrizoate meglumine) given by infusion; the dose of iodine was 42.3 gm per examination.

The incidence of renal function deterioration increased as renal failure became more severe in both diabetics and nondiabetics. The prevalence in a series of 2,360 pyelographies done in a 10-month period was 0.8%. All but 1 of the nondiabetics had recognized renal disease. In 5 it was due to hypertension. Most patients were elderly. Nine were receiving diuretics and 8, antibiotics. Eleven of 16 episodes in nondiabetics were accompanied by oliguria within 24 hours of pyelography. Oliguria was of short duration and never lasted over 72 hours. The serum creatinine concentration peaked in a mean of 3.3 days. Two patients had structural changes of acute tubular necrosis on renal biopsy. Nine patients recovered completely in a mean of 14.8 days. Four patients underwent chronic hemodialysis. The course was similar in diabetics.

Identification of susceptible patients is the first step in prevention of pyelography-induced renal failure. Initial use of radionuclide or ultrasound studies, or both, is indicated in place of pyelography in some high-risk patients if the desired information can be so obtained. If pyelography is necessary, care should be taken with preparation and contrast dose, and patients should be monitored for renal dysfunction after the procedure.

Acute Renal Failure Following Drip Infusion Pyelography. Alejandro Carvallo, Thomas A. Rakowski, Wil-

(4) Ann. Intern. Med. 89:51–54, July, 1978.

liam P. Argy, Jr., and George E. Schreiner[5] (Georgetown Univ.) describe 10 patients in whom acute renal failure followed drip infusion pyelography (DIP). Only 4 had diabetes. The patients were seen in 1972–77 after DIP with Renografin 60 (diatrizoate meglumine). The criterion for acute renal failure was a rise in serum creatinine concentration of at least 2 mg/100 ml over the prestudy level. All patients received 0.5 mg contrast per lb diluted in equal amounts of 5% aqueous dextrose solution.

Mean patient age was 59.4 years. The 4 diabetic patients and 2 others had severe vascular disease. No patient had multiple myeloma. Eight patients had a baseline serum creatinine concentration above 1.5 mg/dl. Nine had proteinuria before DIP. Five patients were clinically volume depleted, and 2 others had fluid overload with severe heart failure and evidence of decreased renal perfusion. Two other patients had received gentamicin. Eight patients had oliguria within 24 hours after the study, and this lasted for up to 5 days. The peak rise in serum creatinine concentration, occurred at 2–15 days. Renal function returned to baseline level in 3 patients in 8–10 days. Of a total of 44 patients on whom data were reviewed, 92.8% were azotemic, and 70.4% had poor renal perfusion before pyelography. Severe vascular disease was present in 78.9%, diabetes in 59.5% and multiple myeloma in 7.2%. Acute renal failure was associated with oliguria in 94.5% of cases.

The chief predisposing factor in acute renal failure that followed DIP in this series was preexistent renal disease against a background of systemic disease. Renal function should be monitored for a few days after DIP. Factors leading to decreased renal perfusion should be corrected if possible before the procedure, and the concomitant use of nephrotoxic drugs should be avoided.nFluid restriction is seldom indicated.

Renal Failure Following Major Angiography. Acute renal failure is known to follow angiography with contrast agents. Richard D. Swartz, James E. Rubin, Brian W. Leeming and Patricio Silva[6] (Boston) undertook a retrospective study of consecutive angiographic procedures done

(5) Am. J. Med. 65:38–45, July, 1978.

(6) Ibid., pp.31-37.

in 6 months in 1976. The 109 patients on whom data were reviewed represented over 90% of cases in the review period. Acute renal failure was defined as a rise in blood urea nitrogen concentration of 50% or 20 mg/dl, an increase in serum creatinine concentration of 50% or 1 mg/dl, or both, occurring within 48 hours of the procedure.

Thirteen cases of renal failure followed angiography and 1 case followed cholangiography. Volume depletion or dehydration was infrequent in this series. The patients had complicated medical or surgical conditions and generally underwent abdominal or renal angiography. Preexistent renal insufficiency was present in 9 of 13 patients in whom renal failure followed angiography. It was mild in all but 1. Four patients had proteinuria. Liver function was abnormal in 6 patients, and 6 had a decreased serum albumin concentration. Eight patients were diabetic. Only 2 patients had notable acute reactions to angiography. Five patients became oliguric. Two patients required dialysis for uremic complications. Renal function recovered in 90% of cases, but 5 patients died in the hospital. Two or more risk factors were present in 11 of 13 patients with renal failure in this series and in 22% of unaffected patients. Five patients with renal failure and only 4 of 90 unaffected patients had combined renal insufficiency and impaired liver function. Hypoalbuminemia was strongly associated with impaired liver function.

Certain conditions, such as diabetes and perhaps proteinuria, may make the kidney more sensitive to injury by a substance that is directly toxic to the nephron. Others, such as renal insufficiency and hepatic insufficiency, increase the blood concentration or prolong the elimination of the toxic substance. Further study may make it possible to defer potentially dangerous procedures where the benefits are questionable and to plan ahead for diagnosis and management of complications where they are expected.

▶ [The previous four articles document that contrast agents can be nephrotoxic. The mechanism of injury is not defined. From these articles one can, however, summarize the following information: Impairment of renal function occurs immediately. Oliguria occurs frequently; its duration is usually short, with recovery by 10 days, but not always. Some patients required dialysis. Nephrotoxicity seems more likely with large or repeated doses. Nephrotoxicity is worse in patients with renal insufficiency, impaired liver function, diabetes mellitus, hypoalbuminemia and proteinuria. Dehydration, selective renal angiography and hypotension do not seem to be causative factors in the toxicity.

Why is the toxicity just now showing up? Have contrast agents changed? Higher doses? Different preparation of patients? Are clinicians now more observant?

A real danger is exposing the patient with unrecognized contrast toxicity to surgery the next day and further renal insults.

Our institution has had a similar experience with nephrotoxicity after large doses of contrast agents. One patient with normal serum creatinine pre X-ray developed typical X-ray evidence of acute tubular necrosis on the 10-minute film. He developed oliguria and a serum creatinine increase to 4 mg/100ml, with resolution by the 10th day.

One of our residents, John Forrest, has been studying contrast nephropathy in our laboratory. In dogs no acute change in renal function was noted with doses of 2, 4, and 6 ml/kg of 60% Renograffin. With an 8 ml/kg dose all had a decrease in the glomerular filtration rate. Preliminary studies show similar findings if a solution without contrast of the same hyperosmolality and electrolyte concentrations is used. Moreau (Radiology 115:329, 1975) biopsied 211 patients within 10 days of excretory urography or renal arteriography. Osmotic nephrosis of the proximal tubular cells was found in 47 (22%). Tubular necrosis was associated with histologic features in 29 of 47. The mechanisms by which contract media may induce osmotic nephrosis remain unclear.–J.Y.G.] ◀

MISCELLANEOUS

Does the Peritoneum Need to Be Closed at Laparotomy? Harold Ellis and Robert Heddle[7] (London) compared the occurrence of burst abdomen and incisional hernia in a prospective randomized study of patients whose laparotomy wounds were sutured in an identical manner, differing only in whether or not the peritoneum was sutured. A two-layer technique of continuous catgut to peritoneum and continuous nylon to sheath was compared with a one-layer technique in which the peritoneal suture line was omitted. The two closure methods were also evaluated in rabbits. The 162 two-layer and 164 one-layer patients were similar in age, sex, type of incision and complications. Slightly more two-layer patients had malignant disease.

Four total wound disruptions (2.5%) occurred in the two-layer group, and 5 (3%) in the one-layer group. Seven patients in each group had an incisional hernia. Ten of the 14 hernias were detected within 3 months of surgery. Over-

(7) Br. J. Surg. 64:733–736, October, 1978.

all wound failure rates did not differ significantly. A total of 140 patients had been followed for at least 6 months. Seven of 21 jaundiced patients had wound failure. All wound failures were associated with jaundice, obesity and/or postoperative complications. Only 2 patients, both with abdominal dehiscence, were on long-term steroid therapy. In the rabbits, there was no significant difference in tensiometric findings or the incidence of adhesions with one- and two-layer closures, and the histologic appearances were similar in the two groups of animals.

This clinical study failed to show obvious differences in the healing of laparotomy wounds with the peritoneum sutured or left open. Comparable results were obtained in the rabbit study. It is concluded that closure of the peritoneum has little relevance to the subsequent strength of the laparotomy scar. A no. 2 double nylon continuous suture is now used to close the full thickness of the abdominal incision apart from the skin, which is sutured separately with interrupted fine nylon. Over 50 abdominal wounds have been closed in this way without a failure.

▶ [This carefully designed study clearly documents that the peritoneum does not need to be closed after laparotomy.–S.S.H.] ◀

Chyluria: Result of Surgical Treatment in 50 Cases. Severe chyluria can cause distressing dysuria, clot colic and wasting. Operation is required in these cases. Henry H. Y. Yu, C. H. Leong and G. B. Ong[8] (Hong Kong) operated on 50 patients with chyluria in 1964–76. Ligation and stripping of the renal lymphatics were carried out in 27% of 185 patients seen in this period with chyluria. The 34 males and 16 females, had an average age of 33.4 years at diagnosis. Twenty-two patients had passed chylous clots, and 3 of them had chylous clot retention requiring catheterization and irrigation. Five patients had dysuria and 4, loin pain. Ten patients had lost weight. Six patients had associated urologic conditions. Two patients had abnormal urograms, 1 from a urothelial tumor and 1 from an upper pole renal cyst. Cystoscopy after a fatty meal showed chylous efflux in 33 of 36 patients. Pedal lymphography demonstrated reflux in all 49 patients so examined.

---

(8)   J. Urol. 119:104–107, January, 1978.

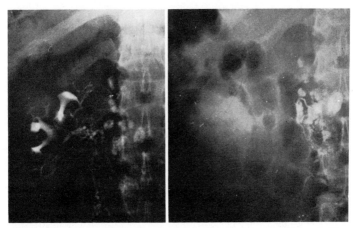

Fig 11 (left).—Preoperative lymphogram showing unilateral renal lymphatic reflux on right side.

Fig 12 (right).—Postoperative lymphogram showing complete disconnection of lymphatics with no evidence of recanalization.

(Courtesy of Yu, H. H. Y., et al.: J. Urol. 119:104–107, January, 1978.)

Only 1 patient had bilateral stripping at one session via the transperitoneal route. Three had bilateral stripping via the extraperitoneal route, 2 at one session. Twenty-six patients were treated for unilateral fistulization. Two patients had wound infections and 1 had prolonged ileus. Three fourths of patients were free from chyluria at followup. Six of 13 with persistent symptoms had had only unilateral stripping despite the presence of bilateral fistulization. Incomplete stripping was shown on postoperative lymphography in the other 7. Complete disconnection of the renal lymphatics of the stripped kidney was demonstrated in 20 patients who underwent unilateral stripping (Figs 11 and 12). Recurrent symptoms from residual renal lymphatics were controlled by dietary restriction.

Until the etiology of chyluria is demonstrated, ligation and stripping of the renal pedicle constitute the treatment of choice. Unilateral stripping gives the best results, even in patients with bilateral reflux. Simultaneous bilateral stripping invariably has led to inadequate stripping.

▶ [As the original article points out, mild cases of chyluria can be treated by substituting medium-chain triglycerides for fat in the diet. Although the authors have a very large experience, it is more likely that their failure of bilateral strippings relates more to surgical technique than to a mysterious factor associated with the bilateral procedure.—S.S.H.] ◄

Management of Intractable Pain in Patients with Advanced Malignant Disease. B. M. Mount, R. Melzack and K. J. Mackinnon[9] evaluated use of the Bromptom mixture to control the chronic pain of malignant disease. The oral narcotic mixture used at the Royal Victoria Hospital in Montreal is shown in the table. Most patients obtain analgesia with 5–20 mg morphine per dose of the mixture, but small or elderly patients may require as little as 2.5 mg. The standard elixir always is given with a phenothiazine. Prochlorperazine usually is highly effective as an antiemetic with little sedative effect; if restlessness or agitation is present, chlorpromazine may be substituted. Expected lengthy survival is not a contraindication. In most cases a pain-free state can be achieved by giving sequential increments in narcotic dose. It is in general wise to change only one component at a time. Dispensation of the morphine mixture and the phenothiazine syrup separately provides greater flexibility in dosage adjustment.

The Brompton mixture and a phenothiazine were evaluated in 90 patients in a palliative care unit and in 238 on general hospital wards or in private rooms. Pain was measured in 92 patients with the McGill-Melzack pain questionnaire. The treatment controlled pain in 90% of patients in the palliative care unit and in 75–80% of those in the wards or private rooms. The mixture produced substantial reductions in sensory, affective and evaluative dimensions

ROYAL VICTORIA HOSPITAL ORAL
NARCOTIC MIXTURE

Morphine, 5 mg. or more
Cocaine, 10 mg.
Ethyl alcohol (98%), 2.5 cc
Syrup, 5 cc
Chloroform water Ad, 20 cc
    given with
Prochlorperazine, 5 mg. or more
(or chlorpromazine, 10 mg. or more)

(9)   J. Urol. 120:720–725, December, 1978.

of pain. Nearly 80% of patients received morphine doses below 20 mg; the overall mean dose was 12.3 mg. The Brompton mixture was, in general, well tolerated. The most common problems were sedation, nausea and vomiting and constipation. Significant tolerance, dependence and respiratory depression were not observed.

When the Brompton mixture is used, dosage can easily be adjusted to meet the patient's needs. Many patients find a syrup easier to swallow than a tablet. The sedative effects usually are transient. Extrapyramidal effects are infrequent with suggested phenothiazine doses. To be effective against the total pain of advanced malignant disease, the Brompton mixture must be used with other treatments. Interpersonal and psychosocial assistance is most helpful.

▶ [The hospice movement and publications such as this show a long overdue concern for improving the quality of life of the terminally ill. The authors' experience suggests that the Brompton mixture can be extremely useful in the management of chronic pain.—S.S.H.] ◀

Urologic Complications of Pelvic Irradiation. There is a strong clinical impression that serious urologic complications are relatively common after curative irradiation of the pelvic viscera. Richard J. Dean and Bernard Lytton[1] (Yale Univ. School of Medicine) evaluated 964 patients who underwent radiotherapy for malignant disease of the pelvic viscera during 1963–68 and were followed for 5–10 years after the completion of treatment. Treatment was for gynecologic tumors in 493 patients, genitourinary tumors in 240, bowel tumors in 172 and various other pelvic malignancies in 59. Either external beam radiotherapy or interstitial therapy with radium plaques or needles was administered. External beam therapy was from a linear accelerator; the usual dose was 6,000 R in 6 weeks.

A total of 203 urologic complications (21%) occurred, but the rate of complications attributable to radiation alone was only 2.5%. Fourteen patients had cystitis, 5 each had hematuria and fistulas and 1 had ureteral obstruction. The complications are summarized in Table 1 and the time of onset of these complications indicated in Table 2. Twelve of 18 patients with cystitis received more than 6,000 R. Four of the 5 with hematuria received more than 7,000 R.

(1) J. Urol. 119:64–67, January, 1978.

TABLE 1.—Pelvic Radiation—Urologic Problems (1963–68)

	No. Pts.	Cystitis	Hematuria	Obstruction	Fistula	Totals
Gynecologic	493	11/18	2/5	1/35	5/11	19/69
Genitourinary	240	2/44	3/20	0/28	0/4	5/96
Bowel	172	0/7	0/4	0/16	0/10	0/37
Other	59	1/1	—	—	—	1/1
Totals	964	14/70	5/29	1/79	5/25	25/203

Number of patients without tumor/total number of patients with symptoms.

TABLE 2.—Time of Onset of Urologic Problems after Pelvic Radiation

	Gynecologic No. Pts. (%)	Genitourinary No. Pts. (%)	Bowel No. Pts. (%)	Totals No. Pts. (%)
Cystitis:				
<6 Mos.	10 (56)	39 (89)	5 (28.5)	54 (78)
>6 Mos.	8 (44)	5 (11)	2 (71.5)	15 (22)
Hematuria:				
<6 Mos.	0	3 (15)	0	3 (10)
>6 Mos.	5 (100)	17 (85)	4 (100)	26 (90)
Fistula:				
<6 Mos.	5 (44)	1 (25)	2 (20)	8 (32)
>6 Mos.	6 (56)	3 (75)	8 (80)	17 (68)
Obstruction:				
<6 Mos.	2 (6)	3 (11)	2 (12.5)	7 (9)
>6 Mos.	33 (94)	25 (89)	14 (87.5)	72 (91)

TABLE 3.—Relationship of Pelvic Radiation Dosage to Urologic Complications

	<4,000R	4,000–6,000R	>6,000R
Cystitis	6 (0)	22 (1)	42 (13)
Hematuria	3 (0)	8 (0)	18 (5)
Obstruction	24 (0)	20 (0)	35 (1)
Fistula	9 (1)	6 (0)	10 (4)
Totals	42 (1)	56 (1)	105 (23)

Numbers in parentheses indicate patients who were free from tumor.

Most patients with fistula received more than 6,000 R, and the 1 with ureteral obstruction received about 8,000 R. The relationship of pelvic radiation dosage to urologic complications is given in Table 3. Thirty of 44 patients with irritative bladder symptoms after treatment for genitourinary tumors had had an open bladder operation before radiotherapy. Nineteen of these 30 patients received more than 6,000 R. Sixteen of 20 patients with hematuria had an open bladder operation, and 14 received more than 6,000 R. About half the gynecologic patients with urinary obstruction or fistulas had radiotherapy before operation, and nearly half of these received more than 4,500 R.

Urologic complications are uncommon after irradiation of the pelvic viscera for malignant disease, in the absence of persistent or recurrent tumor. Intractable cystitis occurred in about 15% of patients treated for bladder cancer, most of whom had evidence of persistent or recurrent tumor and who had received more than 6,000 R or had undergone open bladder surgery before radiotherapy. Urinary fistula formation was associated with tumor in the fistula in 80% of the patients.

▶ [The authors found that only 2.5% of 964 patients who had received pelvic radiotherapy had urologic complications due to radiation alone. However, this is a falsely low figure because patients with recurrent tumor were eliminated from the numerator but not from the denominator. From the data presented we cannot determine how many patients had recurrent cancer; however even if one subtracts only those with cancer and complications, the rate increases to 3.2%. If one were to eliminate all patients who received less than 5,500 R and those with cancer, we suspect that the urologic complication rate would be at least 5% in the high dose cancer-free subgroup.–S.S.H.] ◀

Superiority of Demeclocycline over Lithium in Treatment of Chronic Syndrome of Inappropriate Secretion of Antidiuretic Hormone. Both lithium and demeclocycline interfere with the cellular action of antidiuretic hormone (ADH) and have been suggested as agents for use in long-term treatment of inappropriate ADH secretion. John N. Forrest, Jr., Malcolm Cox, Cornelio Hong, Gail Morrison, Margaret Bia and Irwin Singer[2] compared responses to these agents in 10 patients with chronic inappropriate ADH secretion. Each had a serum sodium value below 130 mEq/L, despite efforts to restrict oral wa-

(2) N. Engl. J. Med. 298:173–177, Jan. 26, 1978.

ter intake to 500 ml daily or less, and inappropriately elevated urine osmolality. Three patients received 600–900 mg lithium carbonate daily. Demeclocycline was given adults in a dosage of 13–15 mg/kg daily. Six patients had lung carcinoma.

All patients showed improvement in the classic plasma and urine abnormalities on demeclocycline therapy. Maximum urine concentrating ability remained submaximal 3 weeks after the drug was stopped. Maximum diluting ability after an oral water load was markedly improved during treatment. Lithium carbonate was not effective when given to 3 patients for 3–5 days before demeclocycline therapy. A patient with a 22-year history of the syndrome was unresponsive to lithium, but long-term demeclocycline therapy was markedly effective.

Demeclocycline is effective in the treatment of chronic inappropriate ADH secretion where severe water restriction is inadequate to control symptoms or unsuccessful because of poor patient compliance. Serious adverse effects of demeclocycline were not observed in this study. All patients but 1 were treated in the hospital. Renal sodium wasting was not observed in balance studies performed during the response to demeclocycline of a patient with long-standing disease. The cause of excessive urinary sodium loss during demeclocycline therapy in patients with cirrhosis and heart failure is unknown.

▶ [The article establishes demeclocycline, which interferes with the action of ADH on the collecting duct at steps before and after intracellular cyclic AMP generation, as the agent of choice to treat inappropriate ADH syndrome. Acute treatment of severe hyponatremia should still be hypertonic saline and furosemide diuresis since demeclocycline takes 5 to 8 days to work.– S.S.H.] ◀

Evaluation of a New Antidiuretic Agent, Desmopressin Acetate (DDAVP), is reported by Mary Ellen Kosman[3] (AMA Dept. of Drugs, Chicago). Aqueous vasopressin is becoming harder to obtain. Vasopressin tannate in oil is given by inconvenient, painful injections and large doses may cause side effects. Lypressin nasal spray has a brief duration of action. The oral nonhormonal agents are ineffective in patients with severe disease. A new synthetic

(3)   J.A.M.A. 240:1896–1897, Oct. 20, 1978.

vasopressin analogue, DDAVP, is available as an aqueous solution for intranasal administration. Structural alterations have increased the antidiuretic/pressor ratio from 0.9 to 2,000 and prolonged the duration of action to 20 hours. Desmopressin reduces urine volume, increases urine osmolality and relieves symptoms of polyuria, nocturia and polydipsia in adults and children with central diabetes insipidus. It has been used successfully in patients with severe, long-standing disease when other antidiuretics were ineffective or not tolerated and also in patients with acute postoperative symptoms. Desmopressin is also of use in evaluating renal concentrating capacity.

Desmopressin is well tolerated, but large doses may cause transient headaches, nausea and a slight rise in blood pressure. Fluid intake should be adjusted during therapy to avoid hyponatremia and water intoxication, especially in infants and elderly patients. Undertreatment is preferable to overtreatment. No organ toxicity has been noted with treatment for up to 3 years. Desmopressin has been given without ill effect to 2 pregnant women. Many believe desmopressin to be the agent of choice for treating central diabetes insipidus. It will probably replace vasopressin tannate in oil for the long-term management of severe disease. Desmopressin is given intranasally through a flexible calibrated catheter. A small dose is used initially. The usual adult dose is 0.1 ml twice daily. For children aged 3 months to 12 years, the usual dosage range is 0.05 to 0.3 ml daily as a single dose or two divided doses.

▶ [Because of its long duration of action and route of administration, DDAVP is clearly a very useful agent in the treatment of diabetes insipidus. We have had occasion to use the drug for diabetes insipidus secondary to pituitary surgery for Cushing's disease.—S.S.H.] ◀

The following review articles are recommended to the reader:

Chan, J. C. M.: Hematuria and proteinuria in pediatric patients: Diagnostic approach, Urology 11:205, 1978.

Dailey, E. T., Rozanski, R. M., Keiffer, S. A., and Dinn, W. M.: Computed tomography in genitourinary pathology, Urology 12:95, 1978.

Friberg, J.: Genital mycoplasma infection, Am. J. Obstet. Gynecol. 132:573, 1978.

Seddon, J. M., and Bruce, A. W.: Cystourethritis, Urology 11:1, 1978.

Siegle, R. L., and Lieberman, P.: Review of untoward reactions to iodinated contrast material, J. Urol. 119:581, 1978.

The Adrenals

Localization of Pheochromocytoma by Computed Tomography. Knowledge of the precise location and extent of pheochromocytoma is important for its safe and expeditious removal. Bruce H. Stewart, Emmanuel L. Bravo, John Haaga, Thomas F. Meaney and Robert Tarazi[4] (Cleveland Clinic) investigated computerized axial tomography (CAT) as an alternative to pyelography and other more invasive procedures for localization of pheochromocytoma. Eleven patients with proved pheochromocytoma underwent pyelography with laminagraphy, selective renal angiography and CAT of the abdomen. Eight patients had a solitary tumor of adrenal origin, 1 had bilateral tumors and 2 had a malignant lesion, which in 1 was extra-adrenal. Only 4 tumors were localized by pyelography. Angiography and computed tomographic scanning each localized 10 tumors. The scan and angiogram each demonstrated 1 tumor that was missed on the other study.

Computed tomographic scanning can show the presence, location and extent of pheochromocytomas as accurately as selective angiography and with less risk. The test is usually not diagnostic in cases of small adenomas, but it appears to be highly accurate in detection of tumors over 2 cm in size, as the vast majority of pheochromocytomas are. The use of CAT should all but eliminate the need for arteriographic studies in preoperative evaluation of pheochromocytoma. Patients with positive biochemical tests are now operated on if the scan satisfactorily localizes the lesion. Nephrotomography and selective angiography are unnecessary unless the scan fails to identify the tumor. Selective vena cava sampling for catecholamines is indicated only when an extra-adrenal tumor is suspected or when a primary adrenal tumor cannot be satisfactorily demonstrated by other techniques.

▶ [Our experience parallels that of Stewart and associates. CT scanning is an

(4) N. Engl. J. Med. 299:460–461, Aug. 31, 1978.

excellent method to visualize adrenal masses larger than 1.5 to 2 cm in diameter and is, therefore, very useful in the evaluation of suspected pheochromocytomas, Cushing's syndrome due to carcinoma or adenoma, and adrenal cysts. It does not always identify adrenal hyperplasia and is not very useful in most cases of primary aldosteronism due to adrenal adenoma because these tumors are usually very small.–S.S.H.] ◄

Incidence of Pituitary Tumors Following Adrenalectomy: Long-Term Follow-up Study of Patients Treated for Cushing's Disease.

Kenneth L. Cohen, Robert H. Noth and Terri Pechinski[5] (Yale Univ.) reviewed information on 21 patients seen in 1951–76 with Cushing's syndrome due to adrenal hyperplasia who underwent total bilateral adrenalectomy without irradiation or exploration of the pituitary. The 19 females and 2 males had a mean age of 30 years at diagnosis. All had multiple clinical features of Cushing's syndrome. All but 1 had normal skull x-rays preoperatively; the exception had a "probably normal" study. Only 1 patient had reduced visual acuity preoperatively. Six patients had formal visual field testing.

Pituitary tumors were documented in 2 patients $1^{1}/_{2}$ and 11 years after adrenalectomy. Visual field tests preoperatively had given equivocal results in these patients. One of 3 patients with headache before adrenalectomy subsequently developed Nelson's syndrome. On follow-up for a mean of 8.5 years, 8 patients have developed pituitary tumors, and 2 others are suspected of having pituitary neoplasia. The diagnosis of tumor was made a mean of 6.5 years after operation. Seven patients had hyperpigmentation, 6 had erosion or enlargement of the sella and 4 had visual field abnormalities. Pathologic confirmation was obtained in 6 cases. Two patients received radiotherapy only.

The incidence of pituitary tumor in this series was 38%. All patients who undergo adrenalectomy alone for Cushing's disease require lifelong follow-up, including yearly sellar tomography and visual field examination. Commercial assays for ACTH may also be of use. The occurrence of pituitary tumors may be circumvented with few side effects by combined pituitary irradiation and adrenalectomy. The present findings raise the question whether adrenalectomy alone is an acceptable treatment for Cushing's disease.

► [Our experience and that of most other centers is that pituitary tumors infre-

(5) Ach.it med 138:575–579, April, 1978.

quently occur after adrenalectomy (10%). Regardless of the true incidence of Nelson's syndrome such patients should be carefully followed. Initial treatment with pituitary radiation or transphenoidal pituitary surgery should always be considered because of the devastating results of Nelson's syndrome.– S.S.H.] ◀

Adrenal Medullary Hyperplasia. Wu, Chieh-ping[6] (Peking, China) has occasionally encountered patients whose clinical condition resembled pheochromocytoma but found at operation, instead of tumor, hyperplasia of the adrenal medulla. Most patients have recovered completely or have shown improvement in hypertension after subtotal or partial resection of the enlarged glands.

Woman, 24, had had a blood pressure of 150/110 mm Hg the previous year, with elevations up to 260/170 mm Hg during attacks, as well as dyspnea, dizziness, nausea and vomiting and numb, cold extremities. Attacks usually lasted several hours. Mental upset and physical exertion appeared to be precipitating factors. Attacks occurred every 3–5 days before admission. The blood pressure was 180/110 mm Hg. Diffuse myocardial ischemia was noted during ECG study. The blood sugar was 148 mg/100

Fig 13.—Hyperplasia of adrenal medulla. Hexatoxylin-eosin; 10 × 5. Section of adrenal gland from a woman aged 24 years. Note increase in thickness of the adrenal medulla, which is at the right half of the field. (Courtesy of Wu, Chieh-p'ing: Chin. Med. J. [Engl.] 4:17–22, January, 1978.)

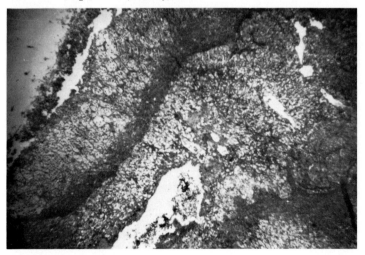

(6) Chin. Med. J. (Engl.) 4:17–22, January, 1978.

ml during an attack. The basal metabolic rate was +39%. A phentolamine test was positive, but no tumor shadow was noted on retroperitoneal pneumography. Both adrenal glands appeared slightly enlarged at exploration. Forty-five percent of the left adrenal and 75% of the right adrenal gland were resected, and hyperplasia of the cortex and medulla of both glands was observed (Figs 13 and 14). Subsequently, the blood pressure stabilized at 120–140/80–100 mm Hg. Paroxysmal hypertension recurred 8 years after operation. Urinary catecholamines were slightly elevated 3 years later.

Seventeen such patients have been operated on to date. The first 3 patients had a diagnosis of pheochromocytoma. Sixteen patients exhibited varying degrees of adrenal medullary hyperplasia, whereas 1 patient had no structural change. Six patients recovered and had normal blood pressures after partial or subtotal adrenalectomy, and 9 others improved. The patient without hyperplasia and 1 other patient failed to improve. Most of the patients had positive phentolamine tests.

Adrenal medullary hyperplasia is an entity requiring further investigation. The clinical manifestations basically

Fig 14.—Hyperplasia of adrenal medulla. Hematoxylin-eosin; 10 × 20. Section of adrenal medulla (same patient as in Fig 13). Swollen, densely packed pheochromocytes with fine basophilic granules. Binuclear cells are occasionally seen. Blood sinusoids are narrowed. (Courtesy of Wu, Chieh-p'ing: Chin. Med. J. [Engl.] 4:17–22, January, 1978.)

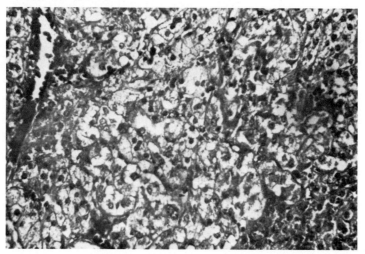

are similar to those of pheochromocytoma. The degree of hyperplasia is not necessarily the same on both sides. There is no specific means of distinguishing the condition from pheochromocytoma at present. Possibly the term "catecholaminism" will prove to be applicable.

▶ [This report is intriguing. We have never recognized a case of adrenal medullary hyperplasia. It will be interesting to see whether this syndrome can be identified in additional centers.–S.S.H.] ◀

Adrenal Cortical Carcinoma. Mark Sullivan, Michel Boileau and C. V. Hodges[7] (Univ. of Oregon) reviewed 28 cases of histologically proved adrenocortical carcinoma seen since 1950. The 18 females and 10 males were followed to death or, for the 4 living patients, from 7 to $15^{1}/_{2}$ years. Mean age at diagnosis was 42 years. Nearly half the patients had node involvement and local invasion or distant metastasis at initial diagnosis, and about a third had node involvement or local invasion. All the males were over age 39 years, and 90% had advanced lesions. Thirteen patients had functional tumors. All but 1 of these patients were cushingoid, virilized or both. Several cases were not diagnosed before operation. Two patients had tumor in both adrenals. The degree of anaplasia generally showed little correlation with function.

Survival was closely related to stage of disease (Fig 15). Survival was poor for patients with node involvement or local invasion or distant metastasis. Radiotherapy seemed to give slight benefit to patients with advanced disease. Multiple chemotherapeutic agents were tried without effect in individual cases. Five patients who appeared to be tumor free postoperatively had recurrences; all but 1 were reexplored and found to have unresectable disease. Metastases were widespread. At least 3 autopsies showed cerebral metastases.

Adrenal cortical carcinoma can occur at any age and can be functional or nonfunctional. Males tend to be older, to have higher-stage nonfunctional tumors and to have shorter survivals. Stage is the most important factor influencing survival, suggesting that operation is the only effective treatment. Among the various antitumor and antihormone agents tried, only mitotane showed much

(7) J. Urol. 120:660–665, December, 1978.

SULLIVAN, BOILEAU AND HODGES

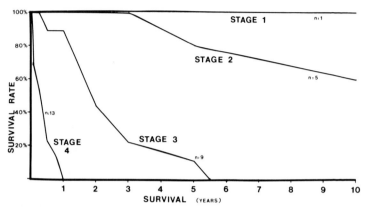

Fig 15.—Survival by stage. (Courtesy of Sullivan, M., et al.: J. Urol. 120:660–665, December, 1978.)

effectiveness. Prolonged follow-up is required. Aggressive evaluation and treatment are necessary for good survival.

▶ [This series confirms that the diagnosis of adrenal carcinoma is made later in men than in women because virilization is more difficult to recognize. It also emphasizes the grim prognosis if the tumor is not resectable and points out the need to develop effective chemotherapeutic agents.–S.S.H.] ◄

Adrenal Scanning and Uptake with [131]I-6 β-Iodomethyl-Nor-Cholesterol. Recently [131]I-6 β-iodomethyl-nor-cholesterol (NP-59) was reported to be a superior adrenal imaging agent. U. Yun Ryo, A. Sidney Johnston, Ilsup Kim and Steven M. Pinsky[8] (Michael Reese Hosp.) determined the minimum effective dose of NP-59 and the minimum time required to obtain a successful image and evaluated the usefulness of adrenal uptake measurements. Fifty-four adrenal scans were made in 50 patients, 42 with NP-59 and 12 with [131]I-19-iodocholesterol. The average dose of NP-59 was 0.78 mc and the dose of [131]I-19-iodocholesterol was 2 mc. A camera with a large field of view and a medium-energy parallel-hole collimator were used with a computer data processor.

The smallest dose of NP-59 injected, 0.3 mc, gave a satisfactory scan. Generally 0.5 mc was sufficient for a satis-

---

(8) Radiology 128:157–161, July, 1978.

factory scan. Smaller doses were adequate in patients with adrenal adenoma or hyperplasia; obese patients required larger doses. Significantly less time was needed to complete the study when NP-59 was used. Functioning adrenal adenomas and hyperplastic glands were imaged in 2 days in many instances. An average of $4^1/_2$ days was required for optimal images in subjects with normal glands or various adrenal diseases, but 5 days or more was required when ^{131}I-19-iodocholesterol was used. Dexamethasone suppression scanning was useful in a few cases. Uptake of NP-59 in 16 glands of patients without adrenal disease averaged 0.13%. Uptake exceeded 0.2% in cases of adrenal hyperplasia, whereas cortical adenomas showed uptake of over 0.28%. Uptake was markedly suppressed by dexametasone in normal adrenals, but not in glands with aldosterone-producing tumors. The study detected adrenal disease correctly in 48 of the 50 patients. One false negative scan and 1 equivocal scan were obtained.

The accuracy of adrenal imaging for detection of adrenal disease and normal glands is far superior to that of adrenal arteriography or venography. However, the scanning agents are not available for routine use, radiation exposure is high and completion of a scan requires a long time. Further, differentiation of hyperplasia from normal adrenals is sometimes difficult. The time required is markedly less when NP-59 rather than ^{131}I-19-iodocholesterol is used.

▶ [Our experience is similar. ^{131}I-6 β-iodomethyl-nor-cholesterol is superior to ^{131}I-19-iodocholesterol as a scanning agent. The former is taken up better by the adrenal and also contributes to greater diagnostic accuracy.–S.S.H.] ◀

The following review article is recommended to the reader:

Cox, M., Sterns, R. H., and Singer, I.: The defense against hyperkalemia: The roles in insulin and aldosterone. N. Engl. J. Med. 299:525, 1978.

The Kidney

Intrarenal Hemodynamics and Renal Function in Postobstructive Uropathy. Chen H. Hsu, Theodore W. Kurtz, Jonathan Rosenzweig and John M. Weller[9] (Univ. of Michigan) used a radioactive microsphere method to determine total renal blood flow (RBF) and intrarenal blood flow distribution after the release of 24-hour bilateral ureteral obstruction (BUO) and unilateral ureteral obstruction (UUO) in the rat. Studies of RBF and renal function were carried out within 3–4 hours after the relief of 24 hours of obstruction. Renal blood flow was measured with use of ^{85}Sr and ^{141}Ce microspheres.

Impaired renal function was observed after the release of 24 hours of both UUO and BUO. Fractional sodium excretion was identical in the obstructed and intact kidneys of UUO rats, whereas massive natriuresis occurred in BUO rats. Renal blood flow in BUO rats, determined after the release of 24 hours of obstruction, was about 60% of control values. Mean RBF in the obstructed kidney of UUO rats after release of obstruction was 78% of the mean RBF of the contralateral unobstructed kidney. No redistribution of intrarenal blood flow was noted in the UUO or BUO animals. Filtration fractions of obstructed kidneys in BUO and UUO rats after release of obstruction were lower than those of controls, suggesting that preglomerular vasoconstriction is primarily involved in the reduction in glomerular filtration rate.

Postobstructive diuresis and natriuresis were observed in the rat after release of BUO but not after UUO in these studies. The disproportionate decrease in glomerular filtration rate and RBF observed is probably attributable to pre-

(9) Invest. Urol. 15:348–351, January, 1978.

glomerular vasoconstriction. Greater renal damage attributable to higher ureteral pressure in BUO rats compared to UUO rats is not responsible for the postobstructive diuresis of the BUO model.

▶ [Clinical postobstructive diuresis is almost always a physiologic response to volume and solute overload and is seen after release of bilateral ureteral obstruction (or solitary kidney); it is seldom life threatening.—J.Y.G.] ◀

Thromboxane A_2 Biosynthesis in the Ureter Obstructed Isolated Perfused Kidney of the Rabbit. In chronic unilateral ureteral ligation, the major change in renal blood flow ipsilaterally is a result of preglomerular vasoconstriction. Production of a potent natural vasoconstrictor substance by the renal cortex could have an important role in the marked reduction in cortical and total renal blood flow in ureteral obstruction. Aubrey R. Morrison, Kohei Nishikawa and Philip Needleman[1] (Washington Univ., St. Louis) attempted (1) to determine whether or not renal thromboxane synthesis occurs, (2) to characterize the site of synthesis and (3) to determine the quantitative production of arachidonic acid (AA) metabolites in the isolated perfused rabbit kidney after ureteral obstruction. A variety of agonists were infused into rabbit kidneys after 3 days of ureteral obstruction.

Infusion of bradykinin, angiotensin II, AA and adenosine triphosphate (ATP) led to release of a substance that contracts rabbit aorta. High doses of AA and ATP led to release of the substance from the contralateral kidney. The substance was labile and disappeared with a half-time of 37 seconds at 37 C, suggesting that the labile constrictor was thromboxane A^2 (TxA^2). Incubation of cortical and medullary microsomal fractions from hydronephrotic kidneys with prostaglandin H^2 yielded a potent labile contractile substance. Enzymatic generation of the substance was inhibited by imidazole, a specific inhibitor of thromboxane synthetase. The primary products formed on incubating microsomes of ureter-obstructed kidneys with ^{14}C-AA were PGE^2 and thromboxane B^2. The TxB^2 zone was abolished when incubations were carried out in the presence of imidazole. Microsomes from the contralateral kidney

(1) J. Pharmacol. Exp. Ther. 205:1–8, April, 1978.

showed comparable rates of synthesis of PGE^2, but formed no TxB^2.

Ureteral obstruction unmasks biosynthesis of TxA^2 in the renal cortex and medulla. This may be important in the alteration of renal blood flow occurring in chronic ureteral obstruction. The data suggest that endogenous TxA^2 synthesis increases renal vascular resistance in this model, but further in vivo studies are needed to elucidate the role of TxA^2 if it is produced in the intact animal.

Effect of Indomethacin on Renal Blood Flow and Ureteral Pressure in Unilateral Ureteral Obstruction in Awake Dogs. Prostaglandin synthesis or release may mediate the immediate transient hyperemic response that follows acute unilateral ureteral occlusion. John T. Allen, E. Darracott Vaughan, Jr. and Jay Y. Gillenwater[2] (Univ. of Virginia) recorded the hemodynamic and ureteral pressure responses to indomethacin, a prostaglandin inhibitor, infused before and during acute unilateral ureteral occlusion in 5 conscious dogs. Indomethacin was given in a bolus of 2 mg/kg, followed by 1 mg/kg/hr for 30 minutes before ureteral obstruction. Studies continued for 8 hours after obstruction. In 6 control dogs only a bolus and infusion of Na_2CO_3 was given.

Ipsilateral blood flow in controls increased significantly on ureteral occlusion and then declined after 1 hour. Control ureteral pressure peaked at 43.7 mm Hg at 2.5 hours and then gradually declined by 8 hours. Indomethacin caused similar reductions in left and right renal blood flows. Ureteral occlusion caused a further fall in ipsilateral renal blood flow. The transient increase in flow seen in control animals was absent. The results are illustrated in Figure 16. Control renal blood flow was significantly less in study than in control animals. Ureteral pressure remained remarkably lower throughout the 8 hour period of ureteral occlusion. The maximum ureteral pressure was 18 mm Hg at 2 hours compared with 42 mm Hg at 2 hours in the control group.

Indomethacin reduced total renal blood flow of both kidneys before ureteral obstruction in these studies and the

(2) Invest. Urol. 15:324–327, January, 1978.

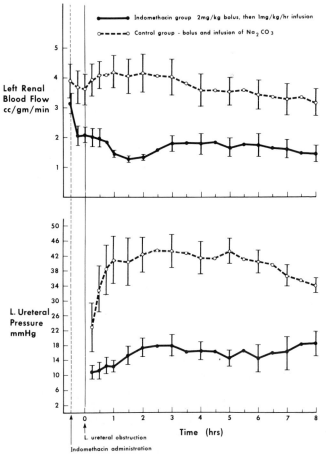

Fig 16.—Responses in ipsilateral renal blood flow and ureteral pressure in the control group *(open circles)* are contrasted with the responses observed in dogs receiving indomethacin *(closed circles)*. Indomethacin treatment caused a significant decrease in renal blood flow ($P < 0.05$), absence of hyperemic response and lower ureteral pressure during the period of ureteral occlusion. (Courtesy of Allen, J. T., et al.: Invest. Urol. 15:324–327, January, 1978.)

transient rise in flow expected after ureteral occlusion was not observed. The initial vasodilatation after ureteral occlusion appears to be prostaglandin dependent. If PGE_2 is responsible, the stimulus for its release is most likely the elevation in intrapelvic pressure. Inhibition of prostaglandin synthesis increases renovascular resistance, possibly through the unopposed action of other renovascular constrictors. The low ureteral pressure noted throughout the time of ureteral occlusion suggests that the increased renal resistance is at the afferent arteriolar level. Recent work has shown exaggerated prostaglandin synthesis and thromboxane A_2 synthesis by the hydronephrotic rabbit kidney.

▶ [This and the preceeding paper give us new information about the renal hemodynamic response to ureteral obstruction. It has been shown that there is a transient (6 hours) renal vasodilation after ureteral obstruction followed by a chronic renal vasoconstriction affecting primarily the afferent arterioles. Allen's study and that by Nishikawa et al. (J. Clin. Invest. 59:1143, 1977) show that the vasodilatation is due to renal prostaglandins (PGE_2). The studies by Morrison's group suggest that a potent labile natural vasoconstrictor, thromboxane A_2, causes the vasoconstriction. These experiments were done with a bioassay system that will need to be confirmed by chemical analysis.

Prostaglandins are formed from arachidonic acid which is converted to PGG_2 and then to PGH_2. Studies on the metabolism of PGG_2 and PGH_2 led to the discovery of two compounds, thromboxanes and prostacyclins, that are chemically unstable and seem to act locally rather than as hormones (by the classical definition of blood-borne messenger). Renal biosynthesis of these compounds has been established.–J.Y.G.] ◀

HYPERTENSION AND VASCULAR DISEASE

Treatment of Renovascular Hypertension with Percutaneous Transluminal Dilatation of a Renal Artery Stenosis. Andreas Grüntzig, Ulrich Kuhlmann, Wilhelm Vetter, Urs Lütolf, Bernhard Meier and Walter Siegenthaler[3] (Univ. Hosp., Zurich, Switzerland) performed percutaneous transluminal dilatation of a left-sided renal artery stenosis in a male patient, aged 61, with hypertension due to atherosclerotic stenosis of the renal artery. The blood pressure ranged from 200/100 to 230/115 mm Hg. A double-lumen catheter was utilized. A dilating catheter with a tipped balloon segment was used to dilate the vessel with a pressure pump. Blood pressure fell to normal 3 hours after the procedure, and increased slightly 2 weeks later, when reserpine and thiazide diuretic therapy was instituted. The total ^{131}I-iodohippurate clearance rose from 237 to 325 ml per minute as a result of improved

---

(3) Lancet 1:801–802, Apr. 15, 1978.

renal plasma flow in the left kidney. The renal plasma flow
rose from 83 to 152 ml per minute.

Percutaneous transluminal dilatation corrected severe
hypertension and improved renal plasma flow in this patient. Further experience will indicate whether this non-
traumatic, inexpensive procedure will be a useful alternative to renal vascular surgery in the management of
renovascular hypertension.

▶ [Percutaneous transluminal dilatation of a renal arterial lesion is an exciting
new method of treating this disease. At present, we still demand the presence of renin criteria that predict reversibility of hypertension after successful
dilatation before recommending the procedure. These criteria are, (1) a high
peripheral plasma renin activity level indexed against sodium excretion, (2)
contralateral suppression of renin secretion by the opposite kidney, (3) an
abnormal renal vein/artery renin relationship from the affected kidney, and
(4) a fall in blood pressure upon administration of antiangiotensin agents.

Of twelve attempts, Dr. Thomas Sos, of our Department of Radiology,
has successfully dilated renal lesions in 7 patients with a fall in blood pressure
in all 7. Clearly long-term follow-up is necessary; however, an impressive fall
in renin secretion occurs within 30 minutes of dilatation.

The technique appears to be particularly suitable for the older patient with
atherosclerotic disease who is at greater risk of complications after revascularization or nephrectomy (J.A.M.A. 231:1148, 1975).

Taken altogether, we are entering an era of tailored therapy for renovascular hypertension whereby patients must be individualized before a specific recommendation for renal arterial revascularization, percutaneous
dilatation, or medical management with the new orally active converting-
enzyme inhibitor, captopril (Prog. Cardiovasc. Dis. 21:195, 1978).–E. Darracott Vaughan, Jr.] ◄

**Ex Vivo Renal Artery Reconstruction Using Perfu-
sion Preservation.** Oscar Salvatierra, Jr., Cornelius Ol-
cott, IV and Ronald J. Stoney[4] (Univ. of California, San
Francisco) found that hypothermic perfusion preservation
facilitates renal revascularization and minimizes ischemic
damage during the ex vivo period. Twenty consecutive patients had 22 renal artery reconstructions by ex vivo techniques in the past 5 years. All but 2 patients were treated
because of uncontrollable hypertension; these 2 had symptomatic renal artery aneurysms in solitary kidneys. A midline transabdominal approach was utilized for complete
mobilization of kidney, renal vessels and ureter. The ureter was divided in only 6 cases. After renal washout, with
Ringer's lactate at 4C, the miniature Belzer preservation

---

(4) J. Urol. 119:16–19, January, 1978.

apparatus was used to perfuse the kidneys with cryoprecipitated plasma. The renal core temperature was consistently
at 10–13 C throughout the procedure. All reconstructions
were done with use of an autogenous artery, usually the
ipsilateral internal iliac artery. Continuous perfusion was
maintained except through the specific small branch vessel
being anastomosed at any given time. All patients had
[131]I-hippurate renal scintiphotography done within 24
hours of reconstruction.

The results are given in the table and an example of a
patient with a solitary kidney in Figure 17. All 18 patients
with previously uncontrollable hypertension had normal
blood pressure after repair. Fibromuscular dysplasia was
the most common renal vascular lesion requiring ex vivo
reconstruction. Only two thrombotic complications occurred postoperatively. Scintiphotography done a day postoperatively showed no evidence of acute tubular necrosis.

Continuous hypothermic perfusion preservation simpli-
fies dissection of the extrarenal vascular tree in ex vivo
renal artery reconstruction and makes possible the accurate identification of injury to minute vessels during dissection. Branch vessel anastomotic leaks are identified and
controlled before the repaired kidney is removed from the
perfusion circuit. Postoperative tubular necrosis can be
avoided. The ureter can be left intact during unilateral ex
vivo artery reconstruction. Every effort should be made to
repair extensive lesions of fibromuscular dysplasia in patients aged 40 or below. Other indications may exist for ex

---

EX VIVO RENAL ARTERY RECONSTRUCTION

Total kidneys (22):	Autograft anastomosis:
Solitary kidneys, 4	To aorta, 8
Previous ipsilateral renal surgery, 6	To renal artery stump, 6
Disease etiology:	To iliac artery, 8
Fibromuscular dysplasia, 19	Ureter management:
Aneurysms, 2	Ureteroneocystostomy, 6
Congenital branch stenosis, 1	Left intact, 16
Arterial autograft:	Complications:
Internal iliac, 20	Acute tubular necrosis, 0
Splenic, 1	Main autograft thrombosis, 1
Common iliac bifurcation, 1	Branch artery thrombosis, 1
Total primary branch anastomoses (57):	
Mean per kidney, 2.6	

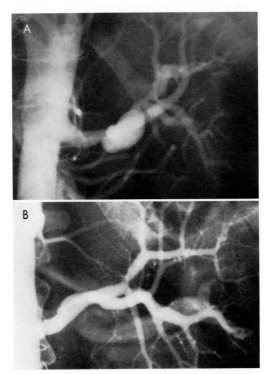

Fig 17.—A, preoperative arteriogram of solitary left kidney shows main renal artery aneurysm and multiple branch vessel stenoses. B, postoperative arteriogram shows patent repair. (Courtesy of Salvatierra, O., Jr., et al.: J. Urol, 119:16–19, January, 1978.)

vivo reconstruction when in situ surgical repair is considered impossible or hazardous.

▶ [It would be interesting to know how many conventional renal revascularizations were done by the same group over the same period. That is, how often is this technique indicated? Other investigators have felt that the indications for extensive bench surgery in patients with renovascular disease is limited (J. Urol. 118:363, 1977). However, the 100% cure rate is unprecedented and probably will not be equaled by alternate techniques.–E. Darracott Vaughan, Jr.] ◀

Surgical Treatment of Renovascular Hypertension in the Pediatric Patient. The results of renal revascularization have been less satisfactory in children than in adults with hypertension, and surgical cure has most often been achieved by nephrectomy. Andrew C. Novick, Ralph A. Straffon, Bruce H. Stewart and Sanford Benjamin[5] (Cleveland Clin., Cleveland, Ohio) reviewed the results obtained in 27 children (14 girls and, 13 boys, aged, 1–18 years) treated surgically for renovascular hypertension during 1955–1977. All had a diastolic blood pressure more than 100 mm Hg. Thirteen patients had perimedial fibroplasia, 11 had intimal fibroplasia and 3 had medial (fibromuscular) hyperplasia. Unilateral right or left renal artery stenosis occurred in 11 and 9 patients, respectively, whereas 7 patients had bilateral disease. Four patients had associated extrarenal arterial disease. A total of 38 operations were done, including 9 aortorenal bypass procedures, 7 splenorenal bypasses and 3 segmental renal arterial resections with reanastomosis. Sixteen ablative procedures were carried out, including 10 primary nephrectomies.

Sixteen patients (59%) were cured, with a blood pressure of 140/90 mm Hg or less 1 year postoperatively. Five others were improved, whereas 6 were failures. Four of 7 children with bilateral renal artery disease failed to gain pressure

VASCULAR PATENCY AFTER REVASCULARIZATION OPERATIONS IN TREATMENT OF RENOVASCULAR HYPERTENSION IN CHILDREN

Operation	No. Performed	Postop. Patency (100%) No. (%)	Comment
Aortorenal bypass with hypogastric arterial autograft	3	3 (100)	All patent
Aortorenal bypass with saphenous vein graft	4	4 (100)	All patent, 1 graft dilatation (200%)
Aortorenal bypass with arterial homograft	2	1 (50)	Same patient, recurrent lt. stenosis
Ex vivo revascularization with hypogastric artery and autotransplantation	1	1 (100)	Performed for branch renal artery disease
Renoaortic reimplantation	2	2 (100)	Same patient, cured
Splenorenal bypass	7	1 (14)	3 graft thrombosis 2 anastomotic stenosis 1 stenosis proximal splenic artery
Resection and reanastomosis	3	0 (0)	3 recurrent anastomotic stenosis

(5) J. Urol. 119:794–799, June, 1978.

control. Renal arterial reconstruction had a favorable outcome in 9 patients. Primary nephrectomy or partial nephrectomy was successful in 7 patients. The results of revascularization procedures are given in the table. Three of the
six operative failures occurred after splenorenal bypass.
The single operative death followed early postoperative
thrombosis of a splenorenal bypass graft to a solitary
kidney.

Renovascular hypertension in children is potentially curable. Currently available data suggest that arterial reconstruction with autogenous vascular bypass grafts represents the optimal surgical treatment in most patients.
Primary nephrectomy should be reserved for patients in
whom renal atrophy and/or severe small vessel disease is
found. Successful renal revascularization with preservation
of renal parenchyma is now possible in most children with
this disease.

▶ [Renal revascularization is clearly the procedure of choice in children with
renovascular hypertension. Nephrectomy is indicated only after failure of revascularization. In fact, with the development of new antiangiotensin agents
such as the orally-active converting enzyme inhibitor captopril, medical management may assume priority over primary nephrectomy in the patient whose
revascularization is impossible.

Despite the surgical complexity, Dr. John C. Whitsell of our vascular surgery group has increasingly utilized renal autotransplantation as the procedure of choice in adults with renovascular hypertension. Perhaps more emphasis should be given to this procedure in children in view of the potential
for late complications of interposition venous or arterial grafts.–E. Darracott
Vaughan, Jr.] ◀

**Renal Vein Renin Concentration in the Hyperten-
sion of Unilateral Reflux Nephropathy.** The
renin-angiotensin system is the likeliest contributor to the
hypertension of unilateral renal disease. R. R. Bailey, C.
U. McRae, T. M. J. Maling, G. Tisch and P. J. Little[6]
(North Canterbury Hosp., Christchurch, New Zealand)
examined the role of this system in the hypertension of
unilateral reflux nephropathy in 23 women and 6 men with
strictly unilateral involvement. Patients were defined as
hypertensive if the mean of 3 supine pressure readings exceeded 140/90 mm Hg. Five of the patients were on anti-
hypertensive therapy. Renal venous renin sampling was
performed after overnight recumbency in 18 cases and af-

(6)   J. Urol. 120:21–23, July, 1978.

ter furosemide stimulation in 11. Radioimmunoassay of generated angiotensin I was carried out. Divided renal function studies were done in 26 cases.

Twelve of the 29 patients were hypertensive; none had malignant hypertension. The renal venous renin ratio exceeded 1.5 in 3 normotensive and 2 hypertensive patients. In 5 normotensive and 3 hypertensive patients the ratio was below 1. Four normotensive patients and 1 hypertensive patient had an increase in mean urinary creatinine concentration exceeding 20% on differential renal function study. One of the normotensive patients had a renal venous renin ratio exceeding 1.5, and the hypertensive patient had a ratio of 1.1.

Hypertension is a common and important complication of reflux nephropathy. Unilateral reflux nephropathy suggests the possibility of surgical cure of the hypertension. The present study indicates that the renin-angiotensin system does not have a primary role in the nonmalignant hypertension associated with unilateral reflux nephropathy. In support of this conclusion, the divided renal function data gave no consistent evidence that the affected kidneys were acting ischemically.

▶ [Patients with hypertension and unilateral renal parenchymal disease rarely exhibit characteristics that implicate the diseased kidney as the source of excessive renin secretion (J.A.M.A. 233:1177, 1975). The authors suggest that patients with unilateral reflux nephropathy also do not have abnormal renin secretion. In contrast, Savage et al. (Lancet 2:441, 1978) have shown inappropriately high plasma renin activity levels in some hypertensive children with reflux nephropathy.

A possible explanation for the discrepancy may be the use of a simple renal vein renin ratio analysis alone in the present study. This type of analysis is limited and is inadequate to identify either unilateral or excessive renin secretion (Cardiovasc. Med. 1:195, 1976).–E. Darracott Vaughan, Jr.] ◀

Revascularization of Totally Occluded Renal Arteries. John M. Barry and Clarence V. Hodges[7] (Univ. of Oregon) report 2 cases of totally occluded renal arteries, showing that there is no correlation between the interval of occlusion and renal viability and that severe hypertension can be corrected by late repair of the arteries. The patients were a woman, 67, with a solitary kidney and hypertensive encephalopathy, and a man, 54, with severe hypertension. The duration of occlusion clinically was 10

(7) J. Urol. 119:412–415, March, 1978.

days and 6 months, respectively, in these cases. Revascularization procedures succeeded in both cases, resulting in
return of renal function and alleviation of hypertension.
One patient underwent renal autotransplantation 6
months after the onset of acute hypertension and 25 days
after angiographic demonstration of total renal artery
occlusion.

These 2 cases and 30 reported cases indicate that the
maximal duration of main renal artery occlusion compatible with subsequent return of renal function is unknown.
The 10-day period of renal artery occlusion in 1 of the present cases is the longest known period of anuria before successful revascularization of a solitary kidney. Occlusion in
these cases was due to embolism and thrombosis at an arteriosclerotic stenosis. Other causes include retrograde
propagation of an aortic thrombosis, aortic dissection and
trauma. Medical management is reasonable when the patient will not survive surgery; when secondary renal hypertension can be controlled satisfactorily; when the other
kidney does not have significant renovascular disease, or
when the inciting cause is not expected to recur. Anticoa-
gulation has succeeded after embolism but is unlikely to
succeed when the occlusion is due to thrombosis at a tight
stenosis. Several surgical options exist, including arteri-
otomy with embolectomy or thrombectomy, aortorenal or
iliorenal bypass, splenorenal anastomosis, saphenous vein
grafting of the renal and superior mesenteric arteries and
renal autotransplantation.

Revascularization of the Ischemic Kidney. After
acute renal artery obstruction, viability of the nephron
may be maintained by collateral blood flow from the capsular and periureteric vessels. Occasionally, if extensive
collateral flow develops, renal function will return spontaneously several months after obstruction. Jonathan B.
Towne and Victor M. Bernhard[8] (Med. College of Wisconsin, Milwaukee) have observed several different mechanisms of acute renal artery obstruction resulting in anuric
renal failure. They included temporary suprarenal placement of an aortic clamp at abdominal aneurysmectomy;
embolism, presumably of cardiac origin, to a solitary kid-

(8)   Arch. Surg. 113:216–218, February, 1978.

ney; and thrombosis of the distal aorta extending to a level proximal to the renal arteries.

Man, 65, with two previous myocardial infarctions, a long history of atrial fibrillation and congestive heart failure had had a left nephrectomy for chronic pyelonephritis. He was anuric shortly after admission, and angiography showed occlusion of the right renal artery 3.5 cm distal to its origin. A renal artery embolectomy was performed and a Scribner shunt inserted. Postoperative angiography showed a patent renal artery and a filling defect in the right lower pole branch. Repeated hemodialysis was necessary postoperatively, and another myocardial infarction occurred with pulmonary edema and hypotension. Thereafter renal function deteriorated, and the patient died 40 days postoperatively of progressive cardiorespiratory problems. At autopsy, the renal artery was patent. Areas of necrosis and hemorrhage were seen in the kidney, and thrombus was found in the peripheral renal arteries adjacent to areas of necrosis.

The duration of ischemia in these patients does not correlate with reversibility or the potential for salvage of the kidney. Renal size also does not correlate with reversibility of the renal ischemia. The potential for salvage depends on the presence of back-bleeding from the kidney once occluding debris is cleared from the distal renal artery. A Scribner shunt should be inserted after renal revascularization, since acute tubular necrosis often develops after successful revascularization. Prompt arteriography and surgical intervention are indicated in these patients.

Renal Vein Valves: Incidence and Significance. Renal venography is now a relatively common procedure. Renal vein valves may be misleading and may interfere with venography. Carl F. Beckmann and Herbert L. Abrams[9] (Boston) analyzed the incidence and characteristics of renal vein valves in 98 renal venograms obtained in 66 patients during the past 8 years. Patients with occlusion of the renal vein by thrombus or with renal venous invasion by carcinoma were excluded. In all patients, precurved renal venous catheters were inserted through the femoral vein into the inferior vena cava. The catheter tip was located in the peripheral segment of the main renal vein under fluoroscopic guidance. In 61 cases, percutaneous transfemoral renal artery catheterization was per-

(9)   Radiology 127:351–356, May, 1978.

formed and renal blood flow deliberately slowed by injection of epinephrine. Renografin was delivered at a rate of 15 ml per second. Fifty-one venograms without and 10 with renal veins valves were compared to determine how often valves account for venograms of inferior quality.

Valves were found in 15% of venograms in 14 patients. In only two right renal venograms were valves close to the entry into the inferior vena cava. In left renal studies of 4 patients, the valves were in the main renal vein. Only one was close to the inferior vena cava. The valves appeared as thin, sharply defined weblike structures; they were bicuspid or tent shaped. Typically, the valves were nonobstructing or only partially obstructing to retrograde flow of contrast material. Two venograms without valves (4%) were rated as poor and 7 (14%) as fair. With valves present, 70% of studies were rated as good and 30% as fair. When renal blood flow was not slowed and valves were present, no venograms were rated as good. When valves were absent, 31% of studies were rated as good.

The presence of renal vein valves may result in venograms of inferior quality, especially when renal blood flow is not slowed by epinephrine. Occasional failures to catheterize the renal vein and its branches selectively may be explained by the presence of competent renal vein valves.

▶ [This is another example of the importance of defining normalcy.—E. Darracott Vaughan, Jr.] ◀

Renal Artery Embolism: Clinical Features and Long-Term Follow-up of 17 Cases. Richard K. Lessman, Steven F. Johnson, Jack W. Coburn and Joseph J. Kaufman[1] (Los Angeles) reviewed the case histories of 17 patients with embolism to major renal arteries who were seen in the past 14 years and followed for up to 10 years. The clinical diagnosis was based on the renal scintiscan and/or renal angiographic findings. Thirteen men and 4 women, with a mean age of 58 years, were affected. Predisposing factors were identified in 16 patients, the most frequent being atrial fibrillation. Five patients had bilateral emboli, and 2 had an embolus to a solitary kidney.

Pain was noted by 13 patients, and nearly half had nau-

(1) Ann. Intern. Med. 89:477–482, October, 1978.

sea and vomiting. Three reported gross hematuria, and 4 a decrease in urine output. Ten of 12 patients were febrile, and 4 had elevated blood pressure. All patients had leukocytosis, and 10 of 12 had significant pyuria. The lactic dehydrogenase serum (LDH) was elevated in every case. In only 4 patients was the diagnosis made on admission. The urogram was abnormal in all 12 patients examined. The perfusion renal scan showed a lack of arterial flow in all but one patient studied. Renal angiography showed major arterial occlusion in all 8 patients studied. Thirteen patients received anticoagulant therapy. Three of the 7 patients with bilateral emboli or embolus to a solitary kidney died within 1 week, 2 of emboli to other organs and 1 of uremia. Two patients with both kidneys present and a unilateral embolus required dialysis, and 1 died. Two patients in this group died of cardiac disease. Three of 5 patients followed for 12–30 months showed reduced renal function.

Renal artery embolism should be considered in patients with heart disease who develop chest or abdominal pain along with reduced renal function, proteinuria or hematuria. Renal scintiscanning is of value in diagnosing renal artery embolism. Renal function may be impaired in unilateral cases. Only 1 of the present patients had corrective vascular surgery. No patient required permanent hemodialysis. Surgery may not be necessary even in bilateral cases. The major risks are embolism to other organs and the underlying cardiovascular disease.

Transcatheter Thromboembolectomy of Acute Renal Artery Occlusion. Acute renal artery occlusion may be a life-threatening event that to now has been remediable only by operation. Victor G. Millan, Melvin H. Sher, Ralph A. Deterling, Jr., Andrew Packard, Jeremy R. Morton and John T. Harrington[2] used an angiographic method of percutaneous disobliteration in 4 patients with a follow-up of 2 years. After acute renal artery occlusion is diagnosed at aortography, the tip of a specially shaped selective catheter with a large lumen is placed in the orifice of the obstructed vessel under fluoroscopic control and advanced to the clot, where strong suction is applied if a

---

(2) Arch. Surg. 113:1086–1092, September, 1978.

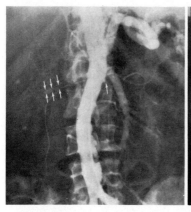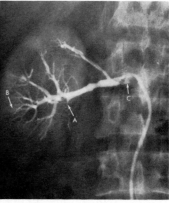

Fig 18 (left).—Abdominal aortogram showing left renal artery stump *(single arrow)* and thrombus within right renal artery *(arrows).*

Fig 19 (right).—Selective right renal arteriogram during process of disobliteration. Some clot *(A)* still remains in lower pole branch. Note filling of reestablished cortical branches *(B).* Note orificial stenosis due to plaque *(C).*

(Courtesy of Millan, V. G., et al.: Arch. Surg. 113:1086–1092, September, 1978; copyright 1978, American Medical Association.)

fresh embolis is present. If thrombosis is present, a no. 3 Fogarty catheter is advanced and the balloon is inflated with contrast material to remove the clot by withdrawal.

Man, 63, with hypertension, arteriosclerotic heart disease, chronic renal insufficiency and two past episodes of acute pulmonary edema, was admitted with florid pulmonary edema and anuria the day after a hemorrhoidectomy. Aortography showed total occlusion of both renal arteries from thrombosis (Fig 18). Transcatheter thrombectomy of both renal arteries was carried out. Atherosclerotic orificial stenoses were confirmed (Fig 19). Renal function was reestablished after five passes in the right renal artery and two in the left. Renal scanning showed decreased renal flow bilaterally on day 7, and direct endarterectomy of both renal orifices was done on day 10, with a Dacron patch across the aorta. Satisfactory renal arterial circulation ensued. Hemodialysis was continued for 5 weeks during resolution of acute tubular necrosis. The patient died of myocardial infarction and cardiac arrest about 2 years after the procedure and was found at autopsy to have patent renal arteries and orifices.

The results of the transcatheter procedure in another patient are shown in Figures 20 and 21. Angiographic throm-

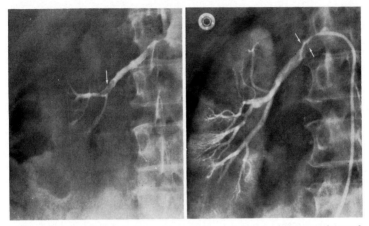

Fig 20 (left).—Thrombus *(arrow)* is well demonstrated by selective right renal arteriogram performed before thrombectomy.

Fig 21 (right).—Restoration of blood flow to most of renal parencyma is shown in this selective right renal arteriogram performed immediately after thrombectomy. Note tight orificial stenosis *(arrows)*.

(Courtesy of Millan, V. G., et al.: Arch. Surg. 113:1086–1092, September, 1978; copyright 1978, American Medical Association.)

boembolectomy can provide safe treatment with low risk; morbidity has not resulted in the 4 patients treated to date. In the presence of orificial stenosis that may later require correction, valuable time can be gained for improvement of the patient's medical state. Restoration of renal function has been prompt. Selective perfusion of the renal artery with a thrombolytic agent after thromboembolectomy may be considered when less than optimal circulation has been restored as a result of residual clot.

Intrarenal Arteriovenous Fistulas: Transcatheter Steel Coil Occlusion. Transcatheter intravascular occlusion offers a nonsurgical alternative to nephrectomy or local or segmental operations for intrarenal arteriovenous fistula. Sidney Wallace, Donald E. Schwarten, Douglas C. Smith, L. Paul Gerson and L. John Davis[3] used the Gianturco stainless steel coil in the transcatheter treatment of 4 patients with intrarenal arteriovenous fistulas. The

(3) J. Urol. 120:282–286, September, 1978.

coil is introduced into the fistula through a selectively placed preshaped, nontapered 7F polytetrafluoroethylene catheter.

Man, 46, had changes of chronic glomerulonephritis in renal angiography. One of two open needle biopsies of the right kidney resulted in considerable bleeding and hematuria and shock ensued. Re-exploration showed a retroperitoneal hematoma of over 2 L on the right. A small renal vein at the hilar area was ligated, but gross hematuria recurred over the next 17 days and necessitated transfusion of 15 units of blood. Repeat angiography showed a large pseudoaneurysm of the upper-pole artery and an arteriovenous fistula (Fig 22). Three steel coils were placed in the feeding interlobar artery, occluding the pseudoaneurysm almost completely. Angiography a day later showed obliteration of the fistula, the pseudoaneurysm and the feeding artery. Another small pseudoaneurysm originating from an inferior branch of the main renal artery was embolized with gelatin sponge. Fever and flank pain occurred for 2 days after the procedure. The patient had no subsequent hematuria and is being maintained on dialysis.

Two fistulas after needle biopsy, a fistula associated with an intrarenal aneurysm and a congenital or cirsoid arteriovenous fistula were treated in this manner. No significant morbidity resulted and renal tissue was conserved

Fig 22.—Arteriovenous fistula after needle biopsy. **A,** right renal arteriogram reveals large pseudoaneurysm with arteriovenous fistula *(arrows)* 18 days after renal biopsy. **B,** angiography after coil occlusion of distal upper-pole artery. (Courtesy of Wallace, S., et al.: J. Urol 120:282–286, September, 1978.)

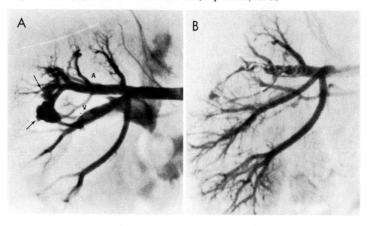

in each case. The complications reported are related to the organ and vascular supply occluded. Transcatheter steel coil occlusion has been used to treat over 75 patients with neoplasms, hemorrhage and arteriovenous fistulas. It has been reported to have been used successfully to treat post-nephrectomy, renal, vertebral, pulmonary, gastroduo-denal and internal iliac arteriovenous fistulas.

▶ [Percutaneous transluminal renal arterial occlusion by a variety of tech-niques now has a secure place in our therapeutic armamentarium. The tech-nique is particulary useful in situations of intrarenal bleeding due to trauma, arteriovenous fistulae or arteriovenous malformations.

The utilization of this technique before nephrectomy in patients with renal cell carcinoma, either to facilitate tumor removal or enhance antibody re-sponse, is less clear.—E. Darracott Vaughan, Jr.] ◀

Simultaneous Balloon Occlusion of the Renal Artery and Hypothermic Perfusion in In Situ Surgery of the Kidney. Intraluminal occlusion of the renal artery with a balloon catheter introduced percutaneously permits transarterial access to the kidney, while the renal circu-lation is interrupted as efficiently as with clamp occlusion. Michael Marberger, Max Georgi, Rolf Guenther and Ru-dolf Hohenfellner[4] (Univ. of Mainz) combined balloon oc-clusion with hypothermic perfusion in an attempt to simplify extensive in situ operations on the renal paren-chyma that require ischemia for a bloodless field.

TECHNIQUE.—Patients are pretreated with oral Dibenzyline for 4 days to prevent vasospasm. A double-lumen 5 F Swan-Ganz catheter is advanced by the Seldinger technique to test occlude the vessel by filling the balloon with 0.2–0.6 ml saline. Only ar-teries 4–10 mm in diameter are suitable for this technique. Hy-pothermic perfusion is begun immediately after balloon inflation at surgery. Ringer's lactate with mannitol added is preferred; the perfusate is cooled to 4–6 C. The renal core temperature is main-tained at 18–25 C throughout ischemia by short phases of high-flow perfusion with long dry intervals.

This technique has been used to clear 31 kidneys (in 30 patients) of complicated calculi requiring extensive nephro-tomies. Four patients had solitary kidneys, and 6 others had total renal function less than 50% of normal. A major-ity of kidneys were infected. The mean ischemia time needed was 54 minutes. Additional clamping of the renal artery was necessary in only 4 cases in which the catheter

(4) J. Urol. 119:463–467, April, 1978.

slipped from the artery during transport of the patient. Blood loss from the perfused kidneys was less than 500 ml in 69% of cases and more than 1 L in 8%. Four kidneys had residual calculi at discharge. Renal plasma flow declined and later increased to more than preoperative values. Hypertension was not noted in patients who were normotensive preoperatively. No patient had progressive loss of total renal function.

Simultaneous balloon occlusion and hypothermic perfusion is a valuable means of performing extensive in situ surgery on the kidney. Along with newer methods of intraoperative radiology and nephroscopy, it provides the basis for removing even the most complicated recurrent calculi. It practically eliminates the need for hazardous extracorporeal workbench operations on infected calculous kidneys.

▶ [The crucial question is whether this elaborate technique affords any advantage over ice slush. The technique failed in 5 of 31 patients and cooling was incomplete in an additional 6. Aside from the added expense and discomfort of the angiographic procedure and the logistic problem of patient transportation with the catheter in place, there is the small, but real, risk of transfemoral arteriography. In the Cooperative Study of Renovascular Hypertension there was a 1.25% major complication rate in 2,089 studies (J.A.M.A. 221:374, 1972). Complications included hemorrhage requiring transfusion or exploration (10), thrombosis (9), and renal injury (6).–E. Darracott Vaughan, Jr.] ◀

Detection of Renal Artery Stenosis by Measuring Urinary N-Acetyl-β-D-Glucosaminidase. N-acetyl-β-D-glucosaminidase (NAG) is a renal tubular enzyme, the urinary activity of which is increased in various nephropathies, including acute renal failure, transplant rejection and glomerulonephritis. M. A. Mansell, N. F. Jones, P. N. Ziroyannis, Susan M. Tucker and W. S. Marson[5] (London) investigated the estimation of NAG as a screening test for underlying renal disease in hypertension. Fourteen patients with angiographically proved renal artery stenosis were studied. Urinary enzyme activity was measured by an automated fluorometric assay technique.

The mean value was 191 nmol/hour/mM creatinine, compared with 76 nmol in 180 control subjects, a significant difference. Ten patients had elevated urinary NAG ac-

(5) Br. Med. J. 1:414–415, Feb. 18, 1978.

tivity. One patient with a normal value had normal urographic and renographic findings at the time of study. Another had two arteries supplying the kidney in question, only one of which was stenotic. All 3 patients with elevated NAG activity who had nephrectomy had normal values after operation.

Urinary NAG estimation detected 10 of 12 patients in this study with stenosis of a main renal artery sufficient to affect renal function, as judged by urography and renography. The measurement is simple and inexpensive. A 24-hour urine collection is not necessary. Results suggest that NAG estimation may serve as a simple, reliable screening test for hypertensive patients to select those in whom detailed study would be more likely to yield positive findings.

▶ [The major problem with the commonly utilized screening tests for renal arterial disease (rapid sequence intravenous urogram–nuclide studies) is an unacceptably high positive rate in patients with essential hypertension. The statement that urinary NAG is increased in "various nephropathies" suggests that the test will not be adequately specific as a screen for renal arterial disease.–E. Darracott Vaughan, Jr.] ◀

TUMORS

Conservative Surgery in Solitary and Bilateral Renal Carcinoma: Indications and Technical Considerations. John M. Palmer and David A. Swanson[6] (Univ. of California, Sacramento) recently managed 7 patients with either solitary or bilateral renal carcinoma. In 4 cases they were able to perform an adequate excision by partial nephrectomy. All these 4 patients are well, and 3 are free of disease on follow-up after 24–32 months. All have had adequate renal function. The pulmonary metastases present in 1 patient have grown slowly. The 3 patients in whom definitive excision was not done have had rapidly progressive malignant disease. More recently, 4 other patients have had operations. Two patients are well after in situ partial nephrectomy for solitary lesion in 1 and bilateral sequential lesions in 1. A 3d patient died of status epilepticus after staged radical nephrectomies for bilat-

(6) J. Urol. 120:113–117, July, 1978.

eral simultaneous lesions, while a 4th with bilateral sequential lesions is recovering from in situ partial nephrectomy.

A survey of similar series indicates a survival of 78% in patients with solitary renal tumors after partial nephrectomy, with a mean follow-up of 52 months. The projected survival for patients having chronic hemodialysis for the same interval is only 65%. Partial nephrectomy, where technically feasible, appears to be the treatment of choice for solitary renal carcinoma. In cases of bilateral disease, the survival after partial nephrectomy appears to be similar to that of patients on hemodialysis. The technical aspects of even extensive partial nephrectomy are not difficult. If tumor recurs in the remaining renal fragment, an opportunity for cure by total excision still exists. Pyelography should be done 4 times in the 1st year after partial nephrectomy and twice in the 2d year. Angiography is done routinely at 12 and 24 months. Surveillance must continue indefinitely. None of the authors' patients have had recurrence of tumor.

▶ [The presence of bilateral simultaneous renal cell carcinomas or the subsequent development of a renal cell carcinoma in a remaining kidney necessitates modification of the traditional surgical therapy to preserve renal function. Our experience was recently reported (Viets et al., J. Urol. 118:937, 1977). In vivo aggressive resection of bilateral renal cell carcinomas has been effective. Satisfactory renal function was obtained in all patients postresection and none has required dialysis. Bench surgery and autotransplantation were unnecessary in our cases.–J.Y.G.] ◀

Natural History of Metastatic Renal Cell Carcinoma: Computer Analysis. Metastatic renal cell carcinoma, especially in the lungs, may have long periods of decreased growth and periods of growth arrest. Regression of metastases undoubtedly has occurred after nephrectomy but patient survival was improved only by several months. Jean B. Dekernion, Kenneth P. Ramming and Robert B. Smith[7] (Univ. of California, Los Angeles) used computer analysis to identify disease factors influencing the survival of patients with metastatic renal cell carcinoma. The study population included 86 patients seen in 1970–76 who did not receive immunotherapy. The 67 men and 19 women had a median age of 59. Forty-five acquired metastases af-

(7) J. Urol. 120:148–152, August, 1978.

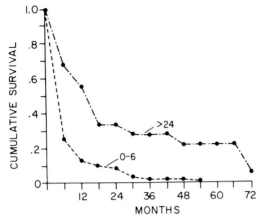

Fig 23.—Cumulative survival of patients with metastatic renal cell carcinoma grouped according to interval between nephrectomy and appearance of metastases (interval free of disease) in months. Patients with 0 interval free of disease were those with metastases at time of original diagnosis. (Courtesy of Dekernion, J. B., et al.: J. Urol. 120:148–152, August, 1978.)

ter nephrectomy. Cumulative survival was 53% at 6 months, 43% at 1 year and 26% at 2 years. The cumulative 5-year survival rate was 13%.

The interval between definitive nephrectomy and the diagnosis of metastasis affected survival (Fig 23). Nearly all patients with local tumor recurrence died within 1 year. Only 20% of those with residual tumor lived 6 months and all died within a year. Patients known to have metastases to regional nodes at the time of nephrectomy had decreased survival. Patients with metastases confined to the lungs had significantly greater survival after the first year of follow-up. The 20 patients having surgery for extirpation of metastatic foci had significantly increased survival at 3 and 5 years over the rest of the population. Survival of patients having palliative nephrectomy was identical to that of the overall study group (Fig 24). Hormonal or cytotoxic drug therapy increased patient survival only slightly. Only 1 patient appears to have had spontaneous regression of pulmonary metastases.

Aggressive treatment of metastases rarely results in long-term cure, but the significant palliation interval ob-

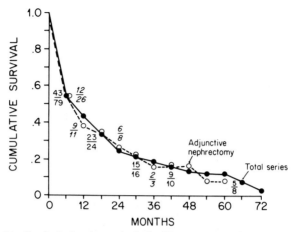

Fig 24.—Survival of patients who had palliative or adjunctive nephrectomy for metastatic renal cell carcinoma compared to entire study population of patients with metastatic renal cell carcinoma. (Courtesy of Dekernion, J. B., et al.: J. Urol. 120:148–152, August, 1978.)

nephrectomy but nephrectomy will not improve survival unless the primary lesion can be completely excised along with any involved regional nodes. Excision of a large primary tumor may be indicated to facilitate systemic therapy in patients with metastases once the treatment has been shown to be effective.

▶ [It is our experience that palliative nephrectomy has not caused regression of distant metastases. However we still do some, especially in those patients who are having problems with pain and bleeding. The 25% 5-year survival with excision of single or multiple pulmonary nodules is impressive.–J.Y.G.] ◀

Radionuclide Imaging of Metastases from Renal Cell Carcinoma by ^{131}I-Labeled Antitumor Antibody. Studies in mouse tumor models have shown that radionuclides linked to antibodies against tumor-associated cell-surface antigens acquire specificity for tumor imaging. Philip Belitsky, Tarun Ghose, Jose Aquino, Joseph Tai and Alan S. MacDonald[8] detected histologically proved metastases of renal cell carcinoma in 6 consecutive patients

(8)   Radiology 126:515–517, February, 1978.

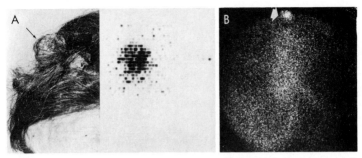

Fig 25.—A, head scan of a patient shows a scalp metastasis from a renal cell carcinoma *(arrow)* 96 hours after intravenous injection of 4 mCi of ^{131}I bound to 100 mg of antitumor globulin. B, gamma camera image of the head 24 hours after ^{131}I-antibody injection also shows the lesion *(arrow)*. (Courtesy of Belitsky, P., et al.: Radiology 126:515–517, February, 1978.)

by radionuclide imaging with "polyvalent" antirenal cell carcinoma globulin bound to [131]I. The antitumor globulin (ATG) preparations were obtained by immunizing goats with renal cell carcinoma from 2 patients. On immunofluorescence assay, they reacted specifically not only with the immunizing tumors but also with histologically similar tumors from other patients.

Four men and 2 women who had had nephrectomy for histologically proved renal cell carcinoma and who were suspected of having metastases underwent ^{131}I-ATG scanning. Localization of ^{131}I-ATG was observed in metastatic lesions in all 6 patients. Examples are shown in Figures 25 and 26. Metastases were observed in the scalp, tibia, mediastinum, peritoneum and pleura and L5. No preferential localization in a BCG-induced abscess in 1 patient was observed. Preferential localization of ^{99m}Tc-sulfur colloid was not observed in any of the lesions.

Labeled antitumor antibodies may have the specificity for tumor imaging that current radiopharmaceuticals lack. Nonspecific trapping of xenogeneic ATG by reticuloendothelial cells in the liver, spleen and lungs, however, limits the usefulness of this method of tumor detection. Purer preparations of antitumor or globulins or their $F(ab)^2$ fragments might improve the results. Further evaluation of the sensitivity and specificity of this

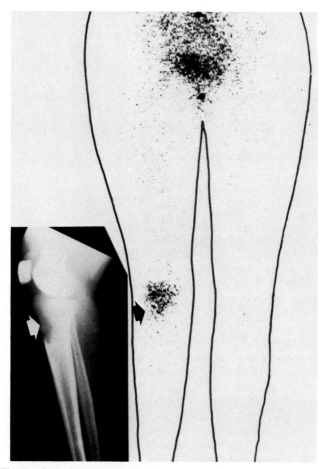

Fig 26.—Scan of the lower half of the body of a patient 48 hours after injection of 3.5 mCi of ^{131}I bound to 100 mg of antitumor globulin, demonstrating localization of the tracer in the osteolytic lesion shown in the radiograph. (Courtesy of Belitsky, P., et al.: Radiology 126:515–517, February, 1978.)

method will require comparison with other tumor-localizing radiopharmaceuticals.

▶ [This preliminary report shows promise in diagnosing metastatic renal cell carcinoma by radionuclide imaging of metastases with a polyvalent antirenal cell carcinoma globulin bound to ^{131}I. Future studies in this area will have to be followed closely.–J.Y.G.] ◀

Bilateral Renal Cell Carcinoma. Douglas E. Johnson, Andrew Voneschenbach and Jack Sternberg[9] (Univ. of Texas System Cancer Center, Houston) diagnosed bilateral renal cell carcinoma simultaneously in 6 patients and sequentially in 4, 3–14 years after the first tumor had been removed by nephrectomy. The patients were among 709 seen in 1947–75 with renal carcinoma, giving an incidence of 1.4%. Malignant disease was simultaneously diagnosed at autopsy in 1 patient who died of generalized disease with a clinically unrecognized primary tumor. The 7 men and 3 women had a mean age of 58.9 years at the initial diagnosis of malignancy. Two patients with simultaneous tumors in whom metastasis was not evident at diagnosis lived more than 3 years. Three of the 4 patients with asynchronously developing renal tumors are alive $1^1/_2$–14 years after diagnosis of the 2d renal malignancy.

The simultaneous appearance of renal carcinoma in both kidneys is an ominous sign, usually indicating a poor prognosis. Where there is no apparent metastasis, bilateral resection operations, either partial nephrectomies or combined nephrectomy and partial nephrectomy, should be considered. The prognosis for patients with asynchronous renal carcinomas has been estimated to be half as good as that of patients with a single lesion. A procedure that preserves renal function is indicated in cases of bilateral renal cell carcinoma, since radical excision and transplantation do not appear to be justified. The behavior of these tumors is unpredictable.

▶ [We agree that an operative procedure designed to conserve some renal function is indicated in bilateral renal cell carcinoma. Renal transplantation or dialysis seems unjustified in view of the poor prognosis (only 10% long-term survival in this series). No bench surgery was required in our cases. Careful preoperative planning is necessary since the kidney with the larger tumor may be more suitable for partial nephrectomy.–J.Y.G.] ◀

Active Specific Immunotherapy of Advanced Renal Cell Carcinoma. The results of treatment of advanced renal adenocarcinoma are poor. The long survival times observed among patients with metastasis and spontaneous regressions of metastatic renal cancer indicate that renal cancer may be immunologically more labile than other types of cancer and so amenable to treatment with immu-

(9) J. Urol. 119:23–24, January, 1978.

nologic methods. H. Tykkä, K. J. Oravisto, T. Lehtonen, S. Sarna and T. Tallberg[1] (Univ. of Helsinki) evaluated specific active immunotherapy after palliative nephrectomy in 31 patients with advanced renal cell carcinoma. Twenty-three comparable patients did not receive immunotherapy. The patients were seen in 1971–73 and had

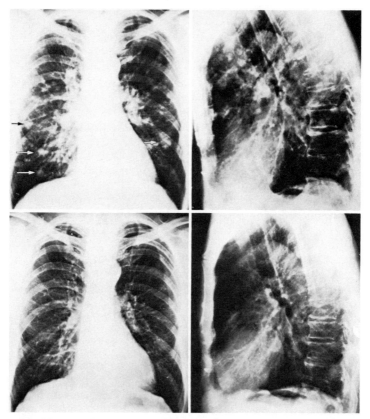

Fig 27 (top).—Multiple metastatic shadows *(arrows)* in both lungs 1 month after nephrectomy.

Fig 28 (bottom).—Same patient 14 months later. No evidence of metastases in lungs. Three years after these films were made patient is still symptomless with no signs of recurrence.

(Courtesy of Tykkä, H., et al.: Eur. Urol. 4:250–258, 1978.)

(1) Eur. Urol. 4:250–258, 1978.

survived operation. No brain metastases had been observed preoperatively. Average ages of the immunotherapy and control groups were 57.7 and 55.7 years, respectively. Eight palliative excisions of metastases were performed in the immunotherapy group and 7 in the control group. Six experimental and 5 control patients received preoperative irradiation of the primary tumor. A "vaccine" prepared from primary tumor and polymerized metastatic tissue was injected intradermally with tuberculin-PPD or *Candida albicans* antigen within a week of nephrectomy and then once a month.

On follow-up for up to 4 years, 7 experimental and no control patients have survived. The statistical 5-year survivals were 23.6% in the immunotherapy group and 4.3% in the control group. The calculated life expectancies were 31.1 months in the immunotherapy group and 15.8 months in the control group, a highly significant difference. None of the 7 surviving patients received preoperative or postoperative radiotherapy. Pulmonary metastases disappeared during immunotherapy in 6 of 16 patients (Figs 27–30). No harmful side effects of immunotherapy were ob-

Fig 29 (left).—Large metastatic shadow *(arrow)* in right lung 5 months after nephrectomy. In preoperative tomogram, shadow had been similar and was considered to be neoplastic.

Fig 30 (right).—Same patient 1 month later. Metastasis *(arrow)* has almost disappeared. Week later, patient died of another disease. Autopsy showed dense area with macrophage infiltration at site of metastasis. No malignant cells were found in this area or elsewhere in this patient.

(Courtesy of Tykkä, H., et al.: Eur. Urol. 4:250–258, 1978.)

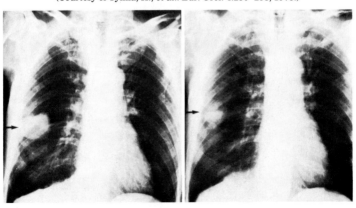

served. Signs of enhancement and autoimmune reactions were not recorded.

Immunotherapy significantly improved survival in this series of patients with advanced renal cell carcinoma, and no side effects were observed. Studies are continuing to determine whether patients most responsive to immunotherapy can be selected and whether indications for operation can be extended.

▶ [The obvious problems in a study of this type are the unpredictable nature of the tumor and in ascertaining whether the control group is comparable. Nevertheless, these results are impressive.–J.Y.G.] ◀

Treatment of Renal Cell Carcinoma with Solitary Metastasis. Michael J. O'Dea, Horst Zincke, David C. Utz and Philip E. Bernatz[2] (Mayo Clinic and Found.) reviewed information on 1,761 patients treated for renal cell carcinoma in 1950–70 and found 330 with metastatic disease, 44 of whom (2.5%) had a solitary metastatic lesion. These 30 men and 14 women had an average age of 56 years. Eighteen presented with renal cell carcinoma and a solitary metastatic lesion, and 14 had symptoms referable to the metastasis. Average time from tumor presentation to appearance of the metastasis in the other 26 patients was 2 years 7 months. The sites of metastasis are given in the table.

Six of 18 patients with synchronous lesions had involvement of a vertebra. The longest survivor was 1 of the 2 who

SITES OF METASTASIS IN 44 PATIENTS WITH RENAL CELL CARCINOMA

	No. Pts.
Brain	14
Spine	8
Lung	7
Rib	1
Bones other than spinal	4
Skin and subcutaneous tissue	3
Contralateral adrenal glands	2
Lymph gland	2
Contralateral ureter	1
Spermatic cord	1
Liver	1
Total	44

(2)   J. Urol. 120:540–542, November, 1978.

underwent nephrectomy, laminectomy and irradiation of the metastatic site. Six patients with brain metastasis survived for an average of 7 years. Aggressive treatment appeared to correlate with better survival in this group. Among the patients with asynchronous lesions, the 8 with a solitary brain lesion did reasonably well except for a postoperative death. Some patients with lung lesions were long-term survivors after aggressive surgical treatment. Six patients lived an average of 43 months after removal of the lung lesion, and 2 are without evidence of disease. Surgery also offered the best survival in patients with metastasis in a bone other than the spine and those with metastases in miscellaneous sites.

Prompt operation has been the policy in most cases of solitary metastasis of renal cell carcinoma. A period of observation may be justified in cases of solitary lung metastasis. It may be necessary to explore the lung later for a further appearance of metastasis.

▶ [The 23% long-term survival rate with aggressive therapy in the asynchronous state justified an aggressive approach.–J.Y.G.] ◀

Histopathology and Prognosis of Wilms' Tumor: Results from the First National Wilms' Tumor Study. J. B. Beckwith and N. F. Palmer[3] (Seattle) report the findings in a detailed histologic analysis of 427 patients entered in the first National Wilms' Tumor Study. Nonanaplastic tumors composed mainly of blastema fared no worse than predominantly epithelial or mixed tumor types, which are presumably more highly differentiated. Tumors composed mainly of differentiated tubules tended to occur in younger patients. Anaplasia contributed heavily to relapse and especially to tumor death.

The presence of large, pleomorphic, hyperchromatic tumor cell nuclei with abnormal multipolar mitotic figures was an unfavorable prognostic factor (table). Only 1 of 25 cases of anaplasia was in a patient under age 2 years, and in this patient the change was focal and not associated with relapse. Sixteen of the 24 older patients relapsed, and 14 died of tumor. The extent of the change was of some significance, but anaplasia was not strongly correlated with the extent of tumor at diagnosis. Anaplasia occurred

(3) Cancer 41:1937–1948, May, 1978.

SIGNIFICANCE OF ANAPLASIA IN NATIONAL WILMS'
TUMOR STUDY*

Degree of Anaplasia	No. Cases	Survivors No.	%	Relapse Free No.	%
Absent	364	338	92.9	305	88.8
Focal	15	9	60.0	8	53.3
Diffuse	10	2	20.0	1	10.0

*This table excludes the 24 sarcomatous patients and also 14 nonsarcomatous patients who died without evidence of tumor.

in the epithelial, stromal and blastemal populations of Wilms' tumor. Usually the stromal compartment exhibited the most extreme cellular atypia. A rhabdomyosarcomatoid pattern predominated in 8 of 24 specimens composed predominantly or exclusively of poorly differentiated stromal cells. A clear cell variant was seen in eleven specimens, and a hyalinizing pattern predominated in two.

In contrast to anaplastic Wilms' tumors, the sarcomatous variants were often seen in younger patients. Seven of ten deaths from tumor in patients less than age 2 years were related to sarcomatous variants. Sarcomas tended to metastasize to bone. Treatment generally failed to prevent relapse in patients with sarcomatous tumors. The extent of tumor at diagnosis influenced the outcome of anaplastic and sarcomatous lesions.

The anaplastic and sarcomatous variants of Wilms' tumor have a very unfavorable prognosis and contribute heavily to the overall mortality from this tumor. Histologic classification into "favorable" and "unfavorable" patterns should be an integral part of future treatment protocols, with more aggressive therapy directed primarily at tumors exhibiting cytologic atypia or a sarcomatous pattern.

▶ [The implications seem clear. Our pathologists must define patients with "unfavorable" patterns and we must treat them more aggressively.–J.Y.G.] ◀

Wilms' Tumor: Prognostic Factors for Patients without Metastases at Diagnosis: Results of the National Wilms' Tumor Study are reported by N. E. Breslow, N. F. Palmer, L. R. Hill, J. Buring and G. J. D'Angio.[4] Multivariate statistical methods were used to

(4) Cancer 41:1577–1589, April, 1978.

SITES OF RECURRENT OR METASTATIC DISEASE FOR 113 RELAPSED PATIENTS

A. Involvement of Individual Sites	No. of pts.	% Of relapses	% Died	
Abdomen	42	37.2	83.3	
Original tumor bed	11		9.7	72.7
Contralateral kidney	11		9.7	63.6
Liver	21		18.6	95.2
Other abdominal	19		16.8	94.7
Lung(s)	92	81.4	53.3	
Unilateral	36		31.9	27.8
Bilateral	42		37.2	76.2
Unspecified	14		12.4	50.0
Brain	6	5.3	66.7	
Bone	13	11.5	76.9	
Other sites*	7	6.2	71.4	

B. Occurrence of Combinations of Sites				
Site combination	No. of pts.	% Of relapses	% Died	
Lung only	55	48.7	34.5	(35.7)†
Abdomen only	17	15.0	70.1	(73.5)
Other site only	2	1.8	50.0	(36.1)
Lung + abdomen	19	16.8	94.7	(88.9)
Lung + other	14	12.4	64.3	(61.9)
Abdomen + other	2	1.8	100.0	(89.0)
Lung + abdomen + other	4	3.5	75.0	(95.9)
TOTAL	113	100.0		

*Includes skull, skin, mediastinum, diaphragm (extra-abdominal). In part B, brain and bone are listed with other sites.

†Figures in parentheses are mortality percentages calculated for each category from fitted model.

evaluate a wide range of factors in predicting relapse and survival in 429 children enrolled in the National Wilms' Tumor Study. Data from several sources were utilized. Of 113 relapses, 83 occurred in the 1st year, 23 in the 2d postoperative year and 4 more in the 25th month. The actuarial figure for long-term disease-free survival is 72.7%. Sites of involvement and mortality rates in relapsed patients are given in the table. Sixty-four relapsed patients have died (Fig 31). An estimated 39.1% of relapsed patients will live 3 years from the time of relapse. The prognosis for patients found to have disease in both lungs or in the abdomen, especially the liver, is not good.

Neither sex nor race had any appreciable effect on relapse. Exclusion of patients with metastatic disease made for a slightly younger age distribution than usual. Patients less than age 2 years at diagnosis had fewer relapses than older children, but the effect of age on mortality was less marked. Overall, combination chemotherapy yielded about one-third fewer relapses than single-agent therapy. With-

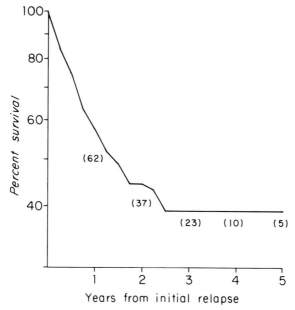

Fig 31.—Survival curve from relapse for 113 relapsed patients. Numbers of patients still alive and being followed at each anniversary are shown in parentheses. (Courtesy of Breslow, N. E., et al.: Cancer 41:1577–1589, April, 1978.)

holding radiotherapy from older patients with localized disease may have increased their rate of abdominal relapse. The very smallest tumors were associated with fewer abdominal relapses and deaths. Capsular penetration affected relapse significantly but less than lymph node involvement or specimen weight. Positive lymph nodes indicated a considerably worsened outlook. Intrarenal vascular invasion had only a small effect on relapse. Direct extension of disease was associated with abdominal relapse and an increased risk of death when relapse occurred. Spillage of tumor during operation had a more adverse effect on survival than on relapse. The presence of anaplastic components or renal sarcoma was an adverse prognostic factor. Strong relationships were evident between most of these variables. Of 17 patients with both unfavorable histology and lymph node metastasis, all relapsed and 15 died.

Age, lymph node status, tumor mass and histologic type are important in determining the likelihood of relapse in patients treated for initially nonmetastatic Wilms' tumor. Treatment with combination chemotherapy is effective regardless of what prognostic factors are operative.

▶ [This excellent article should be copied and placed in one's files. It clearly shows which factors predict relapse and survival in children with Wilms' tumor.–J.Y.G.] ◀

RENAL FAILURE

Reduction of Renal Function by Newer Nonsteroidal Anti-inflammatory Drugs. Aspirin and indomethacin can reduce renal blood flow and glomerular filtration, possibly through inhibiting prostaglandin synthesis. Robert P. Kimberly, Robert E. Bowden, Harry R. Keiser and Paul H. Plotz[5] (Nat. Insts. of Health, Bethesda, Md.) found that three members of another group of nonsteroidal anti-inflammatory drugs, the proprionic acid derivatives, cause similar changes along with a decrease in urinary excretion of immunoreactive prostaglandin E-like material. The observations were made in 3 patients with systemic lupus erythematosus, who took ibuprofen, naproxen and fenoprofen. One patient had a marked rise in plasma potassium concentration, and the others had significant increases. Two patients had a fall in serum sodium levels with an associated weight gain of not more than 2 kg. Two patients showed attenuation of the changes in renal function within several days on continued drug administration. This effect has also been noted with aspirin administration.

The effects of different nonsteroidal anti-inflammatory drugs on renal function in a given patient are not necessarily identical. The factors that determine the different responses and the factors that determine the persistence or attenuation of the changes are unknown. Awareness of the potential for these changes to occur is important in the clinical assessment of renal function in patients taking

(5) Am. J. Med. 64:804–807, May, 1978.

these and perhaps other drugs that inhibit prostaglandin synthesis.

▶ [These data add to the accumulating indirect and circumstantial evidence that prostaglandin metabolism is important in the preservation of renal function. Several chemically unrelated inhibitors of prostaglandin synthesis, including aspirin and indomethecin, can cause substantial reductions of glomerular filtration rate and renal blood flow.–Roscoe R. Robinson and Robert A. Gutman] ◀

Platinum Nephrotoxicity is reviewed by Nicolaos E. Madias and John T. Harrington[6] (Tufts Univ.). Significant evidence from animal studies implicates platinum compounds as nephrotoxic. Clinical trials have indicated that nephrotoxicity is the major limiting source of toxicity of these potent antitumor agents. The biologic handling of platinum is qualitatively similar to that of other heavy metals. The dose-related nature of platinum nephrotoxicity has been confirmed in animal studies. Search for new platinum analogues that are potent and have a therapeutic index superior to that of cis-dichlorodiammineplatinum (II) [cis-DDPt(II)] has produced initially encouraging results. Some organoplatinum coordination complexes may produce less severe renal tubular damage than cis-DDPt(II) when given in roughly equivalent therapeutic doses. Intravenous hydration of patients apparently reduces platinum nephrotoxicity. Einhorn and Donohue reported marked reduction in cis-DDPt(II) nephrotoxicity in patients "prehydrated" with normal saline.

Platinum is clearly nephrotoxic. Both the antitumor and the nephrotoxic activities of the inorganic platinum complexes are critically linked to their molecular configuration. The nephrotoxicity of platinum may be similar to that of mercury. Platinum compounds should not be administered before objective evidence of euvolemia is obtained. The platinum should be given slowly, with saline solution to produce a brisk diuresis. Urine flow probably should be kept at 3 to 4 L/24 hours for the next 2 or 3 days. Whether mannitol or furosemide affords further protection is not yet clear. Until less nephrotoxic platinum complexes are identified, it seems to be advisable to explore the possiblity of using platinum in combination chemotherapy in dosages not associated with significant nephrotoxicity and to avoid

(6)   Am. J. Med. 65:307–314, August, 1978.

other concomitant nephrotoxic insults, especially volume depletion.

▶ [This is an excellent review of a timely topic. Reduction of toxicity should be possible if platinum and mercury compounds have a similar effect on the renal parenchyma.–Roscoe R. Robinson and Robert A. Gutman] ◀

Inosine in Preserving Renal Function during Ischemic Renal Surgery. Inosine provides excellent protection to the kidney during warm ischemia in rats and dogs. Ultrastructural studies of inosine-protected kidneys have shown good preservation of the area of the nephron. J. E. A. Wickham, A. R. Fernando, W. F. Hendry, L. E. Watkinson, H. N. Whitfield, D. M. G. Armstrong and J. R. Griffiths[7] (London) evaluated the use of inosine in 4 patients with staghorn calculi and 1 with bilateral renal tumors who underwent conservative renal surgery under ischemic conditions. A fine cannula was inserted into the

Fig 32.—Serum creatinine concentrations before and after operation and serial measurements of differential renal function in 5 patients. Conversion: SI to traditional units—Serum creatinine: 1 μM/L ≈ 0.01 mg/100 ml. (Courtesy of Wickham, J. E. A., et al.: Br. Med. J. 2:173–174, July 15, 1978.)

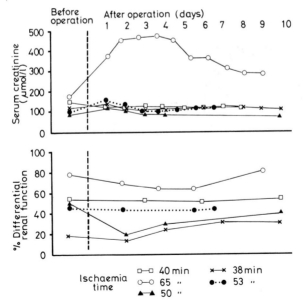

(7) Br. Med. J. 2:173–174, July 15, 1978.

renal artery distal to the clamp and the kidney was perfused with 80 ml of a 2.5% solution of inosine at room temperature. The renal vein was then occluded with a second
bulldog clamp. The serum creatinine values are shown in
Figure 32. Minimal increases in serum creatinine concentration and a slight depression of renographic function resolved within a few days. A transient rise in serum urate
concentration was noted. Reflow of blood on declamping
was faster than after operative protection with hypothermia. No adverse cardiodynamic effects were noted.

These results confirm experimental findings of the protective effect of inosine on the warm ischemic kidney. The
clinical results are as good as those noted in patients having ischemic renal surgery with hypothermic protection,
and the inosine technique is relatively simple. The technique has been used when a bloodless field is required for
conservative renal surgery for up to 75 minutes. Studies
are being done on the effects of inosine combined with hypothermia for more prolonged ischemic surgery and for
preserving cadaver kidneys for transplantation.

▶ [The purine nucleoside, inosine, appears to improve renal function after
experimental warm ischemia. Therefore it was tried in 5 patients whose surgery demanded clamping of the renal artery for over 40 minutes. These preliminary observations are encouraging but cannot yet be viewed as
final.—Roscoe R. Robinson and Robert A. Gutman] ◀

**Acute Renal Failure in Infants and Children: Out-
come of 53 Patients Requiring Hemodialysis Treatment.** Elisabeth M. Hodson, Carl M. Kjellstrand and
S. Michael Mauer[8] (Univ. of Minnesota) used hemodialysis
in the treatment of 53 children with acute renal failure in
the past 10 years. Twenty-three patients had acute tubular
necrosis, 14 after operation and 9 in association with catastrophic medical illnesses. The other 30 had primary
nephrologic disorders. Care was taken to avoid osmolar
changes that could cause the disequilibrium syndrome by
adjusting dialysis efficiency to the level of uremia and to
the patient's size. Most patients with acute tubular necrosis underwent emergency hemodialysis.

Four patients with acute tubular necrosis (17%) and 27
with primary nephrologic disorders (90%) survived. All 4
survivors in the group with acute tubular necrosis were

(8) J. Pediatr. 93:756–761, November, 1978.

postoperative patients. Eight of 11 children who had had cardiac surgery died. No child with medical acute tubular necrosis survived. The 3 deaths in the group with primary nephrologic disease were among the 15 patients with hemolytic-uremic syndrome. All other children with primary nephrologic disorders, including 5 with urologic problems and 5 with acute uric acid nephropathy, survived.

Acute renal failure in infants and children in this series that followed surgical and medical catastrophic illnesses resulted in a mortality of 83%, whereas acute renal failure complicating primary nephrologic disorders was associated with a 90% survival rate. It is not renal failure itself but the underlying disorders that largely determined the outcome in these patients. A clear choice between hemodialysis and peritoneal dialysis for management of acute renal failure cannot be made at present. Hemodialysis is much more efficient and this may be advantageous in treatment of severe pulmonary edema and hyperkalemia. Children with advanced uremia have less risk of disequilibrium on peritoneal dialysis. In experienced hands, hemodialysis is safe even for extremely small children, but peritoneal dialysis is technically simpler to institute and supervise.

▶ [This is a large series from an experienced institution. The principal message is not new but it deserves to be repeated, namely, that acute renal failure does not limit survival nearly so much as does its underlying cause or associated disease processes.—Roscoe R. Robinson and Robert A. Gutman] ◀

Renal Damage with Intestinal Bypass. Ernst J. Drenick, Thomas M. Stanley, Wayne A. Border, Edward T. Zawada, Leslie P. Dornfeld, Tyler Upham and Francisco Llach[9] (Los Angeles) obtained abnormal renal biopsy specimens from 2 intestinal bypass patients who required pyelolithotomies, and then examined renal function and biopsy specimens in 18 patients 7–108 months after intestinal bypass. Electron microscopic studies were made on tissue from 14 patients. All patients were morbidly obese and middle-aged at operation. Renal biopsy specimens were obtained at least 2 or 3 years after operation from all but 2 patients.

Blood urea nitrogen concentrations tended to be low from

(9)   Ann. Intern. Med. 89 (Pt. 1):594–599, November, 1978.

malabsorption and were unreliable indicators of renal function. All but 4 patients had normal serum creatinine concentrations and clearances. All patients studied had moderate to severe hyperoxaluria, with increases up to sixfold above the normal 40 mg/24 hours. Dietary and pharmacologic attempts to reduce oxalate excretion were largely ineffective. Four patients developed oxalate calculi, but a patient with end stage renal oxalosis had had no calculi. All patients had definite morphological abnormality of the renal cortex, but only 8 patients showed oxalate crystal deposit. The most common abnormalities were glomerular hyalinization and periglomerular and interstitial fibrosis. Most patients also had tubular atrophy and an increase in glomerular mesangial matrix. The changes were present as early as 7 months after bypass, but their extent appeared to be unrelated to the interval since operation. Several patients had focal lesions of the peripheral glomerular capillary loops, and similar changes were seen in the peritubular regions. Six of 11 studies showed granular deposits of IgM and C3 in glomerular capillary walls and the mesangium. Circulating immune complex-like material was detected in 6 of 11 patients evaluated by the Clq-binding radioimmune assay.

Annual measurements of urinary oxalate and creatinine clearance in intestinal bypass patients are recommended. If the creatinine clearance declines, renal biopsy may be indicated. The renal lesions appear to be irreversible and they may not be preventable. Immune complex mesangial injury is one apparent factor in bypass nephropathy. If significant damage is found, the bypass should be dismantled.

▶ [We already know of the dangers of oxaluria and stone disease in these patients. It now appears that immunologic mechanisms may be involved in the pathogenesis of associated renal disease. The patients have yet to suffer important renal functional impairment but the possiblity should be kept in mind.–Roscoe R. Robinson and Robert A. Gutman] ◀

Attainment and Maintenance of Normal Stature with Alkali Therapy in Infants and Children with Classic Renal Tubular Acidosis. Elisabeth McSherry and R. Curtis Morris, Jr.[1] (Univ. of California, San Francisco) investigated alkali therapy in 10 infants and chil-

(1) J. Clin. Invest. 61:509–527, February, 1978.

dren, at ages ranging from 8 days to 9.5 years, with classic renal tubular acidosis (RTA). When alkali therapy was begun, 6 (4 infants and 2 children) patients were stunted. Of the others, 2 were too young to have become stunted. Six had RTA as an apparent mendelian dominant trait, whereas 4 had idiopathic RTA. All patients had characteristic clinical features of RTA. None had hyperaminoaciduria. Alkali therapy was given to correct acidosis, as assessed by venous CO_2 content and plasma bicarbonate measurements. Alkali was given every 4 hours to young infants, and 4–5 times daily to the older patients. Metabolic studies were done in 6 children on the same dose of alkali for 3–10 months in whom acidosis occurred.

All patients reached and maintained normal stature on alkali therapy. Mean height increased from the 1.4 to the 37.0 percentile of a normal age- and sex-matched population. Mean height reached the 69th percentile in the 8 evaluable patients. The growth rate increased two- to threefold. Normal height was attained within 6 months in the stunted infants and within 3 years in stunted children. The height attained correlated inversely with the maximal possible duration of acidosis (before treatment) only in those patients in whom therapy was begun after age 6 months and not in those treated earlier. The amount of alkali needed to sustain correction of acidosis increased substantially during the course of treatment in each case. The maximal requirement ranged from 4.8 to 14.1 mEq/kg daily. It was determined principally by the degree of renal bicarbonate wasting.

Impaired growth can be prevented or corrected by alkali therapy that sustains correction of acidosis in infants and children with classic RTA. Optimal growth may require treatment in amounts that maintain a normal plasma bicarbonate concentration. Growth impairment in untreated classic RTA may require an acidosis-dependent impairment of renal conversion of $25(OH)D_3$ to $1,25-(OH)_2D_3$ and perhaps to other biologically active metabolites of $25(OH)D_3$ as well.

▶ [This is a valuable contribution on an important issue, particularly in view of the fact that previous attempts had failed to correct impaired growth. In general, however, previous treatment with alkali had also failed to correct acidosis completely. Full correction of acidosis with larger amounts of alkali may well be required, although the exact mechanistic interplay between the correction of acidosis, and other unmeasured biochemical and physiologic variables, and the correction of impaired growth has yet to be defined.—Roscoe R. Robinson and Robert A. Gutman] ◀

How Important Is Phosphate in Pathogenesis of Renal Osteodystrophy? Eduardo Slatopolsky, W. Ernest Rutherford, Keith Hruska, Kevin Martin and Saulo Klahr[2] (Washington Univ., St. Louis) point out that the pathologic changes in renal osteodystrophy include osteitis fibrosa cystica, which reflects the resorptive effect of increased osteoclastic activity from secondary hyperparathyroidism, and osteomalacia, a defect in bone mineralization that is secondary, at least in part, to changes in vitamin D metabolism. Hypocalcemia, hyperphosphatemia, hypermagnesemia and elevated serum parathyroid hormone (PTH) levels are found in uremia. Phosphate retention plays the major pathogenetic role in the development of secondary hyperparathyroidism in chronic renal failure. Parathyroid hormone plays a key role in the increased phosphaturia per nephron. The serum phosphorus is important in PTH release through inducing changes in ionized calcium. There is no convincing evidence that in early renal insufficiency low levels of $1,25(OH)_2D_3$ or calcium malabsorption play a pathogenetic role in the development of secondary hyperparathyroidism.

Pathogenetic mechanisms of renal osteodystrophy are illustrated in Figure 33. In severe renal insufficiency, secondary hyperparathyroidism is aggravated by the low levels of $1,25(OH)_2D_3$ that impair not only the absorption of calcium from the gut, but also the skeletal response to the action of PTH. Decreased degradation of PTH by the kidney in renal failure contributes to the extremely high levels of PTH often noted in advanced chronic renal insufficiency. Phosphate retention is responsible for the development of secondary hyperparathyroidism. A low-phosphate diet and administration of calcifediol prevent both secondary hyperparathyoidism and osteomalacia in uremic dogs. Skeletal resistance secondary to low levels of circulating

(2)   Arch. Intern. Med. 138:848–852, May 15, 1978.

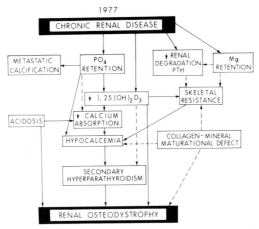

Fig 33.—Diagrammatic representation of pathogenetic mechanisms responsible for development of renal osteodystrophy. Interrupted lines represent hypothetical relationships; PTH indicates parathyroid hormone. (Courtesy of Slatopolsky, E., et al.: Arch. Intern. Med. 138:848–852, May 15, 1978; copyright 1978, American Medical Association.)

$1,25(OH)_2D_3$ is not responsible for the development of secondary hyperparathyroidism early in the course of renal insufficiency.

▶ [This essay is interesting in view of the next two articles. There have been two popular views concerning the mechanism of renal osteodystrophy: one is the "phosphate retention" school and the other has focused on alterations of vitamin D metabolism. This is not too surprising since there are at least two distinct forms of bone disease in patients with renal failure, i.e., osteomalacia and secondary hyperparathyroidism. They may coexist and it is likely that both schools are at least partially correct in their analyses. In this essay, proponents of the "phosphate retention" theory provide a nice summary of some of their elegant work in support of this pathogenetic mechanism. The reduced ability of diseased kidneys to convert 25-hydroxycholeciferol (DHCC), to 1,25-DHCC is considered to be much less important. This conclusion is reached partly because normal blood levels of the vitamin are found in many patients with early renal failure.—Roscoe R. Robinson and Robert A. Gutman] ◀

Deterioration of Renal Function during Treatment of Chronic Renal Failure with 1,25-Dihydroxycholecalciferol. Claus Christiansen, Paul Rødbro, Merete Sanvig Christensen, Birgitte Hartnack and Ib Transbøl[3] com-

---

(3) Lancet 2:700–703, Sept. 30, 1978.

pared the effects of 1,25-dihydroxycholecalciferol $1,25(OH)_2D_3$ and vitamin D_3 in predialysis patients with chronic renal failure. Thirty patients with relatively stable renal function for over a year and no history of renal stone disease or liver or gastrointestinal disorder were included in the study. Thirteen women and 5 men with respective mean ages of 54 and 44 years had a bone mineral content below 90% of normal, a serum calcium concentration lower than the normal mean -1 SD, a serum alkaline phosphatase value higher than the normal mean $+1$ SD or more than one of these. Patients received $1,25(OH)_2D_3$ orally in an initial dosage of 1 μg daily or vitamin D_3 in an initial dosage of 4,000 IU daily. Dosages were adjusted according to the serum calcium concentration. The dosage of $1,25(OH)_2D_3$ usually had to be reduced to 0.5 or 0.25 μg daily.

The patients initially had features of mild renal osteodystrophy. Treatment with $1,25(OH)_2D_3$ increased the serum and urinary calcium and urinary phosphorus values and reduced the serum alkaline phosphatase and both C- and N-terminal immunoreactive parathyroid hormone (iPTH) values. Vitamin D_3 therapy increased the urinary calcium excretion rate and reduced the serum iPTH concentration, especially the C-terminal peptide. Urinary phosphorus excretion was also reduced. Creatinine clearances were virtually unchanged during treatment in both groups. Renal function deteriorated more during $1,25(OH)_2D_3$ therapy than in the preceding 6 months.

Treatment with $1,25(OH)_2D_3$ even in small dosages causes deterioration in renal function more than expected during the spontaneous course of disease. Even mild hypercalcemia is more toxic to renal function than is hyperphosphatemia. Decreased formation of $1,25(OH)_2D_3$ in renal failure can be considered as an important defense mechanism. Treatment with 1α-hydroxylated vitamin D analogues should be restricted to the relatively few patients with severe symptomatic renal osteodystrophy.

▶ [This article should serve as a provocative but preliminary warning. If active vitamin D is given to patients with moderately severe renal disease, one may spare the bones but spoil the kidneys. Any patient receiving vitamin D or its metabolites should be followed carefully.—Roscoe R. Robinson and Robert A. Gutman] ◀

Increased Growth after Long-Term Oral 1α, 25-Vitamin D_3 in Childhood Renal Osteodystrophy.

Russell W. Chesney, A. Vishnu Moorthy, John A. Eisman, Diane K. Jax, Richard B. Mazess and Hector F. DeLuca[4] (Univ. of Wisconsin) studied the effect of long-term treatment with oral 1,25-$(OH)_2D_3$ in children with uremic osteodystrophy for periods of up to 26 months. Six prepubescent patients with chronic renal failure, aged 3 months to 14 years, were studied. Each had previously received vitamin D, oral calcium and oral phosphate binders. Five had congenital renal disorders with lifelong functional impairment. Systemic acidosis was corrected before the study. Single morning doses of 1,25-$(OH)_2D_3$ were given for 4–26 months, along with daily calcium gluconate. The mean serum creatinine concentration rose from 5.3 to 7.9 mg/dl during the study. Three patients received renal allografts after varying periods of treatment. One died of pneumococcal meningitis.

Serum calcium concentrations rose to normal after a month of treatment. Three patients had asymptomatic hypercalcemia, but only 1 patient had more than one episode. The serum phosphorus level increased with treatment, as did the tubular reabsorption of phosphorus. The serum magnesium concentration also increased, and the serum alkaline phosphatase level declined. Serum parathyroid hormone levels decreased during 1,25-$(OH)_2D_3$ treatment. Healing of rickets was noted within 4–12 weeks of the start of treatment, with progressive improvement over the course of the trial. An improvement in bone mineral content was noted on serial photon absorptiometric study of the forearm bones. Height velocity increased from 2.6 to 8 cm per year in the year after treatment in 4 evaluable patients. No acceleration of bone age was observed. Circulating levels of 1,25-$(OH)_2D_3$ increased significantly during treatment.

Oral 1,25-$(OH)_2D_3$ treatment can reverse renal bone disease and increase growth in uremic children. Continuous monitoring of the serum calcium level is necessary. With hyperphosphatemia, it is possible that metastatic calcification could occur. All the present patients had increased

(4) N.'Engl. J. Med.'298:238–242, Feb. 2, 1978.

requirements for phosphorus-binding agents during treatment.

▶ [These data suggest that altered vitamin D metabolism also plays a role in the pathogenesis of renal osteodystrophy. The patients' bones *and* secondary hyperparathyroidism improved with 1,25-vitamin D$_3$ therapy. Moreover the serum level of this vitamin was low at the outset. However, as the authors note, the observed deterioration of renal function may have occurred as a consequence of the natural progression of disease, but it is also possible that it occurred for the same reason as noted in the preceding article–Roscoe R. Robinson and Robert A. Gutman] ◀

Uremic Pruritus: Management and Possible Pathogenesis are discussed by Barbara Gilchrest[5] (Beth Israel Hosp., Boston). Generalized pruritus is common in patients on maintenance hemodialysis. Many first develop pruritus after dialysis is begun for control of chronic renal failure. Most patients notice a marked exacerbation at night and during dialysis. Use of emollients is a reasonable first step. Relatively greasy creams and ointments such as Eucerin and petrolatum are particularly useful. Menthol and phenol may give temporary relief in many cases and can be incorporated into emollients. Alcohol should be avoided. Topical corticosteroid creams and ointments appear to be minimally effective. Oral antihistamine therapy and minor tranquilizers frequently are used, but they provide only modest relief. Subtotal parathyroidectomy has been reported to provide dramatic relief in certain patients with secondary hyperparathyroidism. Lidocaine given intravenously relieves pruritus temporarily.

Recently ultraviolet phototherapy was evaluated for treatment of uremic pruritus. Adults with chronic renal failure requiring hemodialysis who had had intractable pruritus for at least 2 months, not satisfactorily controlled by conventional therapy, were evaluated. Ten patients received midrange ultraviolet light (UVB) therapy twice weekly for 4 weeks and 8 received long-range ultraviolet light (UVA) therapy. Nine UVB-treated patients reported mild or absent pruritus, compared with only 2 of the 8 controls. Three UVB-treated, patients with recurrent pruritus were successfully re-treated with UVB. Eight of 9 responders remained free from pruritus for at least 8 months; 1 died at 6 months, free from pruritus. The only side effects

(5)   Dialysis Transplant. 7:1021–1022, October, 1978.

were mild sunburning and slight tanning. Similar results have been obtained in 24 further patients given UVB phototherapy for uremic pruritus.

The specific cause of uremic pruritus is unknown, but some substance or metabolic change associated with dialysis may be a factor. Ultraviolet phototherapy appears to be a safe and effective treatment. Its ultimate role in the management of uremic pruritus remains to be determined.

▶ [This is a good summary of the conservative management of this difficult clinical problem. Midrange ultraviolet light does appear to be more effective than long-range light for relief of symptoms. It is also 1,000 times more effective in causing sunburn or suntan. The relief of symptoms and tanning may be linked but it must be noted that their coexistence may make further control studies more difficult.—Roscoe R. Robinson and Robert A. Gutman.] ◀

Continuous Ambulatory Peritoneal Dialysis. Robert P. Popovich, Jack W. Moncrief, Karl D. Nolph, Ahad J. Ghods, Zbylut J. Twardowski and W. K. Pyle[6] report results of continuous ambulatory peritoneal dialysis in 9 patients treated over 136 patient-weeks. This approach trades relatively long dialysis sessions 3 days a week for 5 daily 30–45 minute interruptions of activities. Indwelling Tenckhoff long-term peritoneal catheters were placed. Exchanges were with 2 L commercial dialysis solution (Dianeal). The peritoneal cavity was drained by gravity in 15–20 minutes and fresh solution was instilled by gravity in 10 minutes, with the patient using sterile technique to connect the peritoneal catheter to the tubing. Most solutions contained 1.5% dextrose. Dialysis was continued when signs of peritonitis developed, with antibiotics added to the dialysis fluid or given parenterally or orally. Protein intake was increased to 1 gm/kg or above. Potassium intake was 50 mEq daily and sodium intake was 88–200 mEq or more daily.

Renal function is shown in Figure 34. Low-normal serum albumin concentrations were maintained despite fairly extensive protein losses. Patients tolerated the 50-mEq potassium diet well. Three patients have maintained and 6 have increased total body weight. Blood pressure has been readily controlled. Thirteen episodes of peritonitis occurred in the 136 patient-weeks of dialysis. All patients showed resolution of symptoms and clearing of dialysate in 1 or 2

(6) Ann. Intern. Med. 88:449–456, April, 1978.

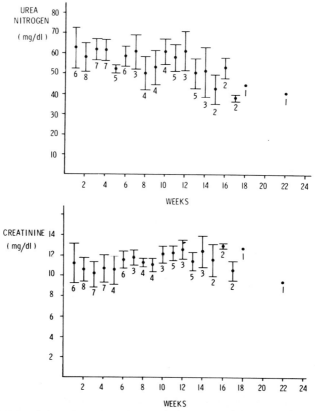

Fig 34.—Mean ± SEM urea nitrogen and creatinine concentrations related to weeks on continuous ambulatory peritoneal dialysis. Numbers below points represent those patients seen in clinics any particular week after continuous ambulatory peritoneal dialysis was started. Mean values are calculated from these same patients. (Courtesy of Popovich, R. P., et al.: Ann. Intern. Med. 88:449–456, April, 1978.)

days. Only 1 patient has required catheter replacement. Most patients reported improved well-being, increased energy and good appetite and were enthusiastic about the treatment. Many increased their activities above the level at which they had performed for years.

Continuous ambulatory peritoneal dialysis provides acceptable control of serum chemistry values and sustained subjective improvement in patients. Large-molecule clearances per week are up to 6 times those obtained with typical hemodialysis. Prolonged interruption of daily activities is unnecessary. Better connecting devices could reduce the occurrence of peritonitis. The cost can be high if premixed solutions at maximum prices are used. The technique does not require maximally efficient clearances of small solutes.

▶ [This technique is clearly effective. It is possible that the greater clearance of larger molecular weight substances is an important advantage but there is no direct proof. Recurrent peritonitis may eventually limit the permeability of the peritoneal membrane for adequate dialysis. Long-term follow-up of a larger group of patients will be necessary before the general applicability of this technique can be established.—Roscoe R. Robinson and Robert A. Gutman] ◀

Chronic Renal Failure in Children. Persons under age 20 years account for about 7% of all patients undergoing dialysis in Ontario and 20% of all who undergo renal transplantation in the United States. J.-G. Mongeau, P. Robitaille and M.-M. Grall[7] (Univ. of Montreal, Canada) reviewed the findings in 77 children with chronic renal failure, seen at one hospital in Quebec during 1970–75. They represent an incidence of 2.5 per 1,000,000 population per year. Chronic renal failure was defined as a serum creatinine concentration more than 2 mg/dl for at least 2 months.

The causes of renal failure are given in the table. Urinary tract malformation was present in over a third of the children. In 75% of 28 patients with bilateral vesicoureteral reflux or a posterior urethral valve, chronic renal failure could have been prevented by earlier diagnosis. All these patients had their malformations corrected, but 6 of 7 with a neurogenic bladder required an ileal conduit. Seven girls with chronic glomerulonephritis presented with nephrotic syndrome. Seven children with the nephritic syndrome were reported to have "end-stage" renal disease, and 3 had interstitial nephritis. The group with congenital malformation of the renal parenchyma included 12 older patients who were severely uremic at diagnosis, and 4 younger children who presented with failure to thrive, gastrointestinal symptoms and vitamin D-resistant rickets. Ten children had hereditary nephropathy. Five of these had cystinosis, and 4 of these received a renal transplant.

---

(7) Can. Med. Assoc. J. 118:907–913, Apr. 22, 1978.

CAUSES OF CHRONIC RENAL FAILURE (CRF)

Cause of CRF	Hôpital Sainte-Justine, Montreal		Hôpital des enfants malades, Paris
	No. (and %) of patients		
Children (aged 0-17 years)			
Urinary tract malformation	28 (36)		57 (21)
Chronic glomerulonephritis	17 (22)		57 (21)
Renal parenchymal malformation	16 (21)		59 (22)
Hereditary nephropathy	10 (13)		61 (23)
Other	6 (8)		36 (13)
Total	77 (100)		270 (100)
Adults (aged 15-64 years)			
Chronic pyelonephritis		144 (30)	
Chronic glomerulonephritis		131 (27)	
Renovascular hypertensive disease		51 (11)	
Polycystic renal disease		33 (7)	
Obstructive nephropathy		28 (6)	
Analgesic nephropathy		23 (5)	
Diabetic nephropathy		15 (3)	
Nephrolithiasis		10 (2)	
Renal hypoplasia		5 (1)	
Other		42 (9)	
Total		482 (101)	

Three children had familial nephritis, and 2 presented with signs of nephronophthisis.

The most frequent causes of chronic renal failure in children in this series were urinary tract malformation, chronic glomerulonephritis, renal parenchymal malformation and hereditary nephropathy. Early renal transplantation is frequently important in these patients, particularly in children with cystinosis.

▶ [This article appropriately emphasizes the opportunities for prevention of renal disease and the increased opportunity for successful rehabilitation with renal transplantation.—Roscoe R. Robinson and Robert A. Gutman] ◀

Quality of Life for Long-Term Survivors of End-Stage Renal Disease. Elva O. Poznanski, Emily Miller, Carlos Salguero and Robert C. Kelsh[8] examined long-term adaptational patterns and the physical and emotional maturation of 18 children and adolescents who survived 2 years or longer after renal transplantation for end-stage renal failure. Semistructured interviews were

(8) J.A.M.A. 239:2343–2347, June 2, 1978.

conducted with the patients and their parents. Most patients had received intrafamilial transplants. Nine patients (group A) had functioning grafts more than 2 years after the transplant, with little evidence of current rejection. Nine (group B) were undergoing short- or long-term rejection and had reduced renal function or had rejected a kidney and received another transplant that was undergoing rejection. Many patients were on intermittent high-dose steroid therapy, and 1 was on continual hemodialysis.

Seven of 9 group A subjects were in school or working full-time, although several were not at grade level. Six group B subjects worked part-time or not at all. A great difference was noted between the groups in capacity to maintain friendships; group B subjects had meager friendships or no friends. Their poor physical status and depression interfered with their capacity to form social relationships. None of these subjects had a heterosexual relationship. Younger patients showed a tendency to accept their height better than older ones. They were more concerned about their facial appearance and weight than about their height. All subjects were concerned about their self-image. Eleven subjects made depressive statements; they clustered in group B, in which only one young person was not depressed. Subjects were unable to talk about rejection until their early 20's, but this issue dominated the parents' thinking.

The quality of life of these young people varied greatly. A realistic assessment of transplant success before surgery would improve the psychologic adaptation of the patients. Routine psychosocial appraisal of recipients at 3-month intervals might also be of use. Particular emphasis is needed on the encouragement of emotional autonomy appropriate to the patient's age. Group interactions might be promoted, and individual counseling might be helpful in selected patients.

▶ [These unusually detailed studies of the degree of rehabilitation underscore the value of a successful renal homograft in young people with renal insufficiency. Unfortunately, renal transplantation also continues to fail with an unfortunately high frequency. The decision can be difficult but, on balance, most might favor an attempt at transplantation in this critical age range.–Roscoe R. Robinson and Robert A. Gutman] ◀

TRANSPLANTATION

Flow and Function in Machine-Preserved Kidneys.

It has been a common practice to discard machine-preserved kidneys with a flow rate less than 100 ml per minute or 80 ml per minute, but there is little objective evidence to support such a policy. Derek Sampson, H. Myron Kauffman, Jr., and Peter Walczak[9] (Med. College of Wisconsin, Milwaukee) reviewed the results of a policy of not discarding kidneys on the basis of flow rates while on the machine in a series of 100 cadaver kidney transplants. In some instances, a period of cold storage preceded machine perfusion. Both the Belzer LI-400 system and the Waters MOX 100 system were utilized, with cryoprecipitated plasma and modified plasmanate, respectively. In both systems, the systolic pressure was adjusted to 60 mm Hg initially. Organs were discarded only if a suitable recipient could not be found.

The table summarizes the results in three groups of kidneys. There was no significant difference in incidence of primary nonfunction according to flow rate on the machine. The duration of acute tubular necrosis tended to be longer with lower flow rates, but this was not significant. Serum creatinine levels in the three groups of kidneys were virtually identical 3 months after transplantation, and function at 1 year was comparable in these groups of kidneys.

PERFORMANCE OF MACHINE-PRESERVED KIDNEYS

| | Flow (ml/min) | | | |
	<80	80–100	>100	P
Range (ml/min)	40–80	80–100	100–300	—
Mean flow (ml/min ± s.d.)	59 ± 11	84 ± 5	154 ± 43	—
No. kidneys	11	14	75	—
No. kidney with primary non-function	1	4	13	n.s.
Mean duration ATN (d ± s.d.)	12 ± 11	7 ± 6	8 ± 1	n.s.
Mean serum creatinine at 3 mth (mg/100 ml)	$2 \cdot 5 \pm 1 \cdot 8$	$2 \cdot 5 \pm 1 \cdot 8$	$2 \cdot 5 \pm 1 \cdot 6$	n.s.

ATN = acute tubular necrosis.

(9) Br. J. Surg. 65:37–40, January, 1978.

Graft function was not related to flow rates on the machine. The duration of acute tubular necrosis was greater when flow decreased during perfusion, but there was no significant difference in serum creatinine levels at 3 months. Most cases of nonfunction were associated with hyperacute or acute rejection. Kidneys with decreasing flow rates were more frequent with use of the Belzer machine than the Waters machine. Kidneys that functioned immediately had a higher rate of accelerated rejection than those which opened up slowly, but the longer term rejection rates were essentially the same.

Flow rates during kidney preservation are not important for graft function after transplantation, justifying a policy of ignoring flow rates in the decision as to whether to transplant a kidney. Such a policy could make available up to 25% more kidneys for transplantation. The development of tubular necrosis, while making early postoperative management a little more difficult, does not lead to impaired function and may even be of some value.

▶ [The perfusion characteristics of cadaver donor kidneys used in clinical transplantation vary tremendously. Every transplant surgeon has noted this variation during simple gravity flushing of the kidneys. Varying degrees of vasoconstriction are evident but, as reported here, correlate poorly with the ultimate outcome. We feel the most important feature in successful organ preservation is maintenance of good renal blood flow prior to donor nephrectomy.–Donald C. Martin] ◀

Value of Urine Cytology in Renal Transplantation. Both lymphocyturia and an increased number of renal tubular cells have been described during acute rejection of a renal transplant. James P. Fidler, Fatima Dajani, M. Roy First, Rino Munda and J. Wesley Alexander[1] (Univ. of Cincinnati) sought to clarify the value of serial urine cytologic examinations in the posttransplant period, particularly in differentiating rejection from nonimmunologic causes of deteriorating renal function. Cytologic study was made of 3,014 urine specimens collected from 132 renal transplant patients over a 42-month period. A total of 217 episodes of deteriorating renal function was evaluated.

Acute rejection was characterized by an increase in number of renal, tubular cells in all cases, and this was the earliest indicator of threatened rejection. Lymphocytes

---

(1)   Transplantation 26:133–135, August, 1978.

were present in the urine in 91% of rejection episodes. Lymphoblasts were found in two thirds of episodes; they were primarily associated with rejection phenomena. Cytologic examination of the urine correctly identified 120 of the 128 episodes of acute rejection diagnosed clinically. Four other episodes in retrospect were not rejections. In 16 episodes with no other associated condition, the urine cytodiagnosis was made an average of 2.4 days before the serum creatinine concentration rose to 0.3 mg/dl. There were 18 false positive cytodiagnoses. Viral infections were present in 13 instances and *Candida* infection of the lower urinary tract in 5. The urine cytologic examination was an excellent prognostic index of the final outcome of rejection. All 18 patients with persistent signs of rejection after antirejection therapy lost their grafts within 1 month.

Correlation between clinical and cytologic diagnoses of acute rejection was generally excellent in this series. False negative cytologic reports were rare. Quantitative cellular differences and the presence of lymphoblasts were often helpful in distinguishing acute rejection, acute tubular necrosis and viral infection. Persistent criteria of rejection after treatment were consistent with a poor prognosis.

▶ [The occurrence of lymphocyturia with renal allograft rejection has been known for at least 15 years. This study documents very well the value of regular and routine examination of the urinary sediment following renal transplantation. Let us never forget the importance of examination of the urine.–Donald C. Martin] ◀

Improved Survival Rates in Presensitized Recipients of Kidney Transplants by Immunosuppression with Maternal Source γ-Globulin. The finding that mixed leukocyte responsiveness (MLR) between maternal cells and those from newborn infants and recipient and donor source cells could be suppressed by serum of the "hosts" suggested that the tolerance observed for "grafts" in these subjects might be related. Robert R. Riggio, Sung J. Kim, Stuart D. Saal, William T. Stubenbord, Jhoong S. Cheigh, Kurt H. Stenzel and Albert L. Rubin[2] (New York Hosp.-Cornell Med. Center) found that 7S immunoglobulins from pooled maternal blood sources almost always blocked MLR between random responder-stimulator cell pairings. The usefulness of this γ-globulin preparation

(2) Lancet 1:233–235, Feb. 4, 1978.

(RPGG) as a graft-enhancing agent was studied in 195 adults who received cadaver kidneys in a 3-year period, 156 as first transplants. Two products from different blood sources were investigated. Patients received azathioprine and prednisone, and the experimental group received 1.6 gm of γ-globulin intramuscularly just before and just after transplantation and then daily for 6 days, weekly for 4 weeks and monthly for 12 months.

The two groups were well matched for factors affecting kidney transplant survival rates, including degree of HLA matching. Differences in graft survival rates were not significant. Nonresponder recipients of first grafts showed no differences at any time. Among responders who received first grafts, the RPGG group had a significantly higher 2-year survival rate than the control group (55.5% vs 28.8%). No serious side effects resulted from use of the globulin solution. No significant differences in actuarial patient survival were observed.

The globulin concentrate significantly improved kidney graft survival in patients in this study with preformed lymphocytotoxic antibodies, but it had no effect in recipients without these antibodies. Host responses may be important in determining the efficacy of RPGG. The γ-globulin preparation appears to alter or suppress immune responses associated with humoral-type rejection, rather than to prevent sensitization. Possibly the graft-prolonging factors in RPGG could be better concentrated. Currently higher intravenous dosages of RPGG are being used for a shorter time.

▶ [A 1-year graft survival of less than 40% in the control group is poor. This low percentage of success with controls would tend to make any investigative procedure look favorable.–Donald C. Martin] ◀

Leukocytosis Is Not a Manifestation of Rejection. It has been suggested that leukocytosis is a manifestation of acute allograft rejection, but some have failed to find a constant association. A. S. Daar, P. J. Morris and D. O. Oliver[3] (Univ. of Oxford) evaluated the leukocytic response to rejection retrospectively in 80 definite rejection episodes that occurred in 50 patients. Forty-four patients received cadaver grafts and 6 living, related-donor grafts. The re-

---

(3) Br. Med. J. 2:1570–1571, Dec. 17, 1977.

jection episodes occurred 4–315 days after transplantation. Rejection was confirmed histologically in 20 episodes. Azathioprine and prednisolone were administered after transplantation. During rejection episodes patients were treated with methylprednisolone intravenously or, in a few, an increased oral dosage of prednisolone. Fourteen episodes resulted in graft loss.

Only 21 rejection episodes (26%) were associated with an increase in the leukocyte count, whereas 27 (34%) were associated with a significant decline in the count. Graft loss from rejection was most frequent in episodes associated with a fall in the leukocyte count and least frequent in those associated with no significant change. Grafts were lost in 4 of the 21 episodes in which leukocyte numbers increased. The differences were not significant.

The leukopenia associated with some renal allograft rejection episodes is probably not due to vigorous antirejection therapy. A more likely explanation is the rejection process itself. Humoral mechanisms and immunologically nonspecific cells are important in mediation of graft damage. Where the marrow has borderline reserves in an immunosuppressed patient and severe systemic manifestations cause further toxic suppression, margination or consumption of leukocytes in the rejecting graft might lead to a fall in the peripheral leukocyte count. Leukocytosis is the least common response to acute allograft rejection. The individual graft prognosis may be poorer when there is a significant fall in the leukocyte count.

▶ [We feel the most important change in the peripheral blood count is the rapid fall in platelets. This can be the sign of an intrarenal coagulopathy associated with a very rapid rejection process and is a very ominous finding which usually requires prompt graft nephrectomy.–Donald C. Martin] ◀

Analysis of Cytomegalovirus Infection and HLA Antigen Matching on Outcome of Renal Transplantation. Several reports indicate that viral infection contributes to renal allograft rejection. Lopez et al. suggested that virtually all rejection is due to cytomegalovirus (CMV) infection. A. G. May, R. F. Betts, R. B. Freeman and C. H. Andrus[4] (Univ. of Rochester) obtained evidence that CMV infection influences graft survival and function as

(4) Ann. Surg. 187:110–117, February, 1978.

much as HLA antigen matching. Fifty-eight consecutive renal transplant patients were analyzed prospectively from 1971, and 27 others retrospectively. The group included 15 parental, 11 sibling and 59 cadaveric transplants. The 85 transplant patients were divided into four groups (Fig 35). Group I consisted of 21 well matched recipients free from CMV (11 cadaver donor). Group II consisted of 5 poorly matched patients free from CMV (all cadaver donor). Group III consisted of 41 well matched patients infected with CMV (25 cadaver donor). Group IV consisted of 18 poorly matched patients infected with CMV (all cadaver donor). Seven of the sibling-sibling transplants were HLA identical. Immunosuppression was with azathioprine and prednisone. Most cadaver-kidney recipients had local irradiation of the transplant as well. Since 1972, acute rejection has been treated with bolus administration of intravenous steroids. The follow-up was 6–120 months.

Sixty of the 85 patients shed virus after transplantation, but only 21 had viremia. The mean time after transplantation when shedding was first detected was 42 days. Forty-four patients had reactivation of CMV that was latent in the patient for months or years. Primary infection after transplantation developed in 15 other patients. Primary infection was frequent in recipients of parental kidneys and rare in CMV seronegative recipients of sibling or

Fig 35.—Allograft survival in all patients grouped by HLA match and CMV infection. (Courtesy of May, A. G., et al.: Ann. Surg. 187:110–117, February, 1978.)

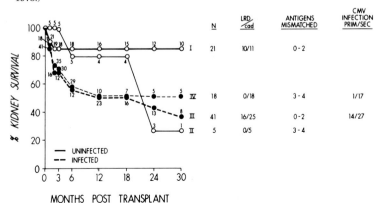

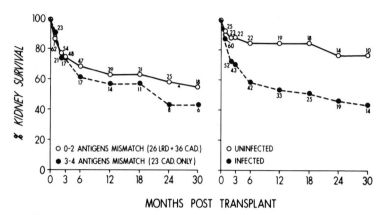

Fig 36.—Allograft survival in all patients grouped by HLA match *(left)* and CMV infection *(right)*. (Courtesy of May, A. G., et al.: Ann. Surg. 187:110–117, February, 1978.)

cadaveric kidneys. Forty-seven grafts, including 27 cadaveric donor grafts, were functioning at follow-up. Graft survival was related to HLA match and CMV infection (Figs 35 and 36). There was a definite descending order of allograft survival from group I to group IV. Lack of presensitization to tissue antigens did not account for the relative success of transplantation in recipients free from CMV infection.

The disparate incidence of CMV infection in sibling, parental and cadaveric transplants is an important factor in differing rates of successful renal transplantation. Primary CMV infection is associated with an increased rate of graft failure, regardless of HLA antigen match. The CMV status of donors and recipients can be determined as quickly as can tissue typing.

▶ [Most clinicians have observed reduced renal function associated with systemic viral infection. To conclude that viral infection is more important than tissue compatibility is to possibly fall prey to the fallacy of *post-hoc ergo propter hoc.* The authors' recommendation of using kidneys from CMV sera-positive donors only for CMV positive recipients is certainly noteworthy.–Donald C. Martin] ◀

Immunologic Factors Determining Survival of Cadaver Kidney Transplants: Effect of HLA Serotyping, Cytotoxic Antibodies and Blood Transfusions on Graft Survival was studied in 510 patients who received primary transplants in 1970–77 by Flavio Vincenti, Robert M. Duca, William Amend, Herbert A. Perkins, Kent C. Cochrum, Nicholas J. Feduska and Oscar Salvatierra, Jr.[5] (Univ. of California, San Francisco). Mixed lymphocyte cultures were used. All kidneys were stored by continuous pulsatile perfusion preservation with cryoprecipitated plasma. Mean patient age was 34 years. No nonviable kidneys were transplanted.

Graft survival was not significantly influenced by race or sex of recipient or donor. Degree of HLA match, previous prenancies and length of time on hemodialysis were not significant factors in graft survival. Graft survival was improved significantly in patients given more than five blood transfusions before transplantation, regardless of the cytotoxic antibody status. The 2-year graft survival rates were 52% for patients given more than five transfusions and 23% for those given none. The groups had similar stimulation indices on mixed lymphocyte culture before transplantation. Administration of blood during transplantation did not appear significantly to improve graft survival at 2 years.

The mechanism of the beneficial effect of blood transfusions on renal graft survival is speculative. The timing of transfusions and the most effective type of red blood cell preparation are uncertain. Transfusions should be used more liberally in prospective cadaver graft recipients on dialysis. Monthly screening for cytotoxic antibodies should be started at the onset of dialysis or in the late phase of chronic renal failure.

▶ [Pretransplant transfusions will result in circulating cytotoxins in many patients. Once again these authors report the presence of cytotoxins does not adversely affect the outcome of first cadaver donor kidney transplants. However, the presence of cytotoxins will obviously make it more difficult to find a kidney for the individual recipient with circulating antibody.–Donald C. Martin] ◀

Improvement of Kidney Graft Survival with Increased Numbers of Blood Transfusions. A higher renal transplant survival rate has been documented in patients pretreated with blood transfusions. Gerhard Opelz and Paul I. Terasaki[6] (Univ. of California, Los Angeles)

(5) N. Engl. J. Med. 299:793–798, Oct. 12, 1978.

(6) Ibid. pp. 799–803.

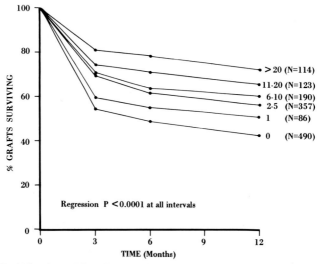

Fig 36A.—Actuarial graft survival rates in recipients of first cadaver kidney transplants separated by the number of pretransplant blood transfusions that the recipients had received. The number of blood units transfused is indicated at the end of each curve. All types of blood products (whole, packed or frozen) were included. Numbers of patients in each subset are given in parentheses. Statistical significance was calculated by weighted regression analysis. (Courtesy of Opelz, G., and Terasaki, P. I.: N. Engl. J. Med. 299:799–803, Oct. 12, 1978.)

have found that multiple tranfusions are more effective than single ones and that pretransplantation transfusion is more effective than transfusion at the time of transplantation only. Study was made of 1,360 cadaver-donor kidney transplants done through 1977.

A striking stepwise increase in graft survival rate with an increase in numbers of transfused blood units was observed. The correlation was maintained throughout the entire follow-up period (Fig 36A). Packed cells accounted for almost 90% of all transfusions. The influence of different blood products on graft survival is shown in the table. Centers with varying results of transplantation all exhibited a significant graft prolongation effect from pretransplant transfusions. Only a slight improvement in graft outcome was attributable to transfusions given during operation. No additional effects on graft outcome attributable to pregnancies was observed. The influence of tranfusions on graft survival in related-donor grafts is less clear.

INFLUENCE OF DIFFERENT BLOOD PRODUCTS ON SURVIVAL OF FIRST
CADAVER-DONOR TRANSPLANTS

No. of Pretransplant Transfusions*	Graft Survival Rate at 1 Yr (% ± SE)		
	WHOLE BLOOD ONLY	PACKED CELLS ONLY	FROZEN BLOOD ONLY
>0	49±7 (48)†	59±2 (495)	48±6 (90)
>5	70±11 (17)	66±4 (189)	50±9 (34)
>10	89±11 (9)	68±5 (99)	48±14 (17)

With the graft survival rate in the 490 patients without any transfusions
(42±2% at 1 yr, Fig 1) taken as a reference point, the following P values are
derived:

P 0 vs >0	NS‡	<0.00001	NS
P 0 vs >5	<0.02	<0.0001	NS
P 0 vs >10	<0.0001	<0.0001	NS

*Patients who had received more than one blood product were not included in
this table.
†Figures in parentheses denote number of patients.

This study confirmed the very powerful effect of blood
transfusions in prolonging renal graft survival. The effect
is proportional to the number of transfusions administered.
Deliberate transfusion trials in prospective transplant recipients should take into account the strong dose dependence of graft prolongation by transfusions. The effect of
deliberate transfusions on an entire population of patients
on dialysis remains uncertain.

**Influence of HLA Matching and Blood Transfusion
on Renal Allograft Survival.** The failure rate of cadaver
kidney transplantation remains high, with rejection causing over 70% of failures. J. Douglas Briggs, John S. F.
Canavan, Heather M. Dick, David N. H. Hamilton, Kenneth F. Kyle, Stuart G. Macpherson, Alistair M. Paton
and D. Michael Titterington[7] (Univ. of Glasgow, Scotland)
examined the influence of various immunologic factors in
a series of 107 consecutive cadaver kidney transplants performed at a single unit during 1969–1975 on 95 patients.
Six patients died early after operation. Three kidneys

(7) Transplantation 25:80–85, February, 1978.

never functioned because of renal artery thrombosis, and 2 because of ischemic damage. Ninety-six transplants in 87 patients were analyzed. The 96 kidneys were either functioning at the time of review (50 cases) or functioned until death of the recipient (8 cases), were rejected (37 cases) or failed at a late stage because of technical reasons (1 case). Of the 87 patients, 58 were male and 29 female subjects, with a mean age at transplantation of 31 years. Twenty-eight patients had bilateral nephrectomy, and 7 had sple-

Fig 37.—Influence of blood transfusion on cumulative graft failure rate from rejection. The overall significance test showed a difference between patients not transfused and those given whole blood ($x^2 = 8.75$, $P < 0.005$) but not between the former group and those given frozen red blood cells. The actuarial method of analysis showed the curves for no blood and whole blood transfusion to differ at all points (at 1 and 3 months and at 1 and 2 years, $P < 0.005$; at 6 months, $P < 0.01$). (Courtesy of Briggs, J. D., et al.: Transplantation 25:80–85, February, 1978.)

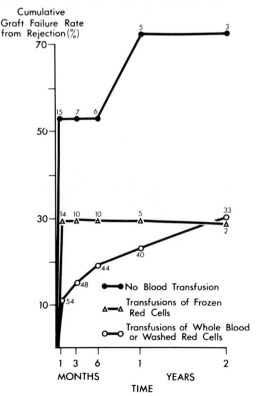

nectomy. Immunosuppression was with prednisolone, azathioprine and, in some cases, antilymphocyte globulin.

The cumulative rate of graft failure from rejection was 22% in the first month and rose to 41% at 2 years, with no further failures over the next 2 years. The 2-year failure rate from rejection was 29% for grafts with less than two HLA incompatibilities, compared with 52% when there were two or more incompatibilities. The presence of HLA antibodies did not adversely affect the survival of first grafts. Patients not transfused before transplantation had a 1 year graft failure rate of 72%, compared with 29% for those given frozen-thawed red blood cells and 23% for those given whole blood. The influence of transfusion on graft failure from rejection is shown in Figure 37. The apparent benefit from transfusion was no greater in patients given over 5 units than in those given less.

Three conclusions can be drawn from this analysis: (1) it adds to growing evidence that HLA matching is beneficial in human renal transplantation (more attention must be given to increasing the numbers of well matched transplants); (2) it suggests that the HLA antibodies induced by blood transfusion are not detrimental to graft survival; and (3) it provides supporting evidence for a beneficial effect of pretransplant blood transfusion on graft survival.

Blood Transfusion and Renal Allograft Survival. R. W. Blamey, M. S. Knapp, R. P. Burden and Maxine Salisbury[8] (Nottingham, England) reviewed 32 first renal transplants with cadaver allografts, performed in 1974–77, to determine how many recipients had received blood transfusions preoperatively. Twenty-one men and 11 women were operated on. Immunosuppression was with prednisolone and azathioprine, and 16 patients received antilymphocyte globulin (ALG) also. Patients undergoing graft rejection were treated with methylprednisolone. Kidneys were matched for ABO group but not for HLA.

A signficant difference in graft survival was found between patients who received transfusion before transplantation and the others. The difference was entirely due to acute rejection within 3 months after transplantation in nontransfusion patients. None of 9 patients with acute re-

(8) Br. Med. J. 1:138–140, Jan. 21, 1978.

jection received preoperative blood transfusions. No significant difference in numbers of rejection episodes occurring after 3 months was observed. Graft survival was not affected by blood group or HLA matching or by transfusion given at or after operation. Administration of ALG did not affect graft survival significantly.

Acute kidney graft rejection was significantly less frequent in patients given blood transfusion before transplantation in this study. If these results are confirmed, raising the overall success rate of first cadaver transplants to 75% by reducing the number of grafts lost from acute early rejection would overcome many problems.

▶ [Improved transplant survival following multiple blood transfusions has been reported throughout the world. The mechanism remains unknown. Hopefully this information can be used as a guide to a more organized manipulation of the immune response.—Donald C. Martin] ◀

Beneficial Effect of Operation-Day Blood Transfusions on Human Renal Allograft Survival. Renal grafts tend to survive better in patients given blood transfusions before operation. C. R. Stiller, B. L. Lockwood, N. R. Sinclair, R. A. Ulan, R. R. Sheppard, J. A. Sharpe and P. Hayman[9] (London, Ont.) studied the effects of transfusion at operation in 56 patients who underwent, cadaver renal graft transplantation more than a year previously. Generally buffy coat-poor blood was transfused before operation, but occasionally whole blood was given. All blood given during or after transplant surgery was buffy coat poor.

The 1-year graft survival rates were 71% for patients given transfusion before operation and 40% in the others. An average of 2.9 units was given patients who received transfusion on the day of operation. About 60% of patients given transfusion before operation and about 40% of the others received blood on the day of operation. The 1-year graft survivals were 79% in patients given transfusions on the day of operation and 44% in others. Transfusion on the day of operation appeared to have benefited patients who did not receive transfusion before operation. Graft survival was not significantly improved by transfusion after operation in patients given transfusion on the day of operation. Patients given no blood on the day of operation or after-

(9)　Lancet 1:169–170, Jan. 28, 1978.

ward had a 1-year graft survival of only 20%. Among patients given no blood at any time, only 1 of 11 grafts was functioning at 1 year.

The effects of transfusion on the day of transplantation may explain the variability in reported effects of preoperative transfusion. The effects of transfusion at transplant operations should be assessed in clinical trials with monitoring of the immune response to ascertain whether patients respond immunologically to antigens in transfused blood or to those in the transplanted kidney. The possibility that postoperative transfusions are beneficial should also be investigated.

▶ [The beneficial role of transfusions weeks and months prior to transplantation is clearly established in large series. This reported benefit of immediate preoperative transfusion is based on a much smaller patient population. Should this data be corroborated with a larger experience, it would greatly simplify the management of patients with regard to the use of transfusions to enhance graft survival. A larger experience is needed to corroborate these findings before they can be universally accepted.–Donald C. Martin] ◀

Technique for Lengthening the Right Renal Vein of Cadaver Donor Kidneys. Robert J. Corry and Stephen E. Kelley[1] (Univ. of Iowa) have used the en bloc technique of organ removal with perfusion of kidneys through the aorta. Subsequent anastomosis of a patch of aorta with more than one renal artery to the recipient's external iliac artery is preferable to suture of small arteries individually. Lengthening of the right renal vein is an added benefit of the en bloc procedure. This vein is commonly short, especially if it is transected distal to its junction with the inferior vena cava. Anastomosis of a short renal vein to the recipient's iliac vein can be difficult, and placement of the graft in ideal position is sometimes impossible. The venotomy in the vena cava is extended to open it just above the right renal vein after the left kidney is removed, and it is closed with a running vascular suture as the kidney is immersed in iced saline. The desired length of vena cava is selected, any excess is removed and the vena cava is then sutured to the iliac vein.

This technique eliminates the problem of the short right renal vein in kidney transplantation. Removal of donor kidneys by the en bloc technique not only insures preser-

(1) Am. J. Surg. 135:867, June, 1978.

vation of multiple arteries, but permits creation of a right renal vein of adequate length.

▶ [Frequently the short right renal vein makes the surgery of transplantation difficult but we have experienced no instance in which it was impossible. Simply using the cuff of the vena cava at the junction of the right renal vein suffices in most cases.–Donald C. Martin] ◀

Cyclosporin A in Patients Receiving Renal Allografts from Cadaver Donors. Cyclosporin A (CyA), a peptide fungous metabolite, has been found to be powerfully immunosuppressive without causing obvious side effects in several animal species. R. Y. Calne, D. J. G. White, S. Thiru, D. B. Evans, P. McMaster, D. C. Dunn, G. N. Craddock, B. D. Pentlow and Keith Rolles[2] (Univ. of Cambridge) carried out a pilot study of CyA as the sole immunosuppressive agent in patients with first cadaver renal allografts from mismatched donors. Cyclosporin A was given intramuscularly, starting on the day of transplantation, in a dosage of 25 mg/kg for the first 2 or 3 days and then at the same dosage orally. All kidneys were from donors with complete irreversible cerebral destruction but intact circulation. They were preserved by flush cooling and ice storage. The cold ischemia time ranged from $1^1/_4$ to 16 hours. In no case was the kidney considered to be well matched.

Seven patients on dialysis with renal failure were treated with CyA as the sole immunosuppressive agent in conjunction with cadaver kidney transplantation. Cyclosporin A inhibited rejection, but there was clear evidence of nephrotoxicity and hepatotoxicity. A cyclophosphamide analogue was added to the CyA treatment in 6 cases. Five patients are out of the hospital with functioning allografts, and 2 of these have received no corticosteroids. One patient required allograft nephrectomy because of pyelonephritis in the graft. Another died of systemic *Aspergillus* and *Candida* infection. No biopsy showed severe or extensive mononuclear cell infiltration of the interstitium, interstitial hemorrhage or other histologic evidence of severe rejection. Ultrastructural study of one specimen showed normal glomerular structure and no evidence of basement membrane abnormality.

Cyclosporin A has a profound immunosuppressive effect in man. A slight increase in hair was noticed in the 2 fe-

(2) Lancet 2:1323–1327, Dec. 23 & 30, 1978.

male patients. Hepatotoxicity has been mild and transient. A direct nephrotoxic effect on the renal tubules or their blood supply seems likely. Further careful study of a limited number of patients is needed before CyA can be recommended in clinical practice.

▶ [Cyclosporin A appears to be a potent immunosuppressive in man. Five of seven functioning grafts is a very favorable result if function continues for at least 1 year. I know of no other immunosuppressive agent which, if used alone, would accomplish this result. The evidence of renal toxicity is a disturbing feature of the use of cyclosporin A in recipients of renal allografts and may ultimately limit its application.–Donald C. Martin] ◀

Cyclosporin A for Treatment of Graft-versus-Host Disease in Man. Cyclosporin A (CyA) is a new fungous cyclic polypeptide that specifically inhibits transforming lymphocytes and depresses hypersensitivity reactions and antibody production. It can prevent organ and skin graft rejection in animals. R. L. Powles, A. J. Barrett, H. Clink, H. E. M. Kay, J. Sloane and T. J. McElwain[3] report a pilot study of CyA treatment in leukemic patients with graft-versus-host disease (GVHD) after marrow transplantation. The 5 patients studied received allogeneic marrow transplants from HLA-identical, mixed lymphocyte culture-compatible siblings. They were nursed in reverse-barrier isolation, ate sterile food and received nonabsorbable antibiotics orally and topical chlorhexidine decontamination of the orifices. All transfused blood products were irradiated. Cyclophosphamide and total body irradiation were used in conjunction with marrow transplantation, and methotrexate was given after transplantation. Cyclosporin A was given orally or intramuscularly.

The acute erythematous skin reaction of GVHD resolved within 2 days in all instances, but 4 of the 5 patients died. Cyclosporin A in high dosages produced anorexia, nausea and a reversible rise in blood urea concentration. All patients who died had liver damage, but the histologic changes were variable.

Cyclosporin A modified the acute skin reaction of GVHD in these patients, but most of them died with liver failure. Apart from suspected liver toxicity, a definite, though reversible, rise in blood urea was observed. No significant histologic changes were seen in the kidneys, except for occasional granular casts in the distal and collecting tubules.

---

(3) Lancet 2:1327–1331, Dec. 23 & 30, 1978.

The place of CyA in marrow transplantation is uncertain, but a trial of the agent is justified for the treatment and postgraft prophylaxis of GVHD in man.

► [Graft-versus-host disease remains a major problem in bone marrow transplantation. Cyclosporin A did not prevent this disease and is associated with disturbing evidence of liver and renal dysfunction. This latter toxicity would seem to be a serious limitation for application to clinical renal transplantation.–Donald C. Martin] ◄

Factors Contributing to Declining Mortality Rate in Renal Transplantation. Nicholas L. Tilney, Terry B. Strom, Gordon C. Vineyard and John P. Merrill[4] (Harvard Med. School) found that recent modifications in the management of renal allograft patients have reduced the mortality at 1 year to 2% among those given related-donor kidneys and to 5% in those given cadaver kidneys. Of 186 patients given allografts since 1974, 7 (4%) have died within a year of operation. The rate of wound infection has been reduced from about 25% in 1972 to 2% since 1976. No progressive fall in mortality was apparent in 1970–74, a period when patients received maintenance azathioprine and prednisone therapy for immunosuppression, in combination with antilymphocyte globulin and high-dosage corticosteroid pulse therapy for rejection episodes. Such treatment failed to influence graft survival.

The intensity of immunosuppressive therapy has been reduced in recent years. At the authors' institution, standard regimens of azathioprine and prednisone are used, with a 3-day corticosteroid pulse given intravenously for episodes of acute rejection, in a dosage of 1 gm daily. A maximum of three such pulses is used in the first 3 months after transplantation. Tapering of corticosteroids has been more rapid since 1973. Other modifications have included intraoperative use of antibiotics, routine used of ultrasound and substitution of needle biopsy for open renal biopsy. Patients receive an intravenous bolus of 2 gm ampicillin, 2 gm oxacillin and 1.5 mg gentamicin per kg on induction of anesthesia. Clindamycin is used instead in patients with penicillin allergy. Subsequently, specific antibiotics are given only as indicated. The biopsy findings are used as a guide to treatment and prognosis. Since 1974, allografts that have failed irreversibly have been removed

(4) N. Engl. J. Med. 299:1321–1325, Dec. 14, 1978.

only if they produce symptoms after corticosteroid withdrawal. At present, about two thirds of failed grafts are left in place.

It appears that the risk of death from complications attendant on renal transplantation can be considerably reduced. This form of treatment of end stage renal failure thus has become an attractive alternative to long-term dialysis for increasing numbers of patients.

▶ [The authors report an excellent record of morbidity and mortality in recipients of renal allografts. The conservative immunosuppressive regimen described has been utilized at many institutions in this country. Nonetheless, a 5% mortality rate in recipients of cadaver donor organs is very good in view of the chronic illness in these patients and the many hazards from cardiovascular and infectious illness in these immune-suppressed individuals. Preoperative antibiotics have been previously shown to have a salutary role in reducing the incidence of wound infection in transplant recipients.–Donald C. Martin] ◀

Perfusion Characteristics of Preserved Canine Kidneys Subjected to Warm Ischemia. A major problem in cadaveric kidney transplantation is the identification of irreversibly damaged kidneys by simple, reliable methods. V. K. Modgill, P. A. Wiggins and G. R. Giles[5] (St. James Univ. Hosp., Leeds, England) investigated commonly used viability assessments in groups of canine kidneys subjected to 0, 15 or 30 minutes of warm ischemia followed by 24 hours of preservation. All kidneys were perfused at 8 C with Perfudex in a total volume of 500 ml for 24 hours. Recipient animals received 4% dextrose-saline, Lasix and mannitol during the anastomoses.

All the kidneys produced urine immediately after revascularization. Changes in perfusate concentrations of acid radicals, lactate, free fatty acids and lactic dehydrogenase (LDH) were assessed at 1 hour and 24 hours. Except for the LDH level at 1 hour, no single parameter detected kidneys that were so damaged as to be non-life supporting. All dogs that received a kidney releasing enough LDH into perfusate to raise the concentration to more than 100 units/L died.

It is difficult to correlate simple perfusate changes with kidney graft viability after 24 hours of perfusion. It seems likely that one of the main problems is a failure to ensure

(5) Br. J. Urol. 50:1–7, February, 1978.

perfusion of the organ in entirety and thus allow the total anaerobic metabolism and cell lysis to reflect the change in perfusate composition.

▶ [The authors cite a worthy objective. It has not yet been reached.–Donald C. Martin] ◀

MISCELLANEOUS

Pregnancy in Patients with Chronic Renal Disease. Robert A. Bear[6] (Toronto) points out that although it is widely thought that pregnancies carry increased maternal and fetal risk in patients with renal disease this concept is not entirely true. Patients with active or inactive systemic lupus erythematosus (SLE), even without clinically evident lupus nephritis, should never become pregnant, since the rate of relapse is probably increased in pregnancy, and rates of abortion, fetal death and prematurity are high. There is a very high rate of exacerbation of SLE post partum. Therapeutic abortion is not indicated in pregnant SLE patients, but prednisone and azathioprine should be given during pregnancy and in the postpartum period. Women with a history of healed idiopathic nephrotic syndrome do not relapse during pregnancy, and the risk of other fetal or maternal complications is not increased. Women with a history of acute glomerulonephritis but no active glomerular disease also tolerate pregnancy well, although they may be prediposed to premature delivery and preeclampsia.

A loose correlation is evident between the severity of underlying renal disease and the maternal and fetal prognosis of pregnancy, but the data are not adequate for definitive counseling of patients with renal disease who wish to become pregnant or for guidelines to precise clinical management after the onset of gestation. Maternal and fetal complications appear to be strikingly increased in patients with about a 50% loss of renal function, with serum creatinine levels exceeding 1.6 mg/dl. Occasionally pregnancies in patients with progressive renal disease have been maintained successfully with frequent hemodialysis,

(6) Can. Med. Assoc. J. 118:663–665, Mar. 18, 1978.

and occasionally patients with end-stage renal disease on long-term dialysis have had uncomplicated pregnancies. Renal transplant recipients usually tolerate pregnancy well, but hypertension and deteriorating renal function have been noted, and dystocia and even uterine rupture may occur. The frequency of fetal abnormalities is increased, and neonatal adrenal suppression and sepsis have been observed. The life expectancy of renal transplant recipients is uncertain, and these patients should be counseled as to the advisability of undertaking pregnancy.

▶ [Kidney function and disease in pregnancy are not well understood by most urologists since we infrequently encounter problems with pregnant patients.

During pregnancy, the kidneys enlarge (Bailey and Rolleston: J. Obstet. Gynaecol. Br. Commonw. 78:55, January, 1971) and ureters dilate due to mechanical and humoral factors. The physiologic dilatation of the urinary tract may persist to the 12th postpartum week (Crabtree: *Urological Diseases in Pregnancy* (Boston: Little, Brown and Co., 1942). Renal function increases 25 to 50% due to an unknown mechanism and, because of increased GFR, serum creatinine normally decreases. Mild proteinuria is normal.

Coexistence of pregnancy with renal disease, regardless of type or severity, alarms physicians who often wish to terminate the gestation. Such views are unduly pessimistic. If function impairment is mild and hypertension absent, the gestation will probably succeed. As renal disease progresses and function declines, ability to conceive and sustain a viable pregnancy decreases. When renal function decreases to serum creatinine levels of 3 mg/100 ml, gestation rarely succeeds. Women with moderately severe kidney disease have delivered viable infants. There are reports of gravidas in whom sudden deterioration of renal function was managed with hemodialysis and pregnancy succeeded. Women undergoing maintenance dialysis have rarely conceived. Women with chronic renal failure are usually amenorrheic and ovulate infrequently. Ovulation and menses reappear about 6 months after successful transplantation.

After transplantation, it is safe to conceive if the patient has had good health for 2 years, no evidence of rejection, hypertension, or calyceal obstruction, serum creatinine of 2 mg/100 ml or less, and no more than 15 mg/100 ml of Prednisone or azathioprine 3 mg/kg daily. There are risks to infants (prematurity, respiratory distress syndrome, congenital anomalies, hypoadrenalism and neonatal sepsis).

The 4 to 7% prevalence of bacteriuria in gravidas is similar to that in nonpregnant females. Pregnant women with confirmed bacteriuria must be treated with an antibiotic since 40% develop symptomatic infections. Symptomatic kidney infections are known to be associated with prematurity. There is disagreement concerning the relationship of asymptomatic bacteriuria to prematurity, to the occurrence of gestational hypertension, and to the development of anemia.

An excellent reference on this subject is Lindheimer and Katz: *Kidney Function and Disease in Pregnancy* (Philadelphia: Lea & Febiger, 1977).–J.Y.G.] ◀

Control of Bleeding after Renal Biopsy with Epsilon-Aminocaproic Acid. Urokinase, a urinary fibrinolytic activator, may prevent clot formation after urinary tract trauma and promote prolonged or recurrent bleeding. Epsilon-aminocaproic acid (EACA) has been used successfully to inhibit urokinase in the treatment of postprostatectomy bleeding and of hematuria in hemophiliac patients. E. Savdie, J. F. Mahony and B. G. Storey[7] (Sydney Hosp., Sydney, Australia) evaluated EACA in 6 patients who had severe or persistent bleeding after percutaneous renal biopsy. Three patients had persistent gross hematuria and 3, perirenal bleeding confined to the retroperitoneal space. All patients had normal clotting studies before biopsy examination. Four were hypertensive but were adequately controlled. Two had advanced renal failure at the time of biopsy investigation. One patient required treatment 5 hours after biopsy for massive perirenal hemorrhage with life-threatening hypotension. The other patients were treated an average of 14 days after biopsy.

The average dose of EACA used was 9.6 gm daily, and the mean duration of treatment was 17.3 days. No patient required further blood transfusion after EACA therapy. Persistent clots formed in the bladder and ureter in 1 patient, which were successfully treated by ureteric catheterization and irrigation. Five patients responded rapidly to EACA therapy with cessation of bleeding. No patient had evidence of disseminated intravascular coagulation or glomerular capillary thrombosis. No patient had renal function deteriorate attributable to EACA therapy. One patient showed radiographic evidence of permanent damage to the biopsied kidney 1 year after the procedure.

Treatment with EACA appears to be useful in accelerating intrarenal hemostasis in selected patients with bleeding after renal biopsy when there is no evidence of intravascular coagulation. The treatment may shorten hospitalization and reduce the needs for blood tranfusion and operative intervention.

► [We have had a good response when using epsilon-aminocaproic acid for idiopathic gross hematuria and its recurrence.–J.Y.G.] ◄

(7) Br. J. Urol. 50:8–11, February, 1978.

Percutaneous Nephrostomy: Series and Review of the Literature. Derek P. Stables, Nathan J. Ginsberg and Michael L. Johnson[8] (Univ. of Colorado) attempted percutaneous nephrostomy on 53 kidneys of 42 patients, 33 adults and 9 children, in 1972–77. The usual indication was supravesical obstruction with azotemia, infection or both. Less common indications were uncomplicated su-

TABLE 1.—INDICATIONS FOR
PERCUTANEOUS NEPHROSTOMIES

Indication	No. Performed	No. Unsuccessful
Supravesical obstruction:		
With infection	15	0
With infection and azotemia	5	0
With azotemia:		
One kidney	10	1*
Two kidneys	16	3†
Without azotemia or infection	3	0
Urinary fistula	4	1‡
Total	53	5

*Catheter dislodgement.
†One placement failure; 2 pelvicaliceal blood clot retentions (same patient).
‡Inadequate from undilated renal pelvis, in absence of ureteral obstruction.

TABLE 2.—UNDERLYING DISEASE

Cause	No. Nephrostomies
Supravesical obstruction:	
Ureteropelvic junction obstruction	6
Duplex kidney, upper moiety obstruction	2
Ureteral or renal pelvic calculus	7
Postoperative edema	4
Postoperative ureteral stricture	5
Postirradiation ureteral stricture	2
Inflammatory ureteral stricture	2
Bladder trabeculation	2
Retroperitoneal fibrosis	2
Retroperitoneal lymphoma or carcinoma	17
Urinary fistula:	
Sigmoid conduit, ureteral fistula	2
Vesicovaginal fistula	2
Total	53

(8) Am. J. Roentgenol. 130:75–82, January, 1978.

pravesical obstruction and urinary fistula (Table 1). The site and cause of obstruction or fistula were variable (Table 2). Currently the pelvicaliceal system is visualized by both ultrasound and fluoroscopy. An 18-gauge sheath is exchanged over a 0.89-mm guidewire for a no. 6.5 F polyethylene catheter under fluoroscopic control. The balloon catheter technique has been was used in the most recent cases.

In the authors series one placement failure occurred. Percutaneous nephrostomy achieved its goal in 91% of cases, and 62% of these patients did not require subsequent operation (Table 3). Major complications occurred in 8% of cases (Table 4).

Azotemia from bilateral obstruction or obstruction in a single functioning kidney has been the most common indication for nephrostomy in this and other series. Other indications include urinary fistula, drug instillation for dissolution of calculi and calculus extraction. The reported overall incidence of major complications is 4%. Minor complications occurred in 16% of the authors' series and in

TABLE 3.—RESULTS OF NEPHROSTOMY AND
FINAL OUTCOME

Result of Nephrostomy and Outcome	No.
Successful, temporary:*	
Definitive surgery	18†
Radiotherapy	5
Chemotherapy	5
Resolution of edema or fistula	6
Passage of calculus	1
Death from underlying tumor	5
Death from incidental disease	1
Patient refused definitive treatment	1
Subtotal	42
Successful, permanent‡	6
Unsuccessful:	
Surgical nephrostomy	2
Surgical nephrostomy and ureteral ligation	1
Surgical nephrostomy and definitive surgery	1
No treatment§	1
Subtotal	5
Total	53

*Drainage period, 6–305 da (mean, 42).
†Two awaiting definitive surgery.
‡Drainage period, 4 mo to 4 yr.
§Placement failure in one kidney of patient with bilateral ureteral obstruction. Nephrostomy of other kidney was successful.

TABLE 4.—COMPLICATIONS

Complication	No. Nephrostomies *
Major:	
Pelvocalyceal blood clot retention	2†
Transient urinary peritonitis	1
Pyelonephritis due to catheter obstruction	1
Subtotal	4 (8)
Minor:	
Retroperitoneal urine extravasation	1
Retroperitoneal hemorrhage (small)	1
Temporary catheter dislodgement	3
Temporary catheter obstruction by debris	3
Subtotal	8 (15)
Total	12 (23)

*Data on 53 procedures; nos. in parentheses are percentages.
†Both procedures in same patient.

15% of reported cases. Percutaneous nephrostomy should be available on a 24-hour basis in all major hospitals. The only contraindication is a severe bleeding diathesis. The procedure does not entirely replace the surgical approach. Surgical nephrostomy is indicated at exploratory laparotomy or other operation and when percutaneous nephrostomy fails.

▶ [Recently with the addition of better instrumentation for catheter insertion and use of fluoroscopic and realtime ultrasound guidance, placement of the catheter is much easier. The urologist must be involved in these procedures and not give them up by default to the radiologist! With the addition of a fluoroscopic unit to our cystoscopic suite, we have been using percutaneous nephrostomy more and more for diagnostic and therapeutic indications. As pointed out in this article, percutaneous nephrostomies have been used to drain a pyonephrosis (although the pus sometimes is too thick to drain), to determine if a hydronephrosis has resulted in regained function, to instill drugs, and to extract calculi. Their precise role in calculi extraction is undetermined.–J.Y.G.] ◀

Experimental and Preliminary Clinical Experience with Thermography for Avascular Nephrotomy. W. Oosterlinck and W. De Sy[9] (Univ. of Ghent) report a simple method for demarcation between different arterial areas, which permits nephrotomies to be carried out with minimal bleeding and subsequent renal ischemia. The thermal gradient between the segment with occluded blood supply

(9)   J. Urol. 120:528–529, November, 1978.

and adjacent ones retaining their blood supply is defined by a liquid cholesterol crystal sheet. The thermographic sheets used are those prepared for detection of veins in cases of difficult venipuncture. They change from brown at 30 C to green at 31 C to blue at 32 C and remain blue up to 37 C. A temperature difference of 2 degrees C produces a striking color difference. The thermographic sheet is pressed on the renal surface after the branch supplying an area in which a nephrotomy may be necessary is occluded and saline at room temperature is poured over the kidney to cool the occluded portion. The results are read after about 30 seconds. The nephrotomy is then done; the pedicle is clamped with or without cooling.

Clear-cut color variations were observed between vascularized and nonvascularized areas in all 6 canine kidneys studied, proving the reliability of the thermographic method. Thermography has been used successfully in 8 patients, 7 undergoing operation for staghorn calculus and 1 undergoing heminephrectomy. Thermography is as rapid as any other method and requires no puncture of an arterial branch. Arterial spasm in the occluded segment is not important with this technique. In some cases of staghorn calculus it may be impossible to determine the area in which nephrotomy will be done before renal cooling is begun. Thermography nevertheless offers a simple and safe expedient for staghorn calculus operations and for less complicated situations, such as heminephrectomy and nephrotomy for caliceal stones.

▶ [In our experience, finding the bloodless line to do a nephrotomy is not always easy. The use of the liquid cholesterol crystal sheet sounds promising.–J.Y.G.] ◀

A Simple Technique for Partial Nephrectomy is described by Alan J. Wein, Victor L. Carpiniello and John J. Murphy[1] (Philadelphia, Pa.). A simple guillotine amputation with individual suture ligation of vessels has been used in partial nephrectomy to obtain improved wound healing and hemostasis.

TECHNIQUE.—The kidney is approached via any standard incision and carefully mobilized. A preoperative angiogram is helpful but not essential. Any segmental artery that appears to supply

(1) Surg. Gynecol. Obstet. 146:620–621, April, 1978.

the part of the kidney to be removed is occluded and, if confirmed, ligated and divided. Occlusion of the main renal artery is not routinely used. The capsule is sharply incised and, with the kidney tightly squeezed manually, a blunt knife handle is used to perform a transverse guillotine resection, and the cut surface is compressed with a sponge for 3–5 minutes. Bleeding points are sutured individually with figure-of-eight 4–0 chromic catgut. The collecting system is closed in a watertight manner with 4–0 or 5–0 chromic catgut. Intravenous indigo carmine with mannitol or furosemide permits identification of any part of the collecting system that requires further suturing. The capsule is closed with interrupted 4–0 chromic catgut sutures. A Penrose drain is placed adjacent to the resection site and brought out through a retroperitoneal stab wound.

Eighty-nine patients have been operated on with this technique in the past 12 years, with no operative mortality and no significant secondary hemorrhage. Postoperative urography has generally shown normal function of the remaining parenchyma. Only one nonfunctioning kidney resulted in a patient who had a lower pole partial nephrectomy along with an opposite pole nephrolithotomy. This technique is recommended whenever partial nephrectomy is indicated.

▶ [Our experience with guillotine partial nephrectomy has been excellent. Enough renal capsule should be left to pull together over the edges and a segmental artery should be ligated when possible. Recently we have also been using a microfibrillar collagen hemostat (Avitene) for added control of bleeding.–J.Y.G.] ◀

Plasmapheresis in Rapidly Progressive Glomerulonephritis. Priscilla Kincaid-Smith and Anthony J. F. d'Apice[2] (Victoria, Australia) point out that plasmapheresis removes abnormal immune reactants; depletion of mediators of the immune response, such as complement components and procoagulants, depends on the composition of the replacement fluid. Theoretically, plasmapheresis should interrupt the cycle in human antibasement membrane disease in which autoantibody provokes further autoantibody production. Removal of the normal feedback inhibition of IgG, however, could result in a rebound peak of antibody production when plasmapheresis is stopped. This is one reason for the concurrent use of immunosuppressive therapy. Vascular access is usually obtained by

(2) Am. J. Med. 65:564–566, October, 1978.

use of arteriovenous shunts. Artificial plasma expanders are not suitable during intensive plasmapheresis. Human albumin-based solutions are most commonly used. Four-liter exchanges have been carried out daily for 4 or 5 days and then every 2 or 3 days. Usually treatment is continued for 1 to 2 weeks after renal function has stabilized.

Renal function has been preserved in 5 of 10 patients with Goodpasture's syndrome and much better results could have been achieved. Two patients responded but relapsed when plasmapheresis was stopped and did not respond adequately to retreatment. One patient died of influenzal pneumonia contracted during the period of plasmapheresis and immunosuppression. Treatment should be started as soon as possible after diagnosis. Anticoagulants should not be used. Meticulous aseptic management of arteriovenous shunts is essential to avoid infection. Optimally patients should be referred to regional centers. Renal function improved in 16 of 22 patients with immune complex-mediated glomerulonephritis. There is little doubt that these results represent a marked improvement over the natural history of disease in patients with diffuse crescents and a rapidly progressive course. Serious complications have been few, compared with the group with Goodpasture's syndrome.

▶ [Goodpasture's syndrome presents with anemia, dyspnea and pulmonary hemorrhage with accompanying fulminating glomerulonephritis. The reported improvement with plasmapheresis combined with immunosuppression in the article are impressive.–J.Y.G.] ◀

Anatrophic Nephrolithotomy in the Solitary Kidney. Despite the successes of anatrophic nephrolithotomy with reconstructive calicoplasty, concern remains that the procedure results in a significant loss of viable renal tissue and that any apparent improvement in function is due to compensatory changes in the contralateral kidney. Allston J. Stubbs, Martin I. Resnick and William H. Boyce[3] (Bowman Gray School of Medicine) examined this question by reviewing 30 patients who underwent anatrophic nephrolithotomy for staghorn calculus disease in a solitary kidney in 1960–76. The 21 women and 9 men were aged

---

(3)   J. Urol. 119:457–460, April, 1978.

22–75 years. Seventeen presented with recurrent infection, 10 with flank pain and 3 with advanced renal insufficiency. All had an infectious and/or identifiable metabolic basis for stone formation, and a predisposing factor was identified in 12 of 27 infected patients. Renal function was significantly impaired in 14 of the 23 patients evaluated, excluding the 3 with severe renal insufficiency. Twenty-nine patients had had nephrectomy, usually for complications of stone disease, and 11 also had had ipsilateral renal surgery.

The operating time averaged nearly 6 hours. Two patients required 5 nephrolithotomies. No patient was anuric postoperatively. The average follow-up period was 6 years. Seven patients died during follow-up, 5 of nonrenal causes. There were no operative deaths. Renal function did not change significantly after operation. Eight of 27 infected patients had positive cultures postoperatively, but 3 of them had cutaneous urinary diversions. Six patients had recurrent calculi; 4 had concomitant urinary infection. Three stones in 2 patients required repeat nephrolithotomy.

Renal function remained stable after anatrophic nephrolithotomy in these patients. Two with end-stage renal disease showed improvement in renal function, and chronic hemodialysis was avoided. The failures probably resulted from underlying urinary tract pathology that was not amenable to surgical correction. These patients are best managed by the complete removal of all calculi and intensive antimicrobial therapy.

▶ [This is a well-controlled demonstration that anatrophic nephrolithotomy done in the best hands does not decrease renal function and may actually increase it in selected cases. Presumably, these cases were done with local hypothermia. Staghorn calculus disease is managed best by surgical removal of the calculi since the majority of the nonoperated patients will eventually develop sepsis and perinephric abscesses (Blandy: J. Urol. 115:505, 1976).–J.Y.G.] ◀

Use of Microfibrillar Collagen Hemostat for Control of Renal Bleeding. Microfibrillar collagen hemostat is an absorbable, modified natural collagen prepared from purified bovine corium. It has a highly open structure producing a very large surface area; it attracts platelets that adhere to the fibrils and triggers aggregation of platelets and thrombus formation. Martin E. Hanisch and W. G. Guer-riero[4] (Ben Taub Hosp., Houston) used microfibrillar collagen hemostat in the treatment of 23 patients with renal trauma, usually from gunshot wounds. Treatment consisted primarily of partial nephrectomy. One patient with an arteriovenous fistula after needle biopsy underwent nephrectomy after application of the hemostat. The material was applied directly to the bleeding source in a dry state after large vessel hemostasis was achieved. Pressure was applied and excess hemostat removed after 3–5 minutes.

The hemostat succeeded in rapidly controlling renal bleeding except in the patient having needle biopsy, in whom persistent hypertension necessitated nephrectomy. No patient had secondary renal bleeding requiring exploration or transfusion. Complications were minimal and usually resulted from the injury or contamination from the colon. No patient has had a renal stone during follow-up (less than 2 years).

A microfibrillar collagen hemostat is effective in the control of small vessel renal bleeding. No significant complications have occurred in renal trauma patients. No stones have developed, but the follow-up has been short. Extreme care is needed to prevent contamination of the renal collecting system with hemostat. No increase in wound infections has been observed. The wound should be adequately drained, and capsular reapproximation or application of minimal live fat to the denuded area is appropriate.

▶ [In our experience microfibrillar collagen hemostat (Avitene) is effective in controlling small vessel bleeding in all sites. The field must be dry immediately prior to application.–J.Y.G.] ◀

The Kallikrein-Kinin System in Bartter's Syndrome and Its Response to Prostaglandin Synthetase Inhibition. Recent studies in patients with Bartter's syndrome have shown renomedullary cell hyperplasia and an increase in urinary prostaglandin E. The vasodilator kallikrein-kinin system has several interrelationships with the reninangiotensin-aldosterone system and with prostaglandins. Joseph M. Vinci, John R. Gill, Jr., Robert E. Bow-

(4)   J. Urol. 119:312, March, 1978.

den, John J. Pisano, Joseph L. Izzo, Jr., Nazam Radfar, Addison A. Taylor, Randall M. Zusman, Frederic C. Bartter and Harry R. Keiser[5] (Natl. Heart, Lung, and Blood Inst., Bethesda, Md.) examined these interrelationships in 7 patients (all women, with a mean age of 30 years) with Bartter's syndrome before, during and after prostaglandin synthetase inhibition with indomethacin or ibuprofen. All patients were hypokalemic and hyperreninemic and had juxtaglomerular cell hyperplasia on renal biopsy, vascular hyposensitivity to infused angiotensin II and conserved sodium normally in response to a low-sodium intake. Twenty-five normal women were also evaluated.

Urinary immunoreactive prostaglandin E excretion was abruptly reduced during prostaglandin synthetase inhibition. Sodium retention and an increase in weight were also noted, and the serum potassium level was elevated. The creatinine clearance was significantly reduced. An early reduction in plasma renin activity was noted. Urinary kallikrein excretion was increased in patients with Bartter's syndrome, and kinin excretion was reduced. All patients but one had elevated plasma bradykinin values. Basal plasma prekallikrein values were normal. Urinary kallikrein was reduced by prostaglandin synthetase inhibition, and urinary kinins were increased. Plasma bradykinin was markedly reduced, whereas plasma prekallikrein was unaffected.

These findings suggest that prostaglandins mediate the low urinary kinins and high plasma bradykinin in Bartter's syndrome and that urinary kallikrein does not control kinin excretion. The high plasma bradykinin may be a cause of the pressor hyporesponsiveness to angiotensin II observed in this syndrome. The findings are most consistent with a defect in tubular reabsorption of NaCl as the most proximate cause of Bartter's syndrome.

▶ [Bartter's syndrome is rare. I have seen only 1 patient with this disease and this patient presented with the symptoms of hypokalemic alkalosis. However, since it involves both the kidneys and adrenals, urologists should be aware of this condition. Urinary kallikrein, which is derived from the kidney, is increased in conditions in which there are excess sodium retaining hormones. Kallikrein is a proteolytic enzyme that generates bradykinin from precursor

(5) J. Clin. Invest. 61:1671–1682, June, 1978.

proteins, kininogens. It is analogous to renin which generates angiotensin I from angiotensinogen. Potassium loss is promoted by the increased distal tubular flow of sodium allowing increased exchange and loss in the urine.–J.Y.G.] ◄

Closed Renal Trauma. Intravenous pyelography is very important in evaluating closed renal trauma. If the information is unsatisfactory, a retrograde study may be done. J. M. Smith and J. Dermot O'Flynn[6] (Dublin, Ireland) have used a conservative approach to blunt renal trauma, performing surgery only for clinical deterioration or when pedicle avulsion is demonstrated. Seventy-six consecutive patients admitted with a diagnosis of blunt renal trauma during 1954–75 were reviewed. Sports injuries accounted for 33 cases, falling accidents for 22 and road traffic accidents for 16. Eight patients did not have obvious hematuria, and 3 had no pain or tenderness on the injured side. No patient had bilateral renal injury.

All patients had intravenous pyelography. Marked narrowing and rigidity of the upper ureter or along the whole length of the ureter on the affected side were frequent findings. This sign disappeared with recovery. Deviation of the bladder, presumably due to severe retroperitoneal bleeding, was noted in 2 patients. Retrograde pyelography was rarely performed. Angiography is indicated where nonfunction is noted on pyelography. It was used only infrequently in the present series. The radiologic studies performed and the findings are given in Tables 1 and 2, and treatment is summarized in Table 3. Exploration was done on clinical grounds only; the main indication was continued deterioration and signs of severe internal hemorrhage. The average hospital stay was 16.3 days. No deaths occurred. Two patients had transient hypertension while hospitalized. Most follow-up pyelograms showed remarkable recovery.

TABLE 1.—RADIOLOGIC INVESTIGATIONS

Intravenous pyelography:	76
Retrograde pyelogram:	13
Renal angiography:	1
Isotope renogram:	1

(6) Br. J. Surg. 64:753–755, October, 1977.

TABLE 2.—Radiologic Findings

Normal:	40	(53%)
Distortion:	12	(16%)
Disruption:	20	(26%)
Non-function:	4	(5%)

TABLE 3.—Treatment

Conservative:	64	(84·2%)
Exploration:		
Nephrectomy	4	(5·3%)
Evacuation haematoma	2	(2·6%)
Interval nephrectomy:		
Hydronephrotic	5	(6·6%)
Interval pyeloplasty:	1	(1·3%)

Permanent distortion and renal damage, when noted, appeared to cause no ill effects.

The vast majority of patients with closed renal trauma can be treated successfully by a conservative approach. The present findings and others reported in the literature do not support a policy of operating immediately on the basis of angiographic results in order to prevent long-term complications.

▶ [Our prejudice and experience are similar. We try to manage closed blunt renal trauma conservatively. Renal angiography and surgery are used if deterioration is present.–J.Y.G.] ◀

Inosine: Clinical Results of Ischemic Renal Surgery. The purine nucleoside inosine has been found to be effective in protecting the kidney during 1 hour of warm ischemia as regards plasma creatinine concentration and survival after ischemia. J. E. A. Wickham, A. R. Fernando, W. F. Hendry, L. E. Watkinson and H. N. Whitfield[7] (St. Bartholomew's Hosp., London) evaluated inosine in patients requiring renal operation for the removal of stones or tumor in a bloodless field. Mean age was 46.9 years. After mobilization of the kidney, a fine cannula was placed in the renal artery distal to an occluding clamp, and the kidney was perfused with 80 ml of a solution containing 2 gm inosine at room temperature. The renal vein then was occluded.

(7) Br. J. Urol. 50:465–468, December, 1978.

The mean period of ischemia was 57.1 minutes (range, 35–75). No adverse cardiodynamic effects were observed and all patients had uneventful postoperative courses. Minimal to moderate serum creatinine elevations resolved within a week in most cases. The contribution of the kidney that was operated on to the total renal function, assessed by radionuclide renography, was virtually unchanged. Some patients had a transient rise in serum uric acid concentration. All patients were well on follow-up for 2–12 months.

The clinical results obtained with inosine are highly encouraging and similar to those in patients operated on under hypothermic protection with comparable ischemia times. The inosine technique is simpler than hypothermia, but the necessary renal artery puncture may be a disadvantage. Studies are continuing on the use of inosine in cadaver kidney retrieval and preservation and its use for more prolonged ischemia. At present, the ischemic period for clinical use with inosine protection should not exceed 1 hour or, at most, 75 minutes.

▶ [The results in these patients were excellent. Although studies in the rat and dog have shown the benefit of inosine in protecting the kidney from ischemia, it would be difficult to do a controlled clinical study to verify this finding. Further studies are indicated.–J.Y.G.] ◀

The following review articles are recommended to the reader:

Baum, N. H., Moriel, E., and Carlton, C. E.: Renal vein thrombosis, J. Urol. 119:1443, 1978.

Bloom, D. A., and Brosman, S.: The multicystic kidney, J. Urol. 120:211, 1978.

Boucher, R., Demassieux, S., Garcia, R., and Genest, J.: Tonin, angiotensin II system: A review, Circ. Res. 41:(Suppl. II):LL–26, 1977.

Carpenter, C. B.: Transplant rejection in HLA-identical recipients, Kidney Int. 14:283, 1978.

Gil-Vernet, J. M., Caralps, A., and Andru, J.: New development in the surgical treatment of renovascular arterial hypertension, Eur. Urol. 3:362, 1977.

Griffith, G. L., Maull, K. I., Coleman, C., and Baehler, R. W.: Acute reversible intrinsic renal failure, Surg. Gynecol. Obstet. 146:631, 1978.

Guttman, R.: Pretransplant evaluation and treatment of donors and recipients, Dialysis Transplant. 7:118, 1978.

Les transplantations renales de l'enfant a propos de 54 cases, J. Urol. Nephrol. (Paris) 84:173, 1978.

Maggio, A. J., and Brosman, S.: Renal artery trauma, Urology 11:125, 1978.

Salvatierra, O., Jr.: Renal transplantation in perspective, Dialysis Transplant. 7:171, 1978.

Symposium on renal failure (eight articles), Postgrad. Med. 64:5, 1978.

Thier, So. O.: Renal insufficiency and hypercalcemia, Kidney Int. 14:194, 1978.

Walker, D., Dennell, R., Garin, E., and Richard, G.: Spectrum of multicystic renal dysplasia: Diagnosis and management, Urology 11:433, 1978.

West, C. D., and McAdams, A. J.: The chronic glomerulonephritides of childhood: Part I., J. Pediatr. 93:1, 1978.

Wright, L. F., and Myers, W. D.: Medical management of home hemodialysis patients, Ann. Int. Med. 89:367, 1978.

The Ureter

DIVERSION

Pyrah Technique for Ileal Conduit Diversion: A 16-Year Experience. The basic methods of ureteroileal anastomosis are the Bricker, Pyrah and Wallace techniques. The Pyrah method consists of suture of the spatulated distal end of the left ureter to the open proximal end of the ileal segment with full-thickness running sutures of 4–0 chromic gut. Roy Witherington and William W. Mims[8] (Med. College of Georgia) evaluated this procedure in 100 patients seen in 1959–75. A 15–20-cm segment of ileum with its distal end about 16 cm from the ileocecal junction is used. The circumference of spatulation of the left ureter equals the circumference of the proximal end of the ileal segment. Patients receive erythromycin and neomycin before operation.

The upper tracts were unchanged or improved in 78% of patients, but deteriorated progressively in 19%. Nearly 30% of patients who had infected urine preoperatively had sterile urine postoperatively. Nine patients had anastomotic leakage and 4 were reoperated on. Eight patients had definite but mild electrolyte imbalance; none required more than minimal conservative therapy. Six patients had prolonged ileus. Four had pelvic abscess; all had had cystectomy. Three cases of significant sepsis occurred in patients who had received preoperative irradiation; a fourth case resulted from anastomotic disruption and pelvic abscess. Eleven patients had progressive chronic pyelonephritis and 2 had unilateral pyonephrosis. Eleven had a definite ureteroileal stricture; 9 underwent surgical revision, but most eventually required nephrectomy because of renal deterioration. Three patients had small bowel obstruction late after operation. One patient had parastomal drainage

(8)   South. Med. J. 71:23–27, January, 1978.

of urine due to an ileocutaneous fistula. Two patients with staghorn calculi required nephrectomy. Complications were more frequent in irradiated patients. Overall operative mortality was 6%.

These results compare favorably with those of other ileal conduit diversions. The Pyrah technique is somewhat shorter than the standard Bricker procedure. Complications were more frequent in patients given preoperative irradiation.

▶ [Our department still uses the Bricker technique with as short a loop as possible. We have had a similar poor experience with irradiated bowel. Recently we have been testing the vascularity of the bowel with fluorescein dye in the operating room before using it for a conduit. A surprising number of the postirradiated patients have segments of the ileum that are poorly perfused and thus should not be used as conduits.–J.Y.G.] ◀

Nonrefluxing Colon Conduit: Experience with 70 Cases. Alex F. Althausen, Kathleen Hagen-Cook and W. Hardy Hendren III[9] (Harvard Med. School) performed 70 nonrefluxing colon conduit urinary diversions on 40 children and 30 adults in 1969–76. There were 36 males and 34 females in the series. The sigmoid colon was used in 51 patients. The ureterocolonic anastomosis was usually done by the tunnel technique of Leadbetter and Clarke. A Mathisen nipple was used in 5 ureters. Transureteroureterostomy or transureteropyelostomy was used 8 times. Most patients had pre-existing urinary diversions, present for 3–14 years, but had had recurrent pyelonephritis, upper-tract deterioration, calculi, persistent bacilluria, deteriorating renal function or bleeding from ileal loop varices. Eleven patients were treated for neurogenic bladder, 9 for exstrophy of the bladder, 4 for tumor requiring pelvic exenteration and 4 for urethral or bladder trauma. The technique is illustrated in Figures 38 and 39. The stoma usually is placed on the belt line or just below it.

Intravenous pyelography in 61 patients showed upper tracts improved or remained stable except in 6 patients. Seven ureters exhibited low-pressure reflux postoperatively. Nineteen of 34 patients became free of persistent urinary infection. Complications are shown in the table. There were no postoperative deaths.

(9) J. Urol. 120:35–39, July, 1978.

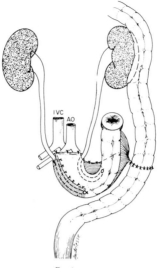

F<small>IG</small>. 1

Fig 38.—Drawing of nonrefluxing colon conduit. The splenic flexure is mobilized to allow end-to-end anastomosis of the descending colon to the rectosigmoid with no tension. The proximal end of the bowel conduit is closed with two layers of absorbable sutures. The colon is rotated clockwise 180 degrees on its mesentery before the conduit is anchored, usually just above the sacral promontory and below the aortic bifurcation. The ureters are mobilized with as much length as possible and with the periureteral adventitia attached. A long tunnel is created in the colon by infiltrating saline into its seromuscular layer. The end of the ureter is anastomosed to the mucosa with 5–0 or 6–0 absorbable sutures. An alternative method of ureterosigmoidostomy can be used when the ureter is not suited for a tunneling anastomosis. A nipple is fashioned from the end of the ureter and a flap of bowel wall. The nipple hangs into the lumen of the conduit and prevents reflux. (Courtesy of Althausen, A. F., et al.: J. Urol. 120:35–39, July, 1978.)

Although the nonrefluxing colon conduit urinary diversion is a longer and more complex procedure, the rate of complications appears to be significantly lower than after ileal loop diversion. It appears to be a better operation than the classical ileal conduit with freely refluxing anastomoses. Incorporation of a nonrefluxing anastomosis between the ureter and bowel appears to be important. A nonrefluxing colon conduit can be joined later to the colon in some patients who have satisfactory upper tracts and normal rectal control.

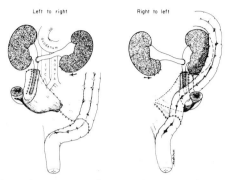

Fig 39.—When only one ureter is long enough to join to the conduit by the tunneling technique, the conduit should be based near the lower pole of the kidney to be drained. The mesentery is not rotated in such instances. Transureteropyelostomy is used to drain the opposite kidney. If the conduit is based near the left kidney it is placed behind the mesentery of the left colon. (Courtesy of Althausen, A. F., et al.: J. Urol. 120:35–39, July, 1978.)

COMPLICATIONS

	No. Children	No. Adults
General surgical:		
Small bowel obstruction	3	1
Wound dehiscence	0	1
Pulmonary embolism	0	1
Wound infection	0	1
Urological:		
Loops		
Parastomal hernia	0	2
Stomal stenosis	0	2
Suture concretions	1	0
Leak	0	1
Electrolyte abnormalities	1	0
Ureter		
Ureterocolic stenosis	4	2
Kidney		
Calculi	0	3
Pyelonephritis	3	2
Bladder		
Pyocystis	0	2
Totals	12	18

▶ [Long-term follow-up is needed to determine whether colon conduits are better than ileal conduits and whether making the colon conduit nonrefluxing is important. It must be remembered that all conduits are open to atmospheric pressure and unless there is obstruction at the stoma, reflux should not occur since the intestinal segments function as conduits rather than reservoirs.–J.Y.G.] ◀

Electrolyte Disturbances after Jejunal Conduit Urinary Diversion. Higher segments of small bowel have been used in patients with bladder carcinoma who require urinary diversion and have received radiotherapy. W. Månsson and E. Lindstedt[1] (Univ. of Lund) performed jejunal loop conduits in 6 patients. The 20 to 30-cm jejunal segments were taken from various parts of the bowel, from just distal to the ligament of Treitz to the jejunoileal transition. Ureterointestinal anastomoses were done with use of the Wallace technique.

Four patients had nausea, vomiting and anorexia 3–4 weeks after diversion. One was lethargic as well. Hyponatremia, hypochloremia, hyperkalemia, acidosis and azotemia were documented. The electrolyte changes were corrected by intensive treatment with fluid, NaCl, sodium bicarbonate and ion-exchange resins. The 3 surviving patients had no electrolyte abnormalities on follow-up 24–31 months after surgery. One had the jejunal loop replaced by a transverse colonic conduit because of obstruction of the ureterointestinal anastomoses. The electrolyte changes are summarized in the table.

Electrolyte changes across the jejunal mucosa explain the disturbances noted when a jejunal loop is used as a urinary conduit. Hyponatremia, hypochloremia and hyperkalemia are noted, and hypovolemia, acidosis and azo-

CHANGES IN CONCENTRATION OF DIFFERENT URINE
PRODUCTS AFTER CONTACT WITH JEJUNAL MUCOSA (%)

Case no.	Na^+	Cl^-	K^+	Creatinine	Urea
3	+19	+23	−18	−12	
4	+3		−27	−18	−54
5	+17	+20	−20	−50	
6	+46		−42	−30	−20

(1) Scand. J. Urol. Nephrol. 12:17–21, 1978.

temia also are typical. The thicker, more voluminous jejunal mucosa, compared to the ileal mucosa, makes ureterointestinal anastomoses more difficult to perform and may contribute to a higher rate of ureteral obstruction and impaired renal function. In patients where the ileum is not suitable, the sigmoid or transverse colon may be more useful as a conduit. Absorption of electrolytes and urea is slower from the colon than from the ileum or jejunum. The jejunum should be avoided.

▶ [Electrolyte disturbances after diversion vary with the intestinal segment used. This information is frequently used on exam questions and is also quite practical in the everyday management of these patients. Patients with ureterosigmoidostomy develop hyperchloremic acidosis. Similar disturbances have been seen in patients with impaired renal function and ileal conduits. After jejunal conduit urinary diversion, hyponatremia, hypochloremia, hyperkalemia acidosis, and azotemia have been reported.–J.Y.G.] ◀

Autosuture Ileal Conduit Construction: Experience in 110 Cases. Anand Karamcheti, Walter F. O'Donnell, Thomas R. Hakala, Frederick N. Schwentker and Felicien M. Steichen[2] (Univ. of Pittsburgh) compared the results of ileal conduit construction with the autosuture technique in 110 patients with those of conventional suture anastomosis in 55. The 133 males and 32 females had a median age of 59 years. Most ileocutaneous ureterostomies were done for carcinoma of the bladder or neurovesical dysfunction. The GIA and TA 55 staplers were used. The GIA is used to create a side-to-side anastomosis and to transect the bowel with simultaneous closure of both bowel ends. The TA 55 instrument places a linear double staggered row of staples and is used for terminal and tangential closure.

An ileal conduit was created as an isolated procedure 88 times with autostaple sutures and 44 times with the conventional suture technique. Seventy-four of these patients had had no previous operation or irradiation. Radical cystectomy was also performed in 33 patients, 18 of whom had had no previous operation or irradiation. Complications in isolated ileal conduit cases are shown in the table. In the group that underwent radical cystectomy, complications were much more frequent in suture cases than in staple cases.

The stapling technique reduced mean operating time by

(2) J. Urol. 120:545–548, November, 1978.

ISOLATED ILEAL CONDUIT COMPLICATIONS

	Staple Technique (88 pts.)	Suture Technique (44 pts.)
	No. (%)	No. (%)
Wound infection	6 (6.8)	7 (15.4)
Low grade fever	10 (11.3)	8 (17.6)
Prolonged ileus	6 (6.8)	7 (15.4)
Wound dehiscence	1 (1.1)	3 (6.6)
Septicemia	2 (2.2)	0 (0)
Ureteroileal disruption	2 (2.2)	1 (2.2)
Ureteroileal stricture	2 (2.2)	1 (2.2)
Subacute internal obstruction	1 (1.1)	1 (2.2)
Pulmonary embolus	0 (0)	1 (2.2)
Atelectasis	3 (3.4)	2 (4.4)
Internal hernia	0 (0)	1 (2.2)
Gastric dilatation	1 (1.1)	0 (0)
Superior mesenteric vein thrombus	1 (1.1)	0 (0)
Deaths	2 (2.2)	4 (9.1)

more than 1 hour in this series and the duration of postoperative ileus by 2 or 3 days. The rate of prolonged ileus was quite low. The mean postoperative hospital stay was reduced by 5 or 6 days. The autostaple technique is an improved method of ileal conduit construction.

REFLUX

Nonoperative Treatment of Vesicoureteral Reflux. Expectant management of reflux whenever possible has replaced early surgical intervention, but the determination of which ureters will stop refluxing or in which ones reflux will result in renal deterioration remains a problem. John J. Mulcahy and Panayotis P. Kelalis[3] evaluated various parameters in 128 children (122 girls and 6 boys, aged 1–16 years when first seen) in whom reflux was followed without surgical intervention. A total of 193 ureters were evaluated by urography, cystoscopy and cystography or voiding cystourethrography. Urinary tract infections were managed with appropriate antibiotics and, if recurrent, by continuous suppressive chemotherapy. Twenty-nine pa-

(3) J. Urol. 120:336–337, September, 1978.

TABLE 1.—Distribution by Age at Which Vesicoureteral Reflux
Ceased (77 Ureters)

Pt. Age When Re-flux Stopped (yrs.)	Totals	Cumulative Totals	Grade of Reflux			
			I	II	III	IV
3	2	2	1	1		
4	5	7	3	2		
5	12	19	3	9		
6	10	29	6	2	2	
7	10	39	5	4	1	
8	13	52	9	3	1	
9	4	56	2	1	1	
10	7	63	4		3	
11	3	66	1	2		
12	6	72	5		1	
13	1	73		1		
Older	4	77	1	2	3	
Totals			40	27	12	0

tients underwent internal urethrotomy, and 29 others sustained urethral dilation.

Reflux persisted in 60% of the ureters followed. Relapse of reflux occurred in thirty-five instances (18%). All patients had normal serum creatinine and/or urea values. In a number of patients, reflux did not stop until adolescence and later (Table 1). There was no particular pattern of age

TABLE 2.—Distribution by Age When the Patient with Persistent
Vesicoureteral Reflux Was Last Seen (116 Ureters)

Pt. Age Last Seen (yrs.)	Totals	Cumulative Totals	Grade of Reflux			
			I	II	III	IV
2	1	1		1		
3	10	11		6	4	
4	13	24	3	3	6	1
5	14	38	4	1	7	2
6	5	43	2	3		
7	14	57	4	5	5	
8	15	72	7	5	3	
9	20	92	10	6	4	
10	8	100	3	3	2	
11	7	107	1	2	4	
12	4	111	3	1		
13	1	112			1	
Older	4	116	3		1	
Totals			40	36	37	3

TABLE 3.—CORRELATION OF PERSISTENCE OR CESSATION OF REFLUX
WITH CONFIGURATION AND LOCATION OF URETERAL ORIFICE AND
PRESENCE OR ABSENCE OF URINARY TRACT INFECTION

	Urine Culture	
	Pos.	Neg.
Normal ureteral orifice (58 ureters):		
Cessation of reflux, 30	16	14
Persistence of reflux, 28	13	15
Moderately abnormal ureteral orifice (69 ureters):		
Cessation of reflux, 25	16	9
Persistence of reflux, 44	25	19
Severely abnormal ureteral orifice (55 ureters):		
Cessation of reflux, 17	8	9
Persistence of reflux, 38	15	23

Six patients (11 ureters) did not undergo cystoscopy.

in the distribution of various grades of reflux (Table 2). Abnormal-appearing ureteral orifices showed persistence of reflux twice as often as cessation of the process (Table 3). There was no apparent difference in this regard between moderately and severely abnormal orifices. Reflux stopped and continued equally in normal-appearing ureteral orifices. The presence or absence of recurrent infection did not appear to influence the maintenance of reflux involving either normal or abnormal ureteral orifices.

No parameters allowing prediction of which ureters will stop refluxing have been identified. Aggressive surgical intervention is indicated for grade IV reflux, but a conservative approach may be taken to lesser reflux, even if radiography shows evidence of renal damage. If there is evidence that reflux is permanent, as with a golf hole orifice, or if subsequent examination shows progressive renal damage, ureteroneocystostomy should be carried out. Serial serum creatinine or urea determinations are not useful in deciding on operative intervention. The chances of reflux stopping spontaneously become less after age 9 or 10 years. The presence of recurrent infection at this time would suggest ureteral reimplantation.

▶ [We operate on all severe cases when they are discovered and observe very mild cases with normal looking orifices. The cases in the middle area are the problem since it is difficult to determine in which cases the reflux will stop. We handle each case of moderate reflux individually, but lean toward surgery. We have had few complications from surgery and in general our philosophy is that reflux is abnormal, allows easy bacterial access to the upper tracts, and sterile reflux can cause ureteral and renal damage. If one side is severe and the other side moderate or mild, we do a Pacquin reimplant on the worse side and an ureteral advancement on the milder side.–J.Y.G.] ◄

Reflux in Complete Duplication in Children. Reflux is the most common abnormality associated with complete ureteral duplication. The lower pole renal segment is affected in 95% of cases. The orifice with reflux may be accompanied by an ectopic orifice, a ureterocele or, rarely, an incompetent upper pole orifice with reflux.

W. E. Kaplan, P. Nasrallah and L. R. King[4] (Children's Meml. Hosp., Chicago) reviewed the results of a nonoperative approach in 59 children seen during 1963–76. About 40% of the children were followed conservatively. Cystograms were repeated at about 6-month intervals. More recently, nuclear cystography has been used.

Duplication was bilateral in 17 of the 46 girls and 13 boys reviewed. Three patients had upper pole reflux. Of the 23 patients treated primarily by surveillance, 11 (48%) are medically stable. Reflux has ceased in 5 of these 11. In 8 patients (35%), reflux continues or antibiotics are needed to control urinary infections. Four patients (17%) required operation after medical management failed. The operations performed in 61% of the patients included ureteroneocystostomy, pyeloureterostomy, ureteroureterostomy and hemi-nephroureterectomy.

When reflux is associated with ureteral duplication, the degree of derangement of the ureterovesical junction is likely to be relatively severe. Management must be individualized, with the response to antibiotics and the social pressures on the child taken into account. Not all patients will improve on medical management, but in about half of the present cases, reflux stopped spontaneously or the children are medically stable with nonoperative surveillance.

► [Ureteral duplication with reflux in only one segment provides nature's own model to study reflux. Interestingly, it is the portion of the kidney with the refluxing segment that sustains the damage.–J.Y.G.] ◄

Renal Scarring and Vesicoureteric Reflux. The relative roles of bacteriuria and vesicoureteric reflux (VUR) in

---

(4) J. Urol. 120:220–222, August, 1978.

the etiology of renal scarring remain to be determined. K. J. Shah, D. G. Robins and R. H. R. White[5] (Birmingham, England) confirmed in a retrospective study of children with urinary tract infection that there is a striking relation between the incidence of scarring and the severity of VUR. Review was made of the case histories of 105 children seen during 1974 with recently diagnosed or previously established urinary tract infection. All were followed for periods of up to 12 years.

An increasing prevalence of grades II–III VUR was found with decreasing age. In infancy, reflux was nearly always severe and affected boys as often as girls. Radiologically scarred kidneys were drained by refluxing ureters in 98% of the patients. The prevalence of scars rose significantly with increasingly severe reflux. Fifteen children showed deterioration of existing scars or new scar formation. Eighteen of twenty affected kidneys were associated with grade III VUR. Two of 5 children who had new scars did so after age 5 years. Urinary tract infection had been diagnosed in all children at the time of presentation, but, since most were subsequently maintained on chemoprophylaxis, only 5 had additional episodes of confirmed bacteriuria before the radiologically observed deterioration.

A highly significant correlation between VUR and renal scarring was confirmed in this study. Only one third of the children showing scar formation or deterioration had demonstrable reinfection during the observation period. The radiographic scar is a late manifestation of renal injury, and normal renal findings on urography does not rule out the scarring process. Fresh scars rarely may develop after age 5 years. At present, the finding of grade II–III VUR must indicate continuous chemoprophylaxis and prolonged follow-up. Cystourethrography is necessary in children of all ages with recurrent infections, even when the urogram is normal. Cystourethrography is a necessary initial investigation in children less than age 5 years because of the increased prevalence of both severe reflux and renal scarring in this group.

▶ [Prospective controlled studies will be needed to determine if sterile reflux can cause scars (reflux nephropathy) in children.–J.Y.G.] ◀

---

(5) Arch. Dis. Child. 53:210–217, March, 1978.

Renal Growth Following Reimplantation of the Ureters for Reflux. The efficacy of reimplantation of the ureter to cure vesicoureteric reflux, the aim of which is to prevent ascending infection and progressive renal scarring, can be determined by measuring renal length on repeated pyelograms and relating the measurements to the patient's age and height. J. D. Atwell and M. R. Vijay[6] (Southampton, England) assessed renal growth 1, 3 and 5 years postoperatively in 17 patients who underwent unilateral or bilateral ureteral reimplantation during 1969–70.

Twenty-six renal units were studied in the 13 females and 4 males, aged 2 years 8 months to 14 years 5 months at operation. The mean follow-up was 6.7 years. Reflux was primary in 14 patients, secondary to paraureteric diverticulum in 2 and due to double ureters in 1. Reflux was present in 25 of the 26 renal units studied. Grade IV reflux was present in 10 patients and grade III reflux in 2.

Renal growth appeared to accelerate following successful ureteral reimplantation, the growth spurt being confined to the 1st postoperative year. Eight patients with unilateral reflux showed equal rates of growth of the reimplanted and the contralateral normal kidneys. The correlation coefficients found were similar to that reported for normal renal growth. Three patients with bilateral reflux had unilateral renal scarring. Scarring does not necessarily prevent renal growth, although there may be a latent period before the rate of renal growth returns to normal.

These findings suggest that successful antireflux surgery results in accelerated renal growth in the 1st year after operation, followed by a longer period of normal renal growth.

▶ [These conclusions seem valid in this small series. There are no data to show what the renal growth would have been had the reflux persisted. The authors' assumption that it would have been impaired is supported by the following two articles.–J.Y.G.] ◀

Effect of Vesicoureteral Reflux on Renal Growth. The choice of adequate therapy for vesicoureteral reflux would be aided if there were a simple and reliable means of detecting subtle renal damage of each kidney from reflux. Seiichi Orikasa, Takao Takamura, Fumiei Inada and

---

(6) Br. J. Urol. 50:367–370, October, 1978.

Ichiro Tsuji[7] (Hokkaido Univ.) studied the effects of primary reflux on renal growth in 62 children and 51 adults. The renal ratio (ratio of renal length to length of L2 plus its disk) was calculated and compared with norms determined in 120 subjects aged 3–60 years. The growth of 76 refluxing kidneys of children was studied over 1–8 years.

The renal ratio was more than 2 SD below the normal mean in 16% of 99 children's refluxing kidneys on initial pyelography (Fig 40). Most of these cases represented grade 3 reflux. Normal growth occurred in 68% of another 76 kidneys with reflux (Fig 41). The renal ratio of 8% fell temporarily below -2 SD, but these kidneys exhibited accelerated growth and regained a normal renal ratio when spontaneous cessation of or improvement in reflux occurred. The ratio in 8% deteriorated gradually to below -2 SD. The renal ratio of 16% of kidneys remained below -2 SD throughout the study. Impaired renal growth was sometimes associated with a normal urogram or sterile urine. Three patients in whom both kidneys were small showed a moderate decrease in total renal function. The renal ratio was below -2 SD in 36% of refluxing adult kidneys. Eight of 23 patients in whom 1 or both kidneys were small were uremic. The 4 patients with 2 small kidneys were uremic. Pathologic study of 4 cases of extremely small

Fig 40.—Renal ratio at initial examination of 99 kidneys in children with reflux. (Courtesy of Orikasa, S., et al.: J. Urol. 119:25–30, January, 1978.)

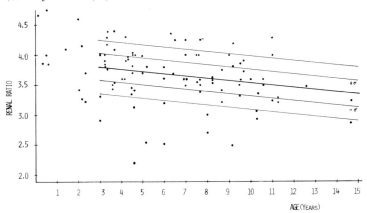

(7)   J. Urol. 119:25–30, January, 1978.

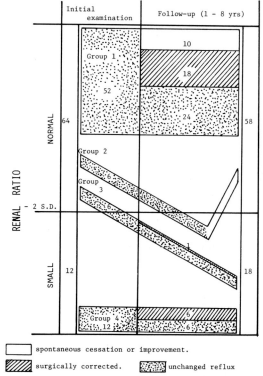

Fig 41.—Renal ratio (renal growth) in relation to reflux in 76 kidneys in children. Open areas indicate spontaneous cessation or improvement; hatched areas represent surgical correction; stippled areas denote unchanged reflux. (Courtesy of Orikasa, S., et al.: J. Urol. 119:25–30, January, 1978.)

kidneys indicated that chronic pyelonephritis or congenital renal dysplasia alone probably was not entirely responsible for the small kidney size.

Measurement of kidney growth yields good indications of whether renal involvement is present and of the efficacy of treatment. When the renal ratio is below -2 SD of normal, an antireflux operation is preferable. Patients with grade 3 reflux or a grade 3 orifice, even if the urine is sterile or the urogram is normal, should be treated surgically before the kidneys become smaller than -2 SD. It is likely that the growing kidney is particularly sensitive to the hydrodynamic effects of reflux, infection or alteration of blood flow, while being readily able to recuperate after elimination of these factors.

▶ [The methodology described by John Hodson to correlate renal growth with the length of the L_2 vertebra plus its disk seems valid.–J.Y.G.] ◀

Growth of Kidneys in Children with Vesicoureteral Reflux. K. Kaas Ibsen, P. Uldall and O. Frøkjaer[8] (Copenhagen) compared renal growth in children who had had vesicoureteral reflux (VUR) for over 1 year with that in a comparable group in which VUR ceased within 1 year. Seventy-six children seen in 1964–74 had a total of 123 refluxing ureters. Thirty-nine evaluable kidneys with VUR for less than a year were compared with 30 that refluxed for over a year. Eleven of the former kidneys were treated with long-term antibiotics and the rest were operated on an average of 3 months after diagnosis. Twelve kidneys with reflux for over a year were eventually operated on. The rest were treated with long-term antibiotics.

More kidneys in the group with reflux for less than 1 year had severe grades of VUR. The groups were similar in age and sex, and in the number of infections occurring between diagnosis and cessation of VUR. Renal growth in the two groups is compared in the table. Absolute growth occurred in most kidneys in both groups. Relative growth decreased in 60% of kidneys with reflux for over a year and in only 30% of those with VUR for less than a year.

The growth of kidneys with persistent vesicoureteral reflux appears to be somewhat slower than that of kidneys with cessation of VUR, even if reflux is more severe in the

GROWTH OF KIDNEYS

	Group A: Kidneys with VUR for less than one year		Group B: Kidneys with persistent VUR for more than one year	
	Absolute	Relative	Absolute	Relative
Increased	33 85%	13 33%	20 66.7%	4 13%
Unchanged	2 5%	14 36%	5 16.6%	8 27%
Decreased	4 10%	12 31%	5 16.6%	18 60%
Total	39 100%	39 100%	30 100%	30 100%

(8)   Acta Paediatr. Scand. 66:741–744, November, 1977.

latter. Most kidneys with persistent VUR appear to grow
well, however, and renal growth should be measured before a decision is made to operate or not to operate.

▶ [The conclusion that kidney growth in children with vesicoureteral reflux is
improved with surgery seems adequately documented in this article. The data
seem more conclusive in view of the fact that the operated group in general
had the more severe grades of reflux.–J.Y.G.] ◀

**Long-Term Follow-up of Surgically Treated Vesi-
coureteral Reflux.** D. M. A. Wallace, D. L. Rothwell and
D. I. Williams[9] (London) followed 83% of 166 patients with
vesicoureteral reflux who were operated on more than 10
years ago, in 1960–67. Patients who had undergone previous upper tract surgery and those with secondary reflux
were excluded from the series, but patients with duplex
systems and paraureteral saccules and diverticula and
those with mild bladder neck obstruction were included.
There were 116 girls and 50 boys in the series.

Five patients had elevated systolic and diastolic blood
pressures preoperatively, and 19 others had a systolic or
diastolic elevation above the 95th percentile for age. Reflux
was bilateral in 92 patients. A satisfactory technique of
ureteral reimplantation was being evolved during the
study period. Follow-up cystograms made 6 months postoperatively showed reflux in the reimplanted ureter in 24
of 158 patients and 8 of these required further operation.
Two of 10 patients with contralateral reflux after unilateral reimplantation required further operation to prevent
reflux. The incidence of further urinary tract infection in
the first 5 years of follow-up was 26%. Twenty-four patients required further operation. A total of 141 patients
was followed-up late, for a mean of 13 years. Eleven patients had hypertension (7.8%) and another 5% had mild
hypertension. All were asymptomatic. Two hypertensive
patients were in renal failure. Seven of 18 hypertensive patients had bilateral renal scarring and 7 had unilateral
scarring. Thirty-eight patients in all had bilateral scarring
and 62 had unilateral scarring. One normotensive patient
was in renal failure. Twelve patients reported recurrent
urinary tract infection and 20 had had occasional urinary
tract infection; all these patients were girls. Thirteen of 98
girls studied had significant bacteriuria.

(9) Br. J. Urol. 50:479–484, December, 1978.

There is a 12.8% incidence of hypertension in patients in whom reflux is treated surgically on follow-up at over 10 years. Since hypertension was diagnosed a mean of 12 years after operation, all patients require close blood pressure surveillance. Patients whose kidneys are unscarred 6 months postoperatively are unlikely to develop hypertension.

In an addendum, the authors report that 2 patients who initially had mild hypertension have had further pressure elevations and will require treatment.

▶ [This study clearly shows that reflux with renal scarring carries significant risk for hypertension and renal failure. Further long-term follow-up studies of patients with reflux are needed.–J.Y.G.] ◀

Delayed Recurrence of Reflux after Initial Success of Antireflux Operation. Arjan D. Amar[1] (Univ. of California, San Francisco) encountered delayed recurrence of reflux in 4 children among 103 who were followed for at least 5 years after ureteral reimplantation for vesicoureteral reflux. Initial success was proved in all cases by 2 cystographic series done 3 months apart after the initial reimplantation. Seventy-three children were evaluated 5 or more years after reimplantation. Reflux recurred after 1 year in 1 patient, 2 years in 2 and 3 years in 1. One had a recurrence in only 1 ureter after bilateral reimplantation. The other 3 had recurrences after unilateral reimplantation. Two patients have had successful reoperation; repeat operation failed in 1 case, and 1 has not had reoperation. Three patients were girls with reflux in kidneys having single ureters, and 1 was a boy having reflux associated with a duplicated ureter.

These cases illustrate the need to follow patients for at least 5 years after the surgical correction of vesicoureteral reflux. Delayed recurrence of reflux of ten can be corrected by a second operation. The ureter should be reimplanted in an area of the bladder that is not weakened by an adjacent diverticulum or in the area where a ureterocele has been excised intravesically. Any associated condition that contributes to increased intravesical pressure on voiding should be corrected to prevent future recurrence of reflux through the reimplanted ureter.

▶ [If the patient is asymptomatic, I do not think routine long-term cystograms

(1)   J. Urol. 119:131–133, January, 1978.

and IVP's are indicated in the clinical setting. However, several centers need to conduct such studies to accurately define the long-term risks.–J.Y.G.] ◄

Ureterovesical Reimplantation in Children: Surgical Results in 491 Children. John W. Coleman and John H. McGovern[2] (New York Hosp.-Cornell Med. Center) reviewed results of reimplantation of 703 ureters in 347 girls and 144 boys up to 1970. Successful results, with elimination of obstruction or reflux at the ureterovesical junction, were achieved in 92% of cases. In 451 children anomalies of the ureterovesical junction were corrected. Forty children represented surgical failures, and 1 child died at operation. Reflux was the chief factor in 576 diseased ureters and junctional obstruction in 127.

Boys less often had junctional anomalies, but they generally had more severe problems when first seen. The role of bladder wall thickness and significant hydronephrosis in the outcome of operation is shown in the table. Children were graded A (normal bladders and minimally altered upper tracts) to D (significant hydronephrosis and a thickened, fibrotic bladder wall). Reflux occurred in only 9 children and 10 reimplanted ureters after use of the Paquin technique. All these children had severely distorted upper tracts. Two are well after corrective repeat reimplantations. Eight of the 703 ureters represented final surgical failures because of reflux after the Paquin technique. Thirty-one boys developed ureterovesical junction obstruction after a first Paquin reimplantation. Fourteen have had a repeat reimplantation, 10 of them successfully. Nine of 16 girls with postoperative junctional obstruction have had repeat reimplantations, 6 with successful results.

SIGNIFICANCE OF BLADDER WALL THICKNESS AND SIGNIFICANT
HYDRONEPHROSIS IN SURGICAL SUCCESS RATE OF URETEROVESICAL
REIMPLANTATION

Group	Males Successful/Total at Risk Reimplantation	Success Rate (%)	Females Successful/Total at Risk Reimplantation	Success Rate (%)
A	4/4	100	166/167	99
B	50/54	92	7/18	39
C	12/14	85	2/2	100
D	1/14	7	1/2	50

(2) Urology 12:514–518, November, 1978.

The success rate of ureteral reimplantation has been maintained in girls and has improved in boys. A good outcome cannot be expected in the child with minimal renal reserve, massively dilated upper tracts and a significantly thickened and fibrotic bladder wall. The Paquin technique of ureteral reimplantation has given successful results in 92% of all cases.

▶ [The Paquin method of ureteral neocystostomy is an excellent method of reimplanting the ureter. We still use this method since "looking outside" the bladder has obvious advantages and keeps one out of trouble. We do not mobilize the bladder as much as described for fear of creating a neurogenic bladder. The bladder is fixed to the psoas muscle to prevent angulation of the reimplant. The tunnel may be started either outside or inside depending on which seems easier. For mild reflux with lateral placement of the orifices, ureteral advancement is an effective procedure.

This group of articles provides data to support the impressions that severe reflux does not spontaneously disappear whereas mild reflux may disappear about 40% of the time. The association of renal scarring with reflux and hypertension with renal scarring is documented. Severe reflux seems associated with decreased renal growth, which improves after successful reimplantation. A small percentage of patients seem to have delayed complications of obstruction and persistent reflux after apparently successful surgery.

Development of a noninvasive screening technique in the nursery to detect moderate and severe degrees of reflux is the major need and opportunity in pediatric urology. This need has been recognized and championed by John Hodson who proposed that if urine refluxed into the tubules and into the systemic circulation, antibodies to the Tamm-Horsfall protein would develop since the protein is found only in the urinary tract and would be recognized as "foreign" to the body. Unfortunately preliminary studies in some centers screening for antibodies to this protein have not helped to identify children with reflux.

There is need for more human data about the long-term effects of reflux. Data from animals, except the pig, are not relevant since their calyceal structures are different from human beings. In patients, only one good prospective controlled study (Scott and Stanfield; Arch. Dis. Child. 43:323, 1968) shows the operated patient does better than the nonoperated patient; renal growth in operated patients was four times that in the nonoperated group.

There is a need to determine why children with severe reflux develop renal damage; perhaps this group has the highest voiding and resting bladder pressures.

An excellent symposium on reflux was published in the May 1979 issue of Kidney International.—J.Y.G.] ◀

MISCELLANEOUS

Treatment of Ureteral Colic with Intravenous Indomethacin. Pressure of urine in the urinary tract above an obstructing ureteral stone tends to increase, and the accompanying high tension in the pelvic and ureteral wall causes severe pain. Increased renal pelvic pressure stimulates synthesis of prostaglandin E_2 in the renal medulla. Indomethacin inhibits prostaglandin synthesis and has an antiphlogistic effect that may improve flow around a ureteral stone surrounded by an edematous wall. Dan Holmlund and Jan-Gunnar Sjödin[3] (Univ. of Umeå) evaluated indomethacin in a prospective, double-blind study of 47 consecutive patients with acute ureteral colic and a verified obstructing ureteral stone. Most indomethacin-treated patients received less than 1 mg/kg body weight; an intravenous dose of 50 mg was used. The placebo was riboflavin given intravenously.

Pain was completely relieved in 21 of 27 indomethacin-treated patients and in 6 of 20 placebo patients, a significant difference. Indomethacin completely relieved pain in 10 of 14 placebo patients who failed to respond to placebo. One of 6 indomethacin-treated patients was relieved after placebo injection. Pain relief usually occurred, within 20 minutes of indomethacin injection. One patient had a recurrence of colic during 4 hours of observation. The 4 patients previously treated with pentazocine during attacks of ureteral colic preferred indomethacin. Pulse and blood pressure were unchanged during and after indomethacin administration. No gastric pain or other side effects were observed.

Indomethacin given intravenously can successfully treat patients with ureteral colic. It acts by reducing the increased pressure of urine above the stone. The effect in general is probably not strong enough completely to relieve severe colic. Indomethacin is as effective as metamizol and is probably less dangerous. The latter has been reported to cause agranulocytosis. Further studies of side effects of intravenous indomethacin therapy are needed before it can be recommended without reservation for patients with ureteral colic.

▶ [The real question of whether or not indomethacin will speed up or slow the passage of the stone is not known (see the article by Allen et al., in the Physiology section of the chapter on the kidney). More studies are needed since the objectives must be to aid the passage of the stone in addition to providing pain relief.–J.Y.G.] ◀

(3)   J. Urol. 120:676–677, December, 1978.

Ureteric Pathology in Relation to Right and Left Gonadal Veins is discussed by B. L. R. A. Coolsaet[4] (Antwerp, Belgium). Extrinsic pressure defects of the ureters are frequently seen on the excretory urogram. Recent work has cast doubt on the concept that dilatation of the ureter in pregnancy is caused by the ovarian vein. A hormonal effect on the ureteric wall has been considered a possible cause of ureteral dilatation in pregnancy. The association of ovarian vein thrombosis, postpartum ovarian vein thrombophlebitis and ureteric obstruction is well recognized. The right side is involved more often than the left. Perivenous fibrosis after ovarian vein thrombophlebitis may be an important cause of the right ovarian vein syndrome during and after pregnancy. After pregnancy the

Fig 42.—Venography of left renal vein. **A,** retrograde filling of dilated left ovarian vein; **B,** filling of pelvic varicosities; **C,** filling of dilated right ovarian vein. (Courtesy of Coolsaet, B. L. R. A.: Urology 12:40–49, July, 1978.)

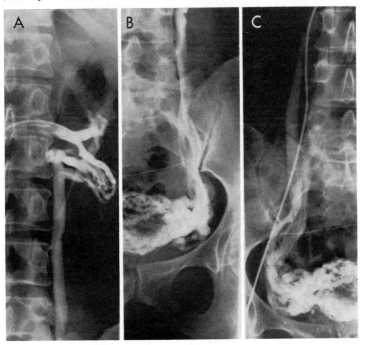

(4) Urology 12:40–49, July, 1978.

right ovarian vein may be dilated because of lack of valves, incompetent valves, vena caval obstruction or retrograde flow down the left ovarian vein (Fig 42). However, enlarged ovarian veins do not in themselves necessarily cause ureteral obstruction (Fig 43). Obstruction due to a congenital pelvic anomaly is illustrated in Figure 44.

Hormonal dependence of the gonadal vein pain syndrome has been described. Retrograde flow in the left gonadal

Fig 43.—**A,** intravenous urogram showing no ureteral obstruction. **B,** gonadal venogram in same patient showing dilated ovarian vein with periureteric varicosities. **C,** intravenous urogram showing bilateral ureteral dilation proximal to first sacral vertebral level, 6 weeks after delivery. **D,** venography shows completely normal right and left ovarian veins. (Courtesy of Coolsaet, B. L. R. A.: Urology 12:40–49, July, 1978.)

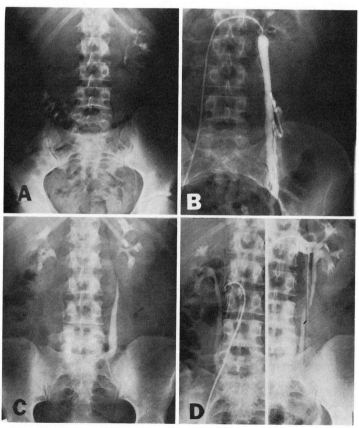

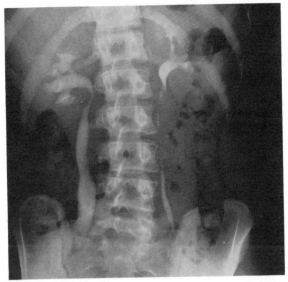

Fig 44.—Urethral obstruction at first sacral vertebral level by pelvic anomaly. At exploration, ovarian vein was situated 1 cm lateral to ureter. (Courtesy of Coolsaet, B. L. R. A.: Urology 12:40–49, July, 1978.)

vein may be due to absence of valves in the vein, incompetent valves, vena caval obstruction, intra- or extraluminal obstruction of the renal vein or abnormal communications between the renal and gonadal veins (canalis renogonadalis). Ureteric varices, when present, are nearly always on the left side. Varices of the ureteric wall usually are an incidental finding in the intravenous urogram. The cause of varices is seldom evident, they may fill from the renal vein via the renoureteral vessels, from below or from dilated lumbar veins. Treatment depends on the hemodynamics. When the gonadal veins have competent valves and there is collateral circulation to the upper renoureteral vessels, ligation of these vessels should be attempted. When the veins fill from below, simple ligation of the gonadal vein will cause collapse of all the periureteric and ureteral varices. Intrarenal varices due to renal vein obstruction may require nephrectomy if there is profuse bleeding from the varices.

▶ [Whether or not and how frequently gonadal veins cause ureteral obstruction is controversial. One should be extremely cautious in attributing pain or ureteral obstruction to the gonadal veins.—J.Y.G.] ◀

Radiographic Features of Ureteral Endometriosis. Endometriosis involving the ureters may be more common than has been thought. Howard M. Pollack (Univ. of Pennsylvania) and John S. Wills[5] (Wilmington, Del., Med. Center) report the findings in 7 cases collected from several hospitals over 9 years. Average age was 41 years. Six patients exhibited hydronephrosis and hydroureter, which in 4 were marked. An area of ureteral narrowing was seen in 6 patients. In 3, medial ureteral angulation was present at the site of narrowing. The strictures usually began abruptly and were smooth. Proof of ureteral involvement was obtained at operation in 6 patients. Two patients had endometriosis within the ureteral wall, 1 with extrinsic involvement also, and 4 had only extrinsic involvement.

Ureteral endometriosis usually is located 2–5 cm from the bladder and involves a short to medium length of ureter. The disease has a predilection for the segment of pelvic ureter projecting within 3 cm of the inferior aspect of the sacroiliac joint, corresponding to the approximate site of the posterior attachments of the uterosacral ligaments. Five strictures in this study were judged to be extremely stenotic, whereas 2 were of moderate severity. The degree of obstructive uropathy was often severe. The excretory urogram was of value in showing the severity of obstruction, its approximate location and the laterality of involvement. It also served as a baseline against which posttreatment studies could be compared. A barium enema study is worthwhile in any patient with suspected endometriosis. The finding of serosal implants provides strong confirmation of the diagnosis.

▶ [Our experience with ureteral endometriosis is limited. If the diagnosis can be established without surgery, estrogen-progesterone therapy should be tried first.—J.Y.G.] ◀

Vein Patch Grafting for Repair of Short Ureteric Strictures. The accepted treatment for short and medium length ureteral strictures has been to split the stricture and splint the ureter for a month or longer, but this approach carries a high risk of infection and requires a long

(5) Am. J. Roentgenol. 131:627–631, October, 1978.

hospital stay. Rolf Pompeius and Rolf Ekroth[6] (Västerås, Sweden) attempted to eliminate these disadvantages by splitting the stricture and covering the defect with a vein patch graft. Four patients, 3 men and 1 woman, aged 38–74 years, had this operation during 1964–1975 and were followed for 6 months to 10 years. The ureteric stricture was split longitudinally and the split continued for 5–10 mm into normal ureter above and below the stricture, and a trimmed piece of spermatic or saphenous vein measuring about 20–30 mm was sutured into the ureteric defect with 5–0 chromic catgut. In 1 patient, a splint was left in the ureter for 10 days.

Man, 41, with a marked tendency to stricture formation, had a stricture after operation for a stone in the lower right ureter. A Boari-Küss plastic procedure was done, but a stricture was present at the anastomotic site 12 years later, and the patient was operated on again. A new stricture had formed after 3 years and a pelvioileovesicostomy was performed. The patient presented with a left hydroureter and a stone 9 years after removal of a stone from the upper left ureter and 3 years after removal of a stone from the lower part of the ureter. The ureteric wall around the stone was about 4–5 mm thick and edematous. A 3–cm graft from the spermatic vein was used, and the ureter was drained for 5 days. Pyelography 4 years later showed a normally functioning left kidney and good function of the right kidney with its ileal ureter.

This method considerably reduces the hospital stay necessary after ureteral stricture repair. Four patients have been treated successfully by vein patch grafting. The method is technically simple. Vein patch grafting is recommended, especially for short strictures.

▶ [The authors report successful repair of short ureteral strictures with vein patch grafting. This seems a worthwhile technique. Ten years ago at our institution a difficult ureteral stricture was corrected with a patch graft of renal capsule (Thompson: J. Urol. 101:487, 1969). For difficult cases the Davis intubated ureterotomy has been successfully used at our institution. Difficulty with ileal replacements has been seen in males with high voiding pressures. Renal autotransplantation is always available for the unusually difficult cases.–J.Y.G.] ◀

Ectopic Ureterocele in the Male Infant is less frequent than in female infants but is more complex. O. Eklöf, G. Löhr, H. Ringertz and B. Thomasson[7] (Stockholm,

(6) Scand. J. Urol. Nephrol. 11:245–247, 1977.
(7) Acta Radiol. [Diagn.] (Stockh.) 19:145–153, 1978.

Sweden) reviewed the findings in 14 boys with a mean age at diagnosis of 25 months and a median age of 6 months. All underwent urographic examination at least once preoperatively, and all but one had a preoperative micturition cystourethographic examination. The mean follow-up was 4.5 years and the median, 2.5 years. Eleven patients presented with urinary infection; 2 had urosepsis. One had urinary retention, and 2 presented with gastrointestinal symptoms due to urinary infection. In 4 patients, the ureterocele involved a ureter of a single collecting system; renal function was abolished in all these patients. Some dilatation was noted in several patients. Four boys had a moderate contralateral lower ureteric obstruction. Eversion of the ureterocele occurred more often in boys. Posterior urethral dilatation due to prolapse of the ureterocele was also frequently noted.

In 1 patient, an erroneous diagnosis of a posterior urethral valve was made, and a transurethral resection was carried out later. Two other patients had fulguration of an erroneously assumed urethral valve at the time of resection of the ureterocele. Three other patients had nephroureterectomy and ureterocele resection for hydronephrosis and very poor function of the reduplicated kidney. Six patients underwent heminephroureterectomy and resection of the ureterocele. Two had only resection of the ureterocele. Functioning of remaining renal tissue improved postoperatively, but some degree of upper tract dilatation often persisted, either on the side of the ureterocele or contralaterally.

The potential behavior of ectopic ureterocele during micturition is shown in Figure 45 and the micturition cystour-

Fig 45.—Potential behavior of ectopic ureterocele during micturition. **A,** tense ureterocele; **B,** compressible ureterocele; **C,** eversion of ureterocele by intussusception into the associated ureter; and **D,** eversion of the ureterocele in a patient with deficient detrusor sheet. (Courtesy of Eklöf, O., et al.: Acta Radiol. [Diagn.] (Stockh.) 19:145–153, 1978.

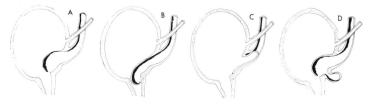

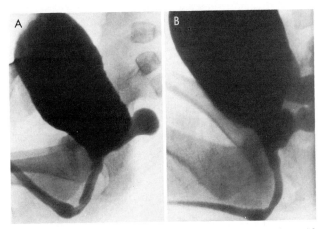

Fig 45.—**A,** micturition cystourethrography appearances in a patient with ureterocele eversion of intussusception into the associated ureter. **B,** after uncapping of the ureterocele. Free reflux to the associated ureter located at the level of previous eversion. (Courtesy of Eklöf, O., et al.: Acta Radiol. [Diagn.] (Stockh.) 19:145–153, 1978.)

ethrographic appearances in 1 patient are illustrated in Figure 46. Eversion may be due to an insufficient detrusor sheet behind the ureterocele or to herniation through the ureteric hiatus of the bladder wall. A broad spectrum of severity of bladder outlet obstruction was encountered in the present patients. More severe obstruction was associated with worse renal function. Supervening infection and, to some extent, the time factor are probably important in progressive deterioration of renal function. Fortunately, the clinical features in male infants with ectopic ureterocele generally call for early examination, which should include urography and micturition cystourethrography.

▶ [Signs and symptoms are more marked in the male than in the female. Most cases were discovered after an episode of bacteriuria, confirming that bacteriuria in male children should be worked up by intravenous urography. Eversion of the ureterocele by intussusception into the ureter is well documented in this article.–J.Y.G.] ◀

Reconstruction of the Urinary Tract in Prune Belly Uropathy. According to John R. Woodard and Thomas S. Parrott[8] (Emory Univ.), the prune belly syndrome is characterized by deficient abdominal muscles, undescended

(8)   J. Urol. 119:824–828, June, 1978.

testes and dilatation of the urinary collecting system. Most patients have intestinal malrotation, and some have a patent urachus. The bladder usually is thick but not trabeculated, and the prostatic urethra is peculiarly large and triangular, but is seldom truly obstructed. Huge, tortuous, dilated ureters with large, flabby renal pelvis are typical. Vesicoureteric reflux usually is present. Hydronephrosis is the rule, and cysts with other dysplastic changes are common. In 56 cases reported during 1950–70, 48 (86%) were treatment or nontreatment failures.

The present authors report on 10 patients, including 7 neonates, with the full-blown syndrome who were treated aggressively during the past 7 years by extensive surgical tailoring of the upper tracts, using primarily the upper ureteral segment, and simultaneous transabdominal orchiopexy.

TECHNIQUE.—Through a midline abdominal incision, the ureter is mobilized and transected at its junction with the bladder (Fig 47). In the neonate, 5–6 cm of proximal ureter is usually

Fig 47.—Surgical photograph of a patient operated on at age 12 days shows excessive ureteral length and adequate spermatic cord length after dissection. (Courtesy of Woodard, J. R., and Parrott, T. S.: J. Urol. 119:824–828, June, 1978.)

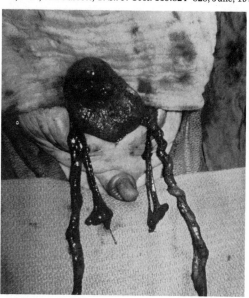

more than adequate to reach the bladder. The proximal ureter is straightened, but may not require tapering. If it is as much as 1 cm wide it is tapered over a 10 F catheter. A modified Paquin technique is used to reimplant the ureter, and splinting ureteral catheters are left indwelling for 10–11 days. A nephrostomy tube usually is left in each kidney. It is advantageous to resect the huge bladder dome before the bladder is closed in layers around a Malecot catheter. The orchiopexy then is completed by tunneling bluntly through the abdominal wall at the external inguinal ring.

The procedure has been tolerated easily in the last 6 patients, including 5 neonates. No mortality or serious morbidity has occurred. All 10 patients have satisfactory drainage of the ureters into the bladder. Only 1 patient has unilateral reflux. None has a serum creatinine over 0.9 mg/dl. Some children have had recurrent bacteriuria, but without evidence of renal involvement. Each child is growing normally and has one or both testes well down in the scrotum with an intact spermatic cord.

This approach has greatly improved the prognosis for longevity of patients with the prune belly syndrome. Adjunctive neonatal orchiopexy may offer a potential for fertility to these patients.

Urinary Tract Reconstruction in Prune Belly Syndrome. Several approaches have been suggested to the management of urinary tract abnormalities in the wide spectrum of involvement seen in prune belly syndrome. Ronald Rabinowitz, Martin Barkin, John F. Schillinger and Robert D. Jeffs[9] (Toronto, Ontario) reviewed the treatment of 25 males seen with the syndrome in 1965–74. Fifteen children required surgery because of uncontrolled infection or progressive loss of renal function. Seventeen of the 27 massively dilated ureters in these boys were associated with reflux; 10 were treated in the first month of life and 6 in the first week.

Loop cutaneous ureterostomy was done in 18 patients. Seven patients later had nontailored ureteral reimplantation and closure of the loop ureterostomy. Only 1 patient improved markedly and 2 continued to deteriorate. In 3 patients ureteral tailoring was done at reimplantation, with good results. Five boys with 8 massively dilated ureters

(9) Urology 12:333–335, September, 1978.

and severely dysplastic kidneys died of progressive azotemia despite adequate diversion and control of infection.
Primary nephroureterectomy for nonfunction and renal
dysplasia was done in 3 patients in whom contralateral
function was satisfactory. Six ureters were reimplanted
primarily with tailoring. The results were uniformly very
successful. The average follow-up after reconstruction was
$4^{1}/_{2}$ years. The results were much better when the ureter
was tailored than when nontailored reimplantation was
carried out.

Children with prune belly megaureters should be evaluated aggressively. Ureteroneocystostomy, if necessary,
should be augmented by a tailoring procedure. The proximal part of the prune belly ureter is functionally and histologically better than the distal portion and it is preferable not to jeopardize subsequent surgery by any type of
diversion if possible.

**Twenty-Five-Year Experience with Prune Belly
Syndrome.** Frederick J. Goulding and Robert A. Garrett[1]
(Indianapolis) reviewed the findings in 30 cases of prune
belly syndrome seen since 1950, with no stillborn deaths.
All males had deficient abdominal wall musculature, bilateral cryptorchism and hydroureteronephrosis. Three patients were females, 2 of whom were alive at follow-up
with normal urinary tracts but absent abdominal musculature. Thirteen of 21 living patients were followed for over
5 years. Two patients are under age 5 at present. Five of
the 6 patients lost to follow-up had adequate renal function
and upper tracts.

Advanced urinary tract dilation in these patients probably deserves at least temporary diversion to insure maturation of renal cortex. In some cases, undiversion may
never be feasible, but most patients who survive the neonatal period come to undiversion. A few children may not
require diversion. Orchiopexy appears to be feasible and
beneficial in a few children with a good life span prognosis.
Nine of 14 patients improved after loop ureterostomy and
3 were unchanged; 5 patients remain in temporary diversion, whereas 4 have had reconstruction with 2 of these
requiring vesicostomy drainage. Two of 3 patients with ne-

(1) Urology 12:329–332, September, 1978.

phrostomy tubes had ureteral tapering and shortening with undiversion and have had a good result. One patient with an ileal loop had stable and adequate function. Patients having suprapubic cystostomy diversion did not improve, but their renal function remained adequate. Five of 9 deaths were due to renal insufficiency. Reflux was present in 85% of males, and about 80% of all patients had some form of lower tract abnormality, most commonly a dilated prostatic urethra. Half the patients had musculoskeletal anomalies; 7 had cardiac and 5, pulmonary anomalies.

The relationship between the genitourinary system and muscular deficiency in prune belly syndrome has not been clearly defined. Not all patients require diversion. If indicated, diversion should be performed early, should be high and preferably should be tubeless. Renal biopsy is done at the same time. Aggressive pulmonary care is necessary in the immediate postoperative period. Use of an operating microscope with microvascular techniques may permit autotransplantation of the testis to the epigastric vessels in future cases.

▶ [These three articles on the management of urologic problems in the prune belly syndrome are excellent. The major recent finding is that orchiopexy done during the neonatal period is technically easy whereas it can be impossible when tried later. It is stated that infection and renal failure await the patient with severe hydronephrosis, based on no controlled series in the era of adequate chemotherapy. Certainly renal function improves in some patients with various forms of temporary diversion in the form of nephrostomy, pyelostomy, cutaneous ureterostomy and vesicostomy. There are no good data to determine which of these methods of diversion is superior. Cutaneous ureterostomies have the disadvantage of requiring a surgical procedure to take it down and sacrificing the best portion of the ureter. The success of aggressive surgical management as advocated by Woodard and Parrott (which is similar to ours) will probably not be achieved by the surgeon who sees an occasional case. These problems should be referred to medical centers.–J.Y.G.] ◀

The following review articles are recommended to the reader:

Pfister, R. C., and Herdenn, W. H.: Primary megaureter in children and adults: Clinical and pathophysiologic features of 150 ureters, Urology 12:160, 1978.

Rabinowitz, R., Burkin, M., Schillinger, J. F., Jeffs, R. D., and Cook, G. T.: The influence of etiology on the surgical management and prognosis of the massively dilated ureter in children, J. Urol. 119:808, 1978.

Rose, J. G., and Gillenwater, J. Y.: Effects of obstruction on ureteral function, Urology 12:139, 1978.

Symposium on the Ureter, Part I, Urology 12:1–14, 1978; Part III, Urology 12:245–289, 1978.

Traitement des stenoses de l'uretre (Twenty papers in French on treatment of urethral strictures), J. Urol. Nephrol. (Paris) 84:55–130, 1978.

Weiss, R. M.: Ureteral function, Urology 12:114, 1978.

The Bladder

NEUROGENIC BLADDER

Percutaneous Radiofrequency Sacral Rhizotomy in Treatment of Hyperreflexic Bladder. Present treatments for hyperreflexic bladder involve several complications, and the external tubes and appliances needed may produce a severe psychologic handicap and be inconvenient to persons with limited physical capabilities. Interruption of sacral nerve roots may reduce bladder irritability and make intermittent clean catheterization feasible. John J. Mulcahy and A. Bryon Young[2] (Univ. of Kentucky) performed percutaneous radiofrequency rhizotomy in 7 patients with hyperreflexic bladder to augment bladder capacity and make intermittent clean catheterization more feasible or to stop precipitous micturition. Various combinations of the S2, S3 and S4 nerve roots were anesthetized with bupivacaine, and urodynamic evaluation was repeated an hour later. When the desired bladder capacity was obtained, the appropriate anterior and posterior roots were ablated by percutaneous radiofrequency electrocoagulation; a 12-gauge needle was advanced under fluoroscopic control. Thermocoagulation at over 70 C was maintained for at least 3 minutes at each site.

In no case was there a change in the urethral pressure profile, and no incontinence resulted. All patients had active anal sphincter contractions after rhizotomy. One patient noticed a slight decrease in intensity of reflex erections after rhizotomy. The other man had been impotent for 4 years and had minimal change in bladder capacity after bilateral ablation of the S2–S4 roots. In 5 patients bladder capacity was increased to a volume at which intermittent catheterization was practical. Rhizotomy abolished leakage in 1 patient in whom urine leaked per urethram despite the presence of a suprapubic tube.

(2) J. Urol. 120:557–558, November, 1978.

These patients have been followed for less than a year after rhizotomy. If bladder spasticity returns, repeat percutaneous rhizotomy or electrocoagulation of alternative pathways would seem to be feasible. Repeat thermal destruction could be done at the same or further sacral levels.

▶ [This technique may or may not avoid the problems associated with rhizotomy after laminectomy, which include recurrence of detrusor hyperreflexia and the occurrence of causalgia-like pain in the sectioned nerve roots.—William E. Bradley] ◀

Treatment of Female Urinary Incontinence is reviewed by R. Turner Warwick[3] (London). Relatively few patients are accurate observers of their own urologic functions. Patient satisfaction alone is a limited criterion for the success of a surgical procedure. Somewhat more than half of the female patients with troublesome incontinence are easily treated by a wide variety of procedures, whereas a small proportion are virtually impossible to cure without some form of variable artificial sphincter.

An incompetent bladder neck mechanism is the primary defect in stress incontinence. Incompetence may result from an intrinsic deficiency or from activity of the detrusor-trigonal-bladder-neck-opening mechanism. Detrusor instability may be relevant to the results of surgery for incontinence, through both loss of bladder neck competence and the rise in intravesical pressure resulting from the detrusor contraction. None of the standard operations for stress incontinence significantly convert an unstable detrusor mechanism to a stable effective mechanism. Accurate detection of detrusor stability in the erect posture may require a subtracted pressure study to identify the significant bladder-neck-opening contractions of a relatively low-pressure detrusor. Although operations that tend to recreate a "posterior angle" may also generally tend to reestablish urinary control, it does not follow that continence results because the angle is reestablished. The urethral pressure profile has proved somewhat disappointing in evaluating sphincter function, especially in the bladder neck area. When continence is restored, it is important to try to assess whether this has been achieved at the bladder neck or at the urethral sphincter level. Although many operations are supposedly directed toward the reestablish-

(3) Urol. Int. 33:101–106, 1978.

ment of continence at the bladder neck level they more commonly seem to achieve it at the urethral sphincter distal to it.

The fundamental need is for the accumulation of basic functional observations rather than the rationalization of treatments adopted on the basis of tenuous evidence.

▶ [The author of this article summarizes his considerable experience and insight into the pathophysiology of stress incontinence. He focuses on the radiographic and pressure correlates of this disability believing that stress incontinence is related to bladder neck incompetence.

Many other studies utilizing urethral pressure profiles have demonstrated that, in whole or in part, true stress incontinence in the female is secondary to loss of smooth muscle tone in the urethra. This conflict in conceptualization awaits the conclusion of future studies.—William E. Bradley] ◀

Role of Adjunctive Drug Therapy for Intermittent Catheterization and Self-Catheterization in Children with Vesical Dysfunction.

Nabil Hilwa and Alan D. Perlmutter[4] (Detroit) report experience with 39 children having vesical dysfunction who were managed by clean intermittent catheterization or self-catheterization and evaluated adjunctive drug therapy. The 26 girls and 13 boys were aged 15 months to 14 years. Thirty children had myelodysplasia (myelomeningocele). All had significant residual urine or chronic retention. The primary indication for intermittent catheterization was incontinence, present in all but 2 children. The other indication was chronic or recurrent urinary tract infection. Five children had had unsuccessful operations to promote bladder emptying. Three boys had perineal urethrostomy after entering the program. A modification of the clean, nonsterile technique of intermittent catheterization was utilized. Catheterization was done on an average of 4 times daily.

Five girls achieved continence day and night without drug therapy, and all but 1 of 16 patients on drug therapy became dry. The drugs used were anticholinergics, anticholinomimetic agents and α-adrenergic agents. There were 2 treatment failures. Only 2 boys were dry without drug therapy, but 8 of 9 became continent on medication. Oxybutynin was the primary agent used to increase bladder capacity. Infection persisted in 11 of 31 patients despite vigorous chemotherapy. Two children who were uninfected

(4) J. Urol. 119:551–554, April, 1978.

initially acquired acute infection after catheterization; both responded to treatment. Lesser grades of vesicoureteral reflux improved on the catheterization program. Hydronephrosis did not progress during treatment, and a majority of affected patients improved. Parenchymal loss did not progress in the 5 children affected.

Although the primary goal of intermittent catheterization was to obtain continence, renal damage induced by infection and reflux was minimized by the intermittent catheterization program. Intermittent catheterization in childhood is a preferred alternative to urinary diversion in cases of neurogenic bladder dysfunction. Complications are uncommon; the commonest in this series was penile edema.

▶ [The advantages of clean self-intermittent catheterization in the management of urinary bladder dysfunction in childhood are further documented by this study. In this report pharmocotherapy was a useful adjunct to the use of the catheter. Whether clean self-intermittent catheterization will continue to be of long-range benefit to these children awaits results of long-term follow-up studies.—William E. Bradley] ◀

Incidence and Consequences of Damage to Parasympathetic Nerve Supply to Bladder after Abdominoperineal Resection of Rectum for Carcinoma. Voiding dysfunction has been observed in 30–50% of patients undergoing abdominoperineal resection of the rectum for carcinoma. Both bladder neck obstruction and pelvic nerve injury have been implicated. J. W. Fowler, D. N. Bremner and L. E. F. Moffat[5] (Edinburgh) evaluated bladder function in 51 patients who underwent abdominoperineal resection for carcinoma in 1972–75. Postvoiding difficulty was the chief reason for referral. A minority of patients were seen for routine postoperative evaluation. Cystometry, where abnormal, was repeated after 1 week and 1 month and then every 3 months for a year. The 36 males and 15 females had an average age of 62 years. All were followed for at least 6 months.

Seven patients had significant bladder symptoms preoperatively and 7 of 27 had significant urographic abnormalities. Thirty-seven patients had abnormal cystometric findings after operation. Seven recovered bladder function after 1 week to 6 months. Ten of 21 patients with normal

---

(5) Br. J. Urol. 50:95–98, April, 1978.

bladder innervation and 25 of 30 with cystometric abnormality had significant voiding difficulty. Seven of the 10 patients with symptoms and normal cystometrograms required transurethral prostatectomy or urethrotomy. Thirteen patients with symptoms and denervated bladders underwent operation and 3 received drug therapy also. Two patients required permanent catheter drainage. Motor denervation was more frequent in patients with invasive and more highly malignant tumors and in those with posteriorly placed tumors. The circumferential site of the tumor seemed to be more important than its distance from the anus. Motor denervation was more frequent when the coccyx was not excised and when the perineal wound was left open. Five of 8 patients with denervated bladders who died had significant genitourinary disease, most commonly cystitis and suppurative pyelitis. One patient died of pulmonary emobolism after prostatectomy.

Mechanical factors may be important in some of these cases. Pelvic infection may destroy nerves that otherwise would recover. Failure to identify the correct plane of dissection in front of the sacrum appears to be the likeliest mechanism of injury. If early postoperative denervation goes unnoticed, rehabilitation of the bladder may be difficult. Severe morbidity may occur even when it is recognized.

▶ [This useful study further documents the incidence of bladder denervation after extensive pelvic surgery. Hopefully this morbidity may be avoided in future procedures by the development of methods for intraoperative identification of the nerve supply to the bladder. Postoperative studies (Andersen et al., Scand. J. Urol. Nephrol 10:789, 1976) for electrophysiologic assessment of bladder innervation would also contribute to evaluation of these patients.–William E. Bradley] ◀

Endovesical Transurethral Electrostimulation in Rehabilitation of Neurogenic Bladder in Children: Four Years' Clinical Experience is reported by D. Berger, K. Berger and N. Genton[6] (Lausanne, Switzerland). Endovesical electrostimulation (ES) was evaluated as a means of offering young patients with neurogenic bladder a balanced bladder and better social and familial adjustment. The goal is modification of receptor excitability to reactivate the process of facilitation of stimuli from the

---

(6) Eur. Urol. 4:33–45, 1978.

bladder wall so that they can reach the CNS by an efferent
vegetative tract. Treatment by ES requires daily catheterization. The usual stimulation parameters are 50–60
pulses per second, 5 to 6 ma and 5 to 6 msec. Sessions
usually last 90 minutes, with two 10-minute pauses.
Eighteen boys and 13 girls aged 1 month to $14^1/_2$ years
were treated in 1973–76. Myclomeningocele was present in
23 patients and meningocele in 4. The only contraindications to ES were abnormal renal function and massive ureteral reflux with severe upper tract dilatation.

Treatment resulted in a major change in bladder and
sphincter function in 64% of all patients, but only 26% had
clinically good results, with continence for over 2 hours,
ability to hold the urine for 15–20 minutes when a clear
urge to void was present and complete micturition. Good
results were obtained in children aged 5 months to 14
years. Micturition is now coordinated with a relatively
good stream in these patients, and they all can initiate
voiding voluntarily, although 3 of the 8 occasionally require the aid of abdominal muscles. Twelve patients had
insufficient results, with a vague urge to void and less
forceful micturition. Ten children did not respond to treatment. Function in 1 child became worse.

The level of the spinal lesion did not appear critically to
influence the outcome of Es in this series. In some cases,
ES probably offers a greater possibility for going beyond
the stage of a balanced bladder than do other treatments.
It permits a certain number of children with neurogenic
bladder to acquire socially efficient continence. Contraindications are complete paraplegia, advanced lesions of the
detrusor, low IQ or a deficient social-familial environment
and renal failure. Children with severe bladder decompensation should not be treated.

▶ [I do not understand the physiologic basis for the effectiveness of this technique. A helpful method for evaluation of patient results would be the inclusion
of a randomized, statistically controlled study.–William E. Bradley] ◀

**Phenoxybenzamine in Neurogenic Bladder Dys-
function after Spinal Cord Injury: I. Voiding Dysfunction.** Pharmacologic blockade of the sympathetically innervated bladder neck and urethral smooth muscle has been
used successfully to promote and maintain bladder empty-

TABLE 1.—LOWER MOTOR NEURON BLADDER WITH OR WITHOUT SYMPATHETIC
INNERVATION

	No. Pts.	Response		
		Excellent	Partial	Unchanged
Retention	6	5	1	0
High residual urine and difficulty straining	4	4	0	0
Totals	10	9	1	0

ing in patients with neurogenic bladder dysfunction. Michael B. Scott and James W. Morrow[7] (Downey, Calif.) evaluated phenoxybenzamine, a long-acting α-adrenergic blocking agent, in 38 male subjects with neurogenic bladder secondary to traumatic cord injury. They had poor bladder emptying after 10–12 weeks of intermittent catheterization or had lost previously achieved bladder balance. Patients with both upper and lower motor neuron bladders were treated. Phenoxybenzamine was begun in a dose of 10 mg daily and increased in 10 mg increments at weekly intervals to a maximum of 60 mg if necessary.

Nine of 10 patients with involvement of the sacral micturition center had an excellent response at an average dosage of 30 mg daily, with good bladder balance, no overdistention and alleviation of symptoms of autonomic dysreflexia (Table 1). One patient with injury between L2 and S2 responded to phenoxybenzamine therapy. Patients with injuries at T10–L2 responded poorly (Table 2). The responses of patients with injuries about T10, who had upper motor neuron bladders with sympathetic hyperreflexia below the level of the lesion, were unpredictable and incon-

TABLE 2.—UPPER MOTOR NEURON BLADDER WITH SYMPATHETIC DENERVATION

	No. Pts.	Response		
		Excellent	Partial	Unchanged
Retention	3	0	0	3
High residual urine	3	0	2	1
Totals	6	0	2	4

(7) J. Urol. 119:480–482, April, 1978.

TABLE 3.—UPPER MOTOR NEURON BLADDER WITH SYMPATHETIC HYPERREFLEXIA

	No. Pts.	Response		
		Excellent	Partial	No Change
Retention	8	2	5	1
High resid-ual urine	13	6	2	5
High resid-ual urine with auto-nomic dys-reflexia	6	5	1	0
Total pts.	21	8	7	6

stant (Table 3). Side effects were infrequent. Two patients had postural hypotension and 6 had temporary lassitude. No patient lost reflex erections.

Phenoxybenzamine was effective in patients with lower motor neuron lesions, upper motor neuron lesions and co-existing autonomic dysreflexia or intact sympathetic inner-vation and upper motor neuron bladders. Responses were unpredictable in patients with upper motor neuron lesions without coexisting dysreflexia. Sympathetic hyperreflexia not resulting in dysreflexia did not appear to have a signif-icant role in detrusor sphincter imbalance.

► [Hopefully the authors will extend their work to include a randomized, sta-tistically controlled study of the benefit of this drug.–William E. Bradley] ◄

Choice of Operation to Promote Micturition after Spinal Cord Injury. Some patients with spinal cord in-jury fail to void and require either permanent catheteriza-tion or surgical treatment to reduce the resistance of the bladder outflow tract. Bladder neck resection is followed by retrograde ejaculation, and internal membranous ure-throtomy may cause erectile impotence. G. J. Fellows, I. Nuseibeh and J. J. Walsh[8] (Aylesbury, Bucks, England) attempted to determine whether the outcome of surgical treatment can be predicted in the individual patient. The findings in 61 male patients operated on during 1974–76 were reviewed. External sphincterotomy was done in 15 patients, bladder neck resection in 22 and both procedures in 24. Thirty-one patients had complete urinary retention.

(8) Br. J. Urol. 49:721–724, 1977.

Cord injury was traumatic in 54 patients and due to benign lesions, with or without surgery on the spine, in 7. One fourth of the patients had incomplete lesions.

The superiority of combined surgery over bladder neck resection alone was just short of statistical significance. A second operation was carried out in all but three of the failures, and there was only 1 patient who failed to void after a second operation. Thus 4 patients out of the original 61 were ultimately assigned to catheter drainage. The outcome was not related to age. Three tetraplegic patients failed to void after bladder neck resection. All patients with an upper sensory level at L1 or below passed urine regardless of the operation done. All three failures of sphincterotomy were in patients with lesions above T6. The overall results of operation were better in patients with absent sacral reflexes. The outcome was not related to the strength of detrusor contractions or to the appearance of the bladder neck at cystography.

The failure rate of bladder neck resection alone in patients with cord injury is unacceptably high. It is probably an inappropriate operation for patients with cervical lesions and for those with maximal urethral closure pressure in excess of 100 cm water. Bladder neck resection should be avoided if the patient is able to ejaculate. Internal membranous urethrotomy appears suitable for patients with lesions at all cord levels. If this operation fails, it can be repeated or, if necessary, a bladder neck resection can then be performed. Combined surgery has the greatest chance of success and should be done if no attempt is to be made to preserve sexual function.

▶ [Hopefully, urodynamic studies will be utilized by the authors in future efforts to restore voiding by the application of pharmocotherapy as a supplement to surgical procedures.–William E. Bradley] ◀

Electric Stimulation in Management of Incontinence in Children. Incontinence in the handicapped child is usually permanent, causes skin changes and complicates social acceptance. C. Godec and A. S. Cass[9] (Gillette Children's Hosp., St. Paul, Minn.) used electric stimulation of the anal sphincter in 45 incontinent boys and 32 incontinent girls. There were 36 cases of myelomeningocele

---

(9)   Minn. Med. 61:157–160, March, 1978.

and 10 of spinal cord injury. Twenty-two subjects had the diagnosis of idiopathic bedwetting. Cord lesions were complete in 22 cases and incomplete in 24. Hydrocephalus that required shunting was present in 26 children with myelomeningocele. Either prolonged or acute maximal functional electric stimulation (FES) was carried out. Prolonged FES was applied via an anal plug with a Mentor Continaid or a 3M Stimulator; a continuous train of stimuli was used. The parameters of stimulation were 1 msec, 20 Hz and 3–8.5 v. Acute maximal FES was applied via an anal plug and needle electrodes inserted into the levator ani muscle; stimulation was at 47–50 v. Each acute maximal application lasted 15–20 minutes; applications were repeated 4–10 times at 2- or 3-day intervals.

Cystometrography showed a spastic bladder in 37 subjects and neurogenic bladder with fibrotic bladder wall changes in 25. Repeat tracings during stimulation showed normal findings in 9 of 36 children with a hyperreflexic bladder and less spasticity in 14. Most children had a rise in anal sphincter pressure on stimulation of the pelvic floor muscles. Criteria for FES, including hyperreflexic bladder function or pelvic floor weakness or both with some innervation of the pelvic floor muscles and an anal sphincter pressure rise over 15 cm water with a maximum of 15 v stimulation, were present in 51 children. Only 31 children used FES. The relapse rates were 21% in the 19 children cured and 22% in the 9 improved. Anal pain and diarrhea did not occur. Autonomic dysreflexia did not occur in any cord-injured child.

A rise in anal sphincter pressure on electric stimulation is a more reliable criterion for FES than a rise in maximum urethral pressure. A success rate of 90% was achieved in selected patients in this study.

▶ [The authors have attempted to demonstrate the benefits of the use of external pelvic floor stimulation in patients with urinary incontinence. A comparison of pharmacotherapy with this treatment would be helpful in assessing effectiveness.–William E. Bradley] ◀

Urethral Sphincteric Responses to Stimulation of Sacral Nerves in the Human Female. M. J. Torrens[1] (Frenchay Hosp., Bristol, England) assessed the urethral

(1) Urol. Int. 33:22–26, 1978.

response to sacral nerve stimulation in 10 female patients undergoing surgical denervation for bladder hyperactivity or perineal pain. Four had neurologic disease, which, however, produced no peculiar urethral responses. The nerves were exposed at sacral laminectomy and stimulated with 0.8-msec square wave pulses at 10 cps and 0–10 v. Bladder and urethral pressures were recorded during stimulation.

Stimuli of 6–8 v were required to provoke bladder contraction. Typically, a brief pressure increase in the urethra, lasting about 3 seconds, was followed by a decline for the duration of stimulation, which tended to lessen with time. The response was noted at all levels from S2 to S4, but sphincter contraction was more prominent at S2 and relaxation at S4. After nerve section, stimulation of the proximal nerve end may produce a slight elevation of urethral pressure but no urethral relaxation or significant bladder contraction. Stimulation of the isolated distal nerve end reproduced the typical response to stimulation of the intact nerve. Urethral relaxation could occur in the absence of significant bladder contraction. Lower voltage stimuli caused sphincteric contraction and higher voltage stimuli, bladder contraction and urethral relaxation.

The urethral relaxation observed on sacral nerve stimulation is integrated peripherally. A parasympathetic inhibitory influence has been postulated. The relaxation does not represent a vesicourethral reflex. The pathophysiology of spontaneous urethral relaxation, which may be termed the unstable or overinhibited urethra, seems well founded.

▶ [Whether the reduction of pressure recorded by the urethral catheter was due to muscle relaxation or to an active dilatation of the urethra by bladder muscle contraction awaits further study. The neuromuscular blocking effects of halothane on smooth muscle should also be assessed.—William E. Bradley] ◀

Urinary Bladder Dysfunction in Multiple Sclerosis is a frequent finding and occasionally is an initial manifestation. William E. Bradley[2] (Univ. of Minnesota) reviewed the findings in 302 patients (216 females) with multiple sclerosis. Their mean age was 41.7 years. Mean duration of disease was 11.2 years. The studies performed included

(2) Neurology (Minneap.) 28:52–58, September, 1978.

gas cystometry, integrated sphincter electromyography, uroflowmetry, urethral pressure profile recording, electrophysiologic tests of bladder innervation, intravenous pyelography and voiding cystourethrography. Sphincter electromyography was done with surface electrodes. Uroflowmetry was performed by a load cell technique. The blood urea nitrogen and serum creatinine concentrations were estimated and urinalysis and urine culture were carried out.

The most common symptoms of bladder dysfunction were urgency, frequency and urge incontinence. All patients had sterile urine cultures. About 97% had abnormal cystometrograms. Detrusor hyperreflexia was found in 62% of patients and areflexia in 34%. Detrusor sphincter dyssynergia or reflex sphincter relaxation was observed in 72% of patients on repetitive sphincter electromyography performed with the patient standing. Urine flow studies were abnormal in 68% of patients. Pressure profiles occasionally showed increased amplitude of the maximum urethral closure pressure. The latency of the evoked anal response from bladder and proximal urethral stimulation was increased in 20% of patients. Nearly two thirds of the patients had complete inability to suppress the reflex on command. The principal radiographic finding was mild pyelectasis, seen in 6.4% of patients, none of whom had evidence of decline in renal function. The voiding cystourethrogram was abnormal in 60.2% of patients. The principal finding was inability to initiate voiding or increased residual urine volume. Management was most often with pharmacotherapy and clean, self-intermittent catheterization. Patients with detrusor hyperreflexia were treated with methantheline and propantheline. Several patients had a limited form of rhizotomy, with initially promising results.

Multiple sclerosis is characterized by detrusor reflex abnormalities, principally hyperreflexia and sphincter disturbance. The dysfunction is best managed by a combination of pharmacotherapy and clean, nonsterile, self-intermittent catheterization. If use of the catheter is impossible, an indwelling catheter and anticholinergic agents offer a reasonable approach to treatment.

Tumors

Tumors of the Lower Urinary Tract in Children. O. Eklöf, B. Brun, I. Claësson, P. -E. Heikel and G. Stake[3] reviewed 37 case reports of lower urinary tract tumors in children seen in Scandinavia and Finland in the past two decades, as well as 3 case reports from Switzerland. The 28 boys and 12 girls had a mean age at diagnosis of 31.5 months. There were 33 patients with embryonic rhabdomyosarcoma, 5 with polyp and 1 each with papilloma and hemangioma. Eleven patients had a palpable tumor, and 11 had urinary retention. Three were incontinent. Urinary infection was present in 8 patients and hematuria in 21. Ten patients had dysuria. Seventeen patients with sarcoma had a history of less than 4 weeks.

Simultaneous radiologic demonstration of the bladder and rectum often aided in assessing the size of the tumor and its relation to adjacent structures. Three sarcomas presented as expanding lesions in the retroperitoneal paravertebral region. Bladder capacity was markedly reduced by grapelike tumor masses in 6 patients. Most patients with sarcoma presented with a localized tumor involving the bladder base around the urethra or close to it. Five tumors had a disklike shape, growing partially extravesically at the bladder base. Four patients had a well-demarcated filling defect in the bladder. Five tumors grew mainly extravesically, displacing and deforming the bladder. All the polyps were round and well demarcated and on urography were usually close to the outlet of the bladder. All polyps were pedunculated. The papilloma resembled an ectopic ureterocele. The hemangioma extended into the bladder and was manifest by phleboliths in the lesser pelvis.

Lower urinary tract tumors in children most often affect male subjects and are manifest before age 5 years. Embryonic sarcoma is the most frequent of the lower urinary tract in children. A small amount of barium contrast aids in demonstrating the relationship of the tumor to the rectosigmoid colon and in assessing the posterior border of a

---

(3)   Acta Radiol. [Diagn.] (Stockh.) 19:171–185, 1978.

pelvic mass. The solitary polyp is the most common benign tumor of the lower urinary tract.

▶ [This review of the radiologic characteristics of pediatric lower urinary tract tumors fills a void in the urologic literature. Although the authors do not discuss treatment, we would like to stress that multimodal bladder sparing therapy should be considered in all children with rhabdomyosarcoma of the bladder or prostate.—S.S.H.] ◀

Carcinoma of the Bladder in Patients Less than 40 Years Old. D. E. Johnson and S. Hillis[4] (Univ. of Texas System Cancer Center, Houston) reviewed the records of 22 patients seen before age 40 years with bladder carcinoma. They represented 1% of patients seen in 1944–75 with malignant neoplasms of the bladder. The 19 men and 3 women had an average age at diagnosis of 35.7 years. The most common symptom was gross hematuria; 7 of these 15 patients also had an irritable bladder. The mean duration of symptoms in 17 cases was 6 months. Cystoscopy showed exophytic lesions in 10 patients and endophytic lesions in 6. Transitional cell carcinoma was present in 17 cases, squamous carcinoma in 3 and adenocarcinoma in 2.

Eleven of 12 patients with superficial (stages O–B1) disease had transurethral resection, and 4 of these had recurrences. One patient with stage B1 disease had radical cystectomy with ileal conduit diversion. Three patients with stage C disease had radiotherapy, cystectomy and ileal conduit diversion. One had partial and 1, radical cystectomy. All 3 patients with regional or disseminated metastases received palliative radiotherapy directed to the primary tumor. Eight of 9 patients with superficial disease are alive after $^{1}/_{2}$–28 years. Eleven deaths resulted directly from the disease. The median survival time of patients who died was 11 months.

Bladder carcinoma should be treated on the basis of the clinical stage of disease in patients under age 40, as in older patients. Treatment must not be compromised in younger patients by postponing necessary radical surgery. The consequences of radical cystectomy, such as impotence, and the problems of urinary diversion may be exaggerated in young patients, but they do not alter the need for such treatment.

---

(4) J. Urol. 120:172–173, August, 1978.

▶ [The authors' recommendation that bladder cancer in young patients should be treated appropriately according to stage is unassailable. However, their conclusion—not mentioned in the abstract—that this disease is equally malignant in young and old individuals is difficult to evaluate since their sample size is small, the series uncontrolled and the patient selection at their institution may be atypical.–S.S.H.] ◀

Saccharin, Cyclamate and Human Bladder Cancer: No Evidence of an Association. Cyclamates were banned by the Department of Health, Education and Welfare in 1970 on the basis of presumed carcinogenic effects in laboratory animals, and saccharin was removed from the list of safe food products in 1972. The relevance of animal tests to human cancer etiology is unclear. Irving I. Kessler and J. Page Clark[5] (Johns Hopkins Univ.) report results of an epidemiologic study designed to elucidate the possible roles of these artificial sweeteners in human urinary bladder cancer. Intake was recorded in 519 patients with histologically confirmed bladder cancer and matching controls in metropolitan Baltimore. The patients were discharged from 19 hospitals in 1972–75. Controls were matched with patients for sex, race, age and current marital status.

The intakes of cyclamate and saccharin did not differ significantly in frequency, quantity or duration in the patient and control groups. This held true after simultaneous adjustment for the effects of smoking, occupation, age, diabetes and a number of other potentially confounding factors. The relative risk of bladder cancer did not increase with increasing exposure to artificial sweeteners.

The findings suggest that neither saccharin nor cyclamate is likely to be carcinogenic in man, at least at the moderate dietary ingestion levels reported by this patient sample. The possibility that one of the substances is carcinogenic whereas the other is protective against cancer is contradicted by the data.

▶ [This carefully controlled epidemiologic case study presents strong evidence that saccharin and cyclamates are not associated with human bladder cancer. Unfortunately this work will not settle the issue. The Canadian investigation which found a significant risk in men (Howe et al., Lancet 2:578, 1977) and studies that show saccharin promotes but does not initiate bladder cancer in rats cannot be ignored.–S.S.H.] ◀

---

(5) J.A.M.A. 240:349–355, July 28, 1978.

Cell Surface Antigen A, B or O(H) as an Indicator of Malignant Potential in Stage A Bladder Carcinoma: Preliminary Report. Although the stage of bladder cancer usually corresponds to the degree of cellular anaplasia, 70% of patients presenting with stage A cancer will have a recurrence, 10–20% at a higher stage, including metastases. Stuart Bergman and Nasser Javadpour[6] (Natl. Inst. of Health) attempted to correlate cell surface antigens with the potential for invasion and metastasis of stages O and A papillary transitional cell bladder tumors. Fourteen patients seen in 1953–70 with stage O or A, grade I or II papillary transitional cell bladder tumors were studied. All were followed to recurrence or for at least 5 years. In blood group O patients, H antigen was assayed by use of a *Ulex europaeus* extract in place of antiserum. Cell surface antigens were detected by the specific red cell adherence (SRCA) test; scoring was from 0 to 4 +.

Three of 5 patients with no recurrences had positive SRCA findings of at least 2 +, while 2 had negative findings. The first 3 patients had blood group A or B, while the 2 with false negative results had blood group O. Six of 9 patients with recurrences were stage A, grade I or II. All had 0 or 1 + SRCA results. Three with recurrence and invasion or metastases had negative SRCA findings. Three patients with recurrences underwent cystectomy, and all but 1 of the others had transurethral resection and fulguration.

There appears to be a relation between the absence of the cell surface antigens A, B or H and recurrence of bladder tumors. No false positive results were obtained when the criterion for positivity was taken as 2 +. Both patients with false negative results had blood group O, and the weaker nature of the H antigen on these cells may have been responsible. Study of a larger group of patients is necessary to determine whether this immunologic dedifferentiation occurs early enough to allow predictions of which patients should have earlier, intensive treatment, or attenuated therapy to avoid excessive treatment when less malignant or benign disease is present.

Prognosis in Early Carcinoma of the Bladder Based on Chromosomal Analysis. In well-differentiated and

(6) J. Urol. 119:49–51, January, 1978.

moderately well-differentiated noninvasive transitional cell carcinoma and submucosal invasive carcinoma, the histopathology is of minimal value in differentiating curative resection from recurrence and ultimate death. William H. Falor and Rose M. Ward[7] (Akron City Hosp., Ohio) performed repeated cytogenetic analysis by the direct, nonculture technique in 53 cases of noninvasive or submucosal invasive well-differentiated carcinoma of the bladder. Patients were followed for 4–101 months. Thirty-three had noninvasive carcinoma, and 20 had submucosal invasive lesions. The 39 men and 14 women were aged 38–91 years. An average of 4 cystoscopies were done in each case.

Abnormal chromosomal markers were present in 33 patients, 32 of whom have had recurrences, resulting in 9 deaths. All but 1 of the 20 patients without markers have been followed for up to 8 years and have remained free of recurrence. In the exceptional case, the mode changed from 69 to 92 8 months after diagnosis, indicating dedifferentiation and development of a new tumor in a bladder prone to neoplasia. The modes were peridiploid in most cases of well-differentiated carcinoma with marker chromosomes. About 40% of the modes in submucosal invasive, moderately well-differentiated carcinomas with marker chromosomes were hypotetraploid. In most cases the marker chromosomes included an A1.

A cytogenetic classification has been developed on the basis of a total of 165 cases of bladder carcinoma. It is based on extent of invasion, the presence or absence of markers and the modal chromosome number. Whether marker chromosomes and/or ploidy are important in stage III and IV tumors or in carcinomas of other cell types remains to be determined.

▶ [Which noninvasive bladder tumors should be treated aggressively is an extremely important clinical problem that is addressed by these two articles. Detection of aplasia or carcinoma in situ in random bladder biopsy is clearly one established criterion of potential invasiveness. Bergman, Javadpour and Lange (J. Urol. 119:52, 1978) have presented very strong preliminary evidence that loss of cell surface antigen A, B or O(H) is a second. Falor and Ward suggest that chromosomal analysis is an almost perfect method of predicting prognosis. Frankly we will remain skeptical until these findings are repeated in a blinded study. Because the methods are difficult, there has

---

(7) J. Urol. 119:44–48, January, 1978.

been no similar experience with tumors from other sites and the results seem "too good."–S.S.H.] ◀

Site of Recurrence of Noninfiltrating Bladder Tumors. Noninfiltrating bladder tumors frequently recur after treatment. B. H. Page, V. B. Levison and M. P. Curwen[8] (North Middlesex Hosp., London) studied 56 patients with noninfiltrating bladder tumor, 29 of whom received radiotherapy. None had previously been treated, and all were initially treated by endoscopic diathermy resection. Diagnosis of noninfiltrating transitional cell tumors was confirmed histologically. All patients were followed by periodic cystoscopy for at least 2 years, the first being done about 3 months after primary treatment. During followup, 2 patients received a course of intravesical thio-tepa, and 1 patient received 2 courses of Epodyl and then underwent cystectomy.

In 75% of the cases, the primary tumor was confined to an area of bladder running upward and outward from a ureteric orifice (typical primary site). Recurrences at this site were found in 20% of the cases but were also frequently found at other sites. The posterosuperior wall of the bladder was the most common site for recurrent tumors; of a total of 238 tumors, 178 were accounted for by 8 of the 21 patients having recurrences at this site. Another striking site for recurrence is the small area of bladder where the air bubble settles, a very rare site for a primary tumor, none being found in this series.

The posterosuperior wall of the bladder is the area of the bladder that is always scraped and prodded by the cystoscope or resectoscope when it lies in neutral position, especially when the bladder is relatively empty. The area of bladder where the air bubble lies may be subject to heat trauma from the action of diathermy on the tissues. The distribution of recurrent tumors in the bladder is consistent with their being caused by implantation of tumor cells scattered by the primary treatment. The site of implantation is probably determined by mild mechanical trauma of the mucosa at endoscopy. Recurrences in the air bubble region may be determined by tumor cells being carried there

(8) Br. J. Urol. 50:237–242, June, 1978.

by gas bubbles and by thermal trauma to the mucosa from the hot gas.

In an addendum, it is stated that Boyd and Bernand (1974) have confirmed the distribution of recurrent tumors in the "vault of the bladder."

▶ [This article presents an intriguing observation. If the authors are correct that recurrences are in part due to implantation at sites of trauma during surgery, then intra- or immediate postoperative chemotherapy or low-dose radiotherapy might be advisable. Gavrell et al. (J. Urol. 120:410, 1978), among others, have recommended this approach.–S.S.H.] ◀

Management of the Urethra in Patients Undergoing Radical Cystectomy for Bladder Carcinoma. Some recommend routine urethrectomy prophylactically in all males undergoing radical cystectomy, whereas others reserve it for patients in whom bladder cancer has involved the bladder neck and/or prostatic urethra.

Shlomo Raz, Gorden McLorie, Stephen Johnson and Donald G. Skinner[9] (Univ. of California, Los Angeles) analyzed the computerized clinical and pathologic findings in 247 patients having radical cystectomy for bladder carcinoma during 1955–76. Of the 174 men, 32 had urethrectomy at the time of or subsequent to radical cystectomy; 7 of these 32 patients had overt urethral carcinoma, and 5 of them died of widespread metastases within 2 years of operation. Ten patients had severe epithelial atypia, and 15 had a normal urethra. Four of the 7 patients with overt urethral carcinoma had no bladder neck or prostatic urethral involvement. Overt urethral carcinoma occurred in 4% of all males having radical cystectomy and severe epithelial atypia in 5.7%.

Current evidence indicates a low rate of overt urethral carcinoma or carcinoma in situ in the remaining urethra after cystectomy. Bladder carcinoma extending to the anterior urethra clearly indicates need for urethrectomy after cystectomy; carcinoma in situ at the distal margin of the specimen also calls for removal of the urethra. Urethrectomy should be done at radical cystectomy only when positive margins or an overt urethral tumor is found, or when there is evidence of carcinoma in situ involving the prostatic urethra. Other patients should be followed by clinical

(9)   J. Urol. 120:298–300, September, 1978.

examination, urethral washings and endoscopy when bleeding occurs, with urethrectomy reserved for those with positive cytology.

▶ [We, as recommended by the authors, perform urethrectomy selectively in males undergoing radical cystectomy. This approach seems justified since our patients have not had urethral recurrences.—S.S.H.] ◀

Segmental Resection in the Management of Bladder Carcinoma. Segmental resection appears to be effective in patients presenting with a first high-grade tumor in a mobile part of the bladder, those in whom more aggressive surgery is imprudent for medical reasons and those in whom complete endoscopic resection cannot be done because of the location of the tumor. The procedure has fallen into disrepute in some circles because of failure to apply it appropriately. K. B. Cummings, J. T. Mason, R. J. Correa, Jr. and R. P. Gibbons[1] (Virginia Mason Med. Center, Seattle) reviewed the results of segmental resection of bladder carcinoma in 101 patients treated in 1945–71. Segmental resection was the first surgical procedure in 73 of these 101 patients, 84% of whom were men. The mean age was 62 years. Segmental resection was done as a definitive procedure in the following conditions: in stage O disease not amenable to complete endoscopic resection; invasive carcinoma that was considered curable; and 8 cases of medical contraindications to more aggressive surgery.

The 5-year survival rate was 79% in stage A cases, 80% for stage B1, 45% for stage B2 and 6% for stage C. Combined rates for stages O–B1 and stages B2–C were 83% and 28% respectively. Only 7% of stage O–B1 patients had a history of antecedent tumor, compared to 59% of those with stages B2 and C disease. The correlation of high grade with high-stage disease was significant. Half the recurrences appeared within a year after segmental resection. Increased tumor grade was noted in 40% of patients with multiple recurrences. Survival was significantly compromised in patients with high-stage disease who had involvement of the bladder base. Many patients with higher-grade disease appeared to benefit from added radiotherapy. No operative deaths occurred, but there were 3 vesicocutaneous fistulas, 1 colovesical fistula and 1 recurrence in the

---

(1) J. Urol. 119:56–58, January, 1978.

suprapubic tube tract. Bladder function was compromised significantly in 18% of patients. Cystectomy was performed in 9% of cases.

Contraindications to segmental resection include high-grade and high-stage tumors of the trigone and/or ureteral orifice, invasive carcinoma of the bladder neck in females and transitional cell carcinoma that appears to be a field-change mucosal disease.

▶ [We feel segmental resection should be used cautiously. The authors' survival rate for stage B tumors is much higher than that of most other surgeons. We had been struck by the frequency of extravesical pelvic recurrence after partial cystectomy and therefore recommend low-dose (1,000 rad) preoperative radiation.–S.S.H.] ◀

Effect of Intravesical Thio-TEPA on Normal and Tumor Urothelium. Peter T. Nieh, James J. Daly, John A. Heaney, Niall M. Heney and George R. Prout, Jr.[2] (Boston) investigated intravesical thio-TEPA instillation in a group of 55 patients seen during 1974–77 with biopsy-proved transitional cell carcinoma of the bladder limited to the lamina propria (Marshall stages O and A). Thirty-two patients with residual tumor after transurethral resection/biopsy received two courses of four weekly instillations of either 30 or 60 mg thio-TEPA in 30 or 60 ml water, respectively. Thirty-seven patients in a prophylactic group received monthly instillations of thio-TEPA or no treatment. Twenty-three of these patients were previously untreated.

Results in the therapeutic group are given in Table 1. Twelve of 15 patients who responded to therapeutic thio-TEPA entered the prophylactic regimen. Bone marrow depression or hematuria required a delay in treatment in 7 patients. Results in the prophylactic trial are given in

TABLE 1.—THERAPEUTIC GROUP—32 PATIENTS

Thio-Tepa

	30 Mg.			60 Mg.			Totals
	Subtotal	Visible	Non-Visible	Subtotal	Visible	Non-Visible	
Pts. entered	16	12	4	16	10	6	32
Completed protocol	13	9	4	14	8	6	27
Response (%)	6 (46)	4 (44)	2 (50)	9 (64)	4 (50)	5 (83)	15 (56)

(2) J. Urol. 119:59–61, January, 1978.

TABLE 2.—PROPHYLACTIC GROUP—37 PATIENTS

	Control	30 Mg.	60 Mg.	Total No. Pts.
Pts. entered	18	10	9	37
Incomplete, died or refused treatment	4	4	3	11
Completed more than 3 months	14	6	6	26
Recurrence (%)	9 (64)	4 (67)	3 (50)	16 (62)

Table 2. No patient showed worsening of atypia during treatment with thio-TEPA. Improvement in atypia was not related to the gross tumor response. The presence of large, often fused, surface cells with vacuolated cytoplasm and enlarged hyperchromatic nuclei did not influence the response rate. Apart from patients with persistently positive urine cytology, urine cytologies did not correlate with the response to thio-TEPA.

The overall response rate to therapeutic thio-TEPA in this study was 56%. Patients with microscopic residual tumor showed better response and less toxicity than those with gross residual tumor. Prophylactic thio-TEPA did not reduce recurrence rates. Eradication of microscopic disease with a short course of weekly thio-TEPA instillations may improve the results of monthly prophylaxis. The thio-TEPA effect may represent increased turnover and decreased cohesiveness of atypical or frankly malignant urothelium, leading to increased sloughing of the affected surface cells. The high rate of falsely negative urine cytologies after thio-TEPA treatment emphasizes the importance of cystoscopic surveillance of these patients at frequent intervals.

▶ [This planned, prospective, randomized study is an improvement over the retrospective, anecdotal type of investigation. Nevertheless, because of the variables in timing, frequency of treatment and dose as well as the small numbers in each subgroup, it is difficult to draw any firm conclusions except that thio-TEPA is effective in some patients. The negative results in the prophylactic group should be interpreted cautiously.—S.S.H.] ◀

Treatment of Advanced Bladder Cancer with Cis-diaminedichloroplatinum (II NSC 119875): Pilot Study. New methods of administering cis-diaminedichloroplatinum (CDDP) have prevented most of the renal and auditory toxicity from this agent. Claude Merrin[3] (Roswell Park Meml. Inst.) evaluated the therapeutic action of CDDP in transitional cell carcinoma of the bladder in a pilot study of 19 patients seen in 1975–77 with histologically proved bladder lesions. The average age was 68.1 years. Of the 19 patients, 14 had stage D disease, 3 had stage C and 2 stage B. Most had had previous treatments that had failed. Patients received 1 mg/kg CDDP, weekly for 6 weeks and then every 3 weeks, as a slow infusion lasting 6–8 hours. The drug was given in a mannitol-KCl-5% dextrose in one-third normal saline solution. At least 3 consecutive doses constituted an adequate trial.

Complete clinical remission occurred in 1 stage D patient who died 6 months later of a myocardial infarction. Seven stage D patients and 1 with stage B disease had partial objective remissions (lesion decrease of 50%). Two patients had minimal objective remissions (25% decrease). One stage D patient had a subjective response (disappearance of pain). The overall objective response rate was 47%. The average duration of the responses was 4.8 months. The average total dose of CDDP given was 630 mg. Six patients had tinnitus, and 1 had significant deterioration in hearing. Five patients had mild to moderate myelosuppression; 4 of these had received full pelvic irradiation. Four patients had elevated serum uric acid levels. All patients had nausea and vomiting during CDDP infusion; antiemetics and an antiallergic agent gave some relief.

These results appear to be more promising than those reported by other workers. A higher average total dosage was used in this study. It seems that CDDP is the most effective drug available for treating bladder cancer. Its value may be increased by its future use in combination with other drugs and in adjuvant programs, and its use in earlier stages of the disease.

▶ [It seems clear that several chemotherapeutic agents including cyclophosamide, adriamycin, and platinum derivatives produce occasional *temporary* objective responses in patients with advanced bladder cancer. However, to date, no single agent or combination is effective enough to be significantly helpful in routine clinical practice. The author's claim that his results are better than Yagoda's is not statistically valid.—S.S.H.] ◀

(3) J. Urol. 119:493–495, April, 1978.

URODYNAMICS

Signs of Compensation and Decompensation in Bladder Outlet Obstruction. Residual urine is a sign of decompensation in any type of mechanical voiding disorder, whereas detrusor hyperactivity is considered a sign of compensation. It is important to correct outlet obstruction at the stage of "reversible compensation," but it is not clear what severity of compensation must exist to necessitate surgical treatment. H. Palmtag and H. Heering[4] (Univ. of Heidelberg, Germany) attempted to define the role of outlet obstruction in patients presenting with various subjective symptoms and those without complaints. Combined videographic cystourethrography with simultaneous pressure-flow measurement was carried out in 45 men with prostatic enlargement of varying degrees. Twenty-five women and 25 children were also examined to evaluate possible different detrusor reaction depending on age and sex. All had obstructive infravesical changes without a neurogenic component.

Residual urine was significantly increased in patients with complete retention and slightly reduced in those without symptoms. Average peak flow rates were similar in all groups, except in patients with complete retention. Detrusor activity was increased in men with frequency of urination and somewhat increased in those patients with complete retention. Compliance was low in subjects with frequency and high in the "hypoactive-retention" group. Nonprovocative bladder instability could be found in patients with low compliance or with hyperactivity but never in those with hypoactivity. Only one female subject reported a poor stream; 10 had increased frequency and dysuria. Complete retention in men could derive from hyper- or hypoactivity. The results of surgery were much better in patients in the hyperactive compensated stage. Only 1 of the 25 children with outlet obstruction had a large volume of residual urine. Flow rate was reduced only in patients with severe obstruction, and extreme hypoactivity was not found in children. Some, however, had considerable alterations of the upper urinary tract from urethral obstruction.

(4) Urol. Int. 33:53–59, 1978.

The total micturitional picture is of importance in differentiating compensation from decompensation in patients with bladder outlet obstruction. Residual urine alone cannot be used to decide if an outlet obstruction must be treated because of decompensation of the system. Voiding efficiency, as a product of pressure and flow, may help define the state of the system. A normal flow rate does not exclude extreme hyperactivity, and complete decompensation can occur in a short time, especially in young patients.

▶ [This article suffers from a variety of deficits. The patient population is poorly described (What was the cause of outlet obstruction in the 25 women studied?). Unsubstantiated statements are made (Infection leads to edema which leads to trabeculation). Nevertheless, the interesting concept of "voiding efficiency" as the product of pressure and flow is introduced and correlated with bladder compensation or decompensation. Hydrodynamically, P × F is equivalent to energy/time or power. The authors attempt to show that "efficient" obstructed bladders are compensated and "inefficient" obstructed bladders are decompensated. However, there is a great deal of overlap between the two groups and "voiding efficiency" seems as poor a measurement of bladder compensation as is residual urine determination.—Carl A. Olsson] ◀

Effect of Oral Bethanechol Chloride on the Cystometrogram of the Normal Male Adult. Bethanechol chloride may be useful in alleviating postoperative urinary retention and in treating chronic hypotonic bladder dysfunction. The drug is most effective when given subcutaneously in doses of 5–10 mg; its efficacy when used orally has been documented mainly by anecdotal case reports. Alan J. Wein, Philip M. Hanno, Dennis O. Dixon, David M. Raezer and George S. Benson[5] (Univ. of Pennsylvania) studied the effects of different oral doses of bethanechol chloride on the cystometrograms of 20 men aged 18–70 with normal bladder function. Drug efficacy was assessed by carbon dioxide cystometry. Patients received placebo or bethanechol chloride in a dose of 25, 50 or 100 mg. Two cystometric sessions were held at least 18 hours apart in a double-blind design. Cystometry was done at intervals from 1 to 4 hours after drug administration.

No significant dose-response relationship was found for any parameter. The presence of a voluntary detrusor contraction and its cystometric height did not appear to be influenced by bethanechol administration. It was not possible

(5) J. Urol. 120:330–331, September, 1978.

to determine whether a given patient received bethanechol or placebo or to distinguish between different drug doses. No significant side effects were observed in any patient given bethanechol.

Oral bethanechol chloride in doses up to 100 mg does not significantly affect the CO_2 cystometrogram of the normal adult male. It cannot, however, be concluded from these findings that the doses used have no effect on the smooth muscle of the bladder of a normal male subject. A study that uses simultaneous measurements of intravesical pressure, urinary flow and urethral resistance as comparative parameters is needed to determine whether oral bethanechol chloride affects voiding beneficially.

▶ [Objective analyses of drug effectiveness are long overdue in the growing field of "uropharmacology." This excellent double-blind study demonstrated that bethanechol chloride, administered orally, had no definite effect on cystometrograms in a population of normal men. This study should be repeated in patients with neurogenic bladder dysfunction, since the *denervated* bladder may respond differently. However, the study does lend support to increasing skepticism regarding the usefulness of bethanechol. Our experience has been that, while bethanechol injection may induce voiding in patients with short-term urinary retention (post-operative), we rarely achieve correction of true neuropathic voiding dysfunction with oral bethanechol alone.—Carl A. Olsson] ◀

Comparative Study of Water Cystometry and CO_2 Cystometry. J. Nordling, S. Hebjørn, S. Walter, T. Hald and H. D. Christiansen[6] (Univ. of Copenhagen) compared the results of medium-fill water cystometry and rapid-fill CO_2 cystometry in 102 consecutive patients (64 women) with a mean age of 56 years. Water cystometry was performed at an inflow rate of body-warm saline of about 30 ml per minute. Carbon dioxide cystometry was carried out through the same Foley catheter at a constant inflow rate of 200 ml per minute. Representative results are shown in Figures 48 and 49. The cystometric diagnoses were identical in 90 cases and different to a clinically relevant degree in 3. Three patients exhibited detrusor hyperreflexia on water cystometry and normal results with CO_2. Four patients had high-compliance, and 4 had low-compliance bladders. Compliances in these patients were 21 ± 5.3 by water cystometry and 20 ± 15 by CO_2 cystometry.

Carbon dioxide cystometry gives results as valid as those

(6) Urol. Int. 33:60–67, 1978.

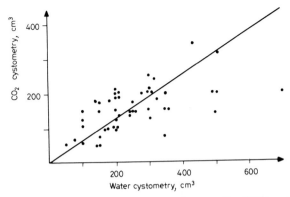

Fig 48.—Corresponding values of volume at first sensation (FS) to void in patients with normal cystometrograms. Straight line is graphic expression of converting formula: FS at CO_2 cystometry = 0.64 × FS at water cystometry. (Courtesy of Nordling, J., et al.: Urol. Int. 33:60–67, 1978.)

Fig 49.—Corresponding values of cystometric bladder capacity in patients with normal cystometrograms. Straight line is graphic expression of converting formula: capacity at CO_2 cystometry = 0.73 × capacity at water cystometry. (Courtesy of Nordling, J., et al.: Urol. Int. 33:60–67, 1978.)

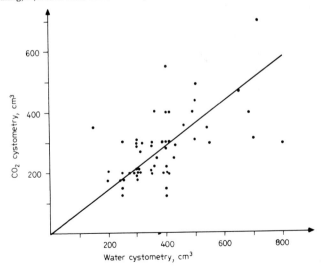

of water cystometry. Volumes at first desire to void, bladder capacity and bladder compliance are about 50% higher on water cystometry in normal subjects. In cases of detrusor hyperreflexia, no important differences in bladder volume at first uninhibited detrusor contraction or in highest intravesical pressure during detrusor contraction are observed. The lower sensitivity of CO_2 cystometry in demonstration of detrusor hyperreflexia is marginal. Carbon dioxide cystometry is easy and very timesaving. Total filling times are about $13^{1}/_2$ hours with water and about $2^{1}/_2$ hours with CO_2. Rapid-filling CO_2 cystometry is an entirely satisfactory method when compared with conventional water cystometry.

▶ [This is an excellent study showing nearly 100% diagnostic correlation between the two forms of cystometry. Therefore, the convenience of gas cystometry is achieved without any alteration in diagnostic accuracy. It should be emphasized that individual cystometric parameters are different with the two techniques, and this should be borne in mind when carrying out sequential cystometric evaluations in individual patients at various times during the course of their disease or therapy.—Carl A. Olsson] ◀

Effect on Bladder Pressure of Sudden Entry of Fluid into the Posterior Urethra. The possibility that entry of fluid into the urethra may initiate bladder contraction has been controversial for over a century. The stimulus for opening of the bladder neck after a detrusor contraction in the unstable bladder has not been clearly identified. Stimulation of stretch receptors in the bladder wall or visceral peritoneum by the rise in intraabdominal pressure has been postulated.

J. R. Sutherst and M. Brown[7] (Univ. of Liverpool) attempted to determine whether fluid entering the posterior urethra causes reflex contraction of the bladder. In 50 consecutive female patients with a mean age of 51 years, continuous medium-fill cystometry was performed with the patient supine, normal saline at 37 C being instilled at a rate of 50 ml/minute. An attempt was made to provoke detrusor contraction by asking the patient to cough while standing with a full bladder. Forty-two patients were studied because of incontinence.

In no case did any change in intrinsic bladder pressure follow the injection of saline, even when detrusor contrac-

(7) Br. J. Urol. 50:406–409, October, 1978.

tions had been provoked by cystometry alone. Forty-three patients reported feeling the injection, but 31 of these reported a slight "pricking" sensation or a "pins and needles" feeling. The sensation was the same when the bladder was full to capacity as when its volume had been reduced to 150 ml. Twelve patients considered the injection painful. Seven of these and also 3 patients without pain on saline injection were shown to have urethritis.

Whatever the type of urinary incontinence in the female, entry of fluid into the posterior urethra does not cause any detrusor activity. The bladder remains stable despite rapid injection of a considerable volume of fluid. The concept that fluid in the posterior urethra initiates the micturition reflex appears to be either unfounded or not important when assessing patients for treatment.

▶ [This study addresses an important question regarding the etiology of bladder instability in the female. It is known that a variable percentage of females with urethral insufficiency also have bladder instability which is often reversed following urethral suspension. Does the entry of fluid into the proximal urethra result in detrusor contraction in these women? This study clearly demonstrates that entry of fluid into the posterior urethra is *not* responsible for the initiation of detrusor activity.—Carl A. Olsson] ◀

Urethral Pressure Profilometry: Assessment of Urethral Function by Combined Intraurethral Pressure and EMG Recording. Jens T. Andersen and William E. Bradley[8] (Univ. of Minnesota) studied the effect of the somatic innervated urethral sphincter on segmental intraurethral pressures by combining urethral pressure profilometry with intraurethral recording of electromyographic (EMG) activity of the striated periurethral musculature. Special silicone rubber catheters were used. The functional profile length (FPL) and maximum urethral closure pressure (MUCP) were the parameters of clinical interest. Carbon dioxide was infused at a rate of 150 ml per minute.

The female urethral pressure profile assumes a parabolic shape (Fig 50), whereas the male profile exhibits a plateau-like rise throughout the prostatic urethra before the MUCP is reached at the membranous urethra (Fig 51). In patients with sphincter spasticity due to cord injury, high MUCPs are recorded with concurrent, widespread, high EMG activity at the area of the MUCP. A significant re-

(8)   Urol. Int. 33:40–49, 1978.

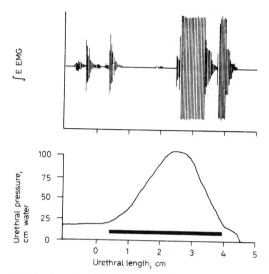

Fig 50.—Combined urethral EMG and CO_2 pressure profile from healthy female. Bar indicates functional profile length. Pressure profile has almost parabolic shape and maximal EMG activity is found at membranous urethra. (Courtesy of Andersen, J. T., and Bradley, W. E.: Urol. Int. 33:40–49, 1978.)

Fig 51.—Combined EMG and CO_2 urethral pressure profile in healthy male. Bar indicates functional profile length. Contour of male pressure profile is completely different from that of female profile. (Courtesy of Andersen, J. T., and Bradley, W. E.: Urol. Int. 33:40–49, 1978.)

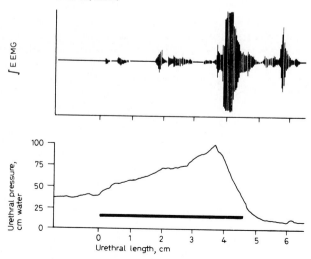

duction in the MUCP and a decrease in the periurethral
EMG follow sphincterotomy. Prostatic enlargement causes
an increase in the FPL with no significant change in the
MUCP. In primary stress incontinence in females, shortening of the FPL and a decrease in MUCP are apparent.
After fiber tape suspension of the urethra, the most consistent finding is an increase in FPL with a variable increase
in the MUCP (Fig 52). Some patients with primary stress
incontinence have normal profile parameters with an
empty bladder, but marked reductions in MUCP with a

Fig 52.—*A,* combined EMG-CO_2 pressure profile from female with primary
stress incontinence. Note low maximal urethral closure pressure and sparse EMG
activity. *B,* combined profile from same patient after bladder neck suspension.
Functional length is increased. Bars indicate functional profile length. (Courtesy of
Andersen, J. T., and Bradley, W. E.: Urol. Int. 33:40–49, 1978.)

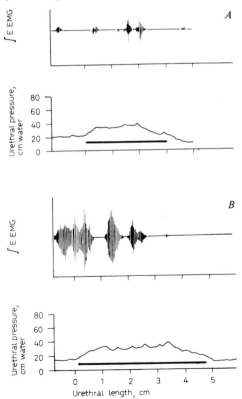

CLINICAL APPLICATIONS OF COMBINED URETHRAL EMG AND CO_2 PRESSURE PROFILOMETRY

Neurogenic dysfunction of the periurethral striated sphincter
  Pelvic floor spasticity

Anatomical urethral dysfunction
  Stress incontinence
  BPH/bladder neck obstruction
  Post-prostatectomy incontinence
  Post-TURP incontinence
  Posttraumatic incontinence

Control of therapy
  External spincterotomy
  Artifical urinary sphincter
  Pharmacological treatment

---

bladder volume of 150 ml CO_2. Only half the patients tested with phentolamine showed a reduction in the proximal part of the pressure profile. An increase in EMG activity in the proximal urethra was seen in patients who responded to α-adrenergic blockade. This had no effect on the intraurethral pressure.

Clinical applications of these studies are summarized in the table. The studies have principal diagnostic value in neurogenic and anastomical disturbances of urethral function. The studies are also of use in controlling surgical, prosthetic or pharmacologic treatment of urethral disorders. Microdrip transducers may eliminate the need for catheter infusion.

▶ [This contribution suffers from the same problem inherent in any study of infusion urethral pressure profilometry. Bladder filling has a definite effect on urethral pressure measurement, at least in individuals with detrusor hyperreflexia. It should be pointed out that there is another school of thought regarding urethral pressure studies in patients with stress urinary incontinence. Such studies carried out by microtransducer technique (without infusion) show no difference in urethral pressure profilometry (UPP) parameters before and after successful urethral suspension operations. Thus, the preoperative decrease in MUCP and shortening of FPL reported by these and other authors with infusion UPP may represent artifacts caused by bladder filling in patients with unstable bladders. The concept that sphincterotomy results in decreased periurethral EMG activity is new to us. This finding reported by the authors may also be artifactual, relating to poor contact of the surface electrodes with the urethral wall following sphincter incision.–Carl A. Olsson] ◀

MISCELLANEOUS

Urologic Aspects of Vesicoenteric Fistulas. Culley C. Carson, Reza S. Malek and William H. Remine[9] (Mayo Clinic and Found.) reviewed 100 consecutive cases of vesicoenteric fistula seen during 1967–74. The 71 men and 29 women had a mean age of 58 years. Symptoms had been present for a mean of 14 months. All patients had microhematuria and leukocyturia. Urine culture in 96 showed significant urinary tract infection in 91. *Escherichia coli* was the most common offender.

Roentgenologic studies showing air or barium in the bladder or contrast medium in the bowel suggested a fistula (Table 1). The cystoscopic findings are given in Table 2. The cause of fistulization was colonic diverticulitis in 51% of the patients, colorectal adenocarcinoma in 16%, Crohn's disease in 12% and bladder carcinoma in 5%.

TABLE 1.—ROENTGENOLOGIC PROCEDURES

	Suggestive of Fistula %
Cystogram	35
Upper gastrointestinal series	21
Barium enema	20
IVP	18
Plain abdominal film	2

TABLE 2.—CYSTOSCOPIC FINDINGS IN 87 PATIENTS

	No. Pts.
Fistula	28
Localized inflammation	14
Bullous edema	13
Feces	10
Erythema	9
Particulate matter	9
Granulation tissue	8
Cystitis	5
Mass	4
Other	4
Normal	20

(9) J. Urol. 119:744–746, June, 1978.

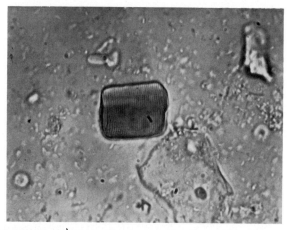

Fig 53.—Undigested muscle fiber in urine of patient with fistula. Note characteristic striations of rhabdomyocyte. (Courtesy of Carson, C. C., et al.: J. Urol. 119:744–746, June, 1978.)

All but 5 patients were treated surgically. About two thirds of those with inflammatory bowel disease had a one-stage bowel resection and fistula closure. Most of the other third had a two-stage procedure: bowel resection and diverting colostomy followed by restoration of bowel continuity. Seven patients died postoperatively, and 9 had major complications. Of 93 patients followed for a mean of 44 months, 6 (6.5%) had recurrent fistulas. Three of these patients had Crohn's disease, and 3 had carcinoma of the prostate, colon or endometrium.

Vesicoenteric fistula is so rare that it is often overlooked. Routine urinalysis may occasionally show characteristically striated muscle fibers (rhabdomyocytes) from undigested food residue in these patients (Fig 53). Retrograde or voiding cystography seems to be more successful than intravenous pyelography in demonstrating the fistulous communication. Thorough cystoscopy has been the most successful diagnostic procedure. Results of surgery have been most gratifying. Neoplastic fistulas do not imply a hopeless prognosis. Surgical intervention is indicated in clinically operable patients with vesicoenteric fistula.

▶ [This very large series provides a wealth of information about the presentation, evaluation and treatment of vesicoureteric fistulas. The surgical results are excellent. However, occasionally patients may resolve fistulas without operation if they are treated by oral and/or intravenous hyperalimentation.–S.S.H.] ◄

How to Manage Colovesical Fistula. F. D. Nemer, T. H. Sweetser, Jr., S. M. Goldberg, E. G. Balcos, J. L. Schottler and C. E. Christenson[1] (Univ. of Minnesota) reviewed information on 16 men and 10 women who were operated on for colovesical fistula. Diverticular disease was responsible in 18 cases. The predominant features were fecaluria, terminal pneumaturia and chronic urinary tract infection. Cystoscopy demonstrated 16 of 22 fistulas and cystography, 8 of 22. Proctosigmoidoscopy was diagnostic in 4 cases and pyelography in 3. Barium enema study showed the fistula in only 3 cases.

Two patients died during emergency operation. One had peritoneal carcinomatosis and 1 died of sepsis and hypovolemia shortly after transverse colostomy. Seven patients had staged procedures, with good results. There were no deaths and only one major complication, small bowel obstruction. No deaths or complications occurred among the 17 patients having one-stage resection. The techniques used included wide local excision of the tract and surrounding bladder wall, simple excision of the fistula and closure of the bladder with running or interrupted sutures. No patient had leakage of the bladder closure. Ureteral catheters were routinely used to aid in difficult pelvic dissections. Bladder continuity was tested by instillation of saline-methylene blue solution.

The choice of a one-stage or multiple-stage procedure for colovesical fistula depends on the cause and extent of disease, the degree of bowel obstruction and the presence of systemic toxicity from bladder, intestinal or peritoneal infection. A conservative approach is used in dealing with an extracolonic pelvic collection or extensive inflammatory involvement of other pelvic viscera. An aggressive single-stage approach is recommended for patients with a nonobstructed, well-prepared colon, a mature fistulous tract and no systemic toxicity.

► [This article as well as the preceding one points out that the majority of colovesical fistulas can be repaired with a one-stage operation, but in complicated situations a two-stage procedure is preferable.–S.S.H.] ◄

(1) Geriatrics 33:86–87, October, 1978.

Exstrophy of the Bladder: Treatment by Trigonosigmoidostomy—Long-Term Results. W. Gregoir and C. C. Schulman[2] (Brussels, Belgium) reviewed the results of treatment of bladder exstrophy by trigonosigmoidostomy in 25 patients. There were 2 female patients in the series, and the average age was 6 years. The average follow-up period was 10 years. The operation was done as primary treatment in 23 patients and after failure of attempted bladder reconstruction in 2. Indications included a normal pyelogram and competent anal sphincter and the absence of reflux. The vesical trigone is implanted in the sigmoid colon without any cutaneous diversion.

Urography has been the most valuable postoperative study. Two patients had renal stones, which in 1 patient caused ureteric obstruction. Another patient experienced bilateral hydronephrosis and severe parenchymal infection due to reflux. About half the patients had transient hyperchloremia and a reduction in bicarbonate. The rate of infection was surprisingly low; antibiotics were administered for only a short period. Two patients required additional surgical treatment. Most patients were incontinent at night for several months postoperatively. One patient died of ruptured esophageal varices, and 1 was a complete failure. There were 18 good, and 4 satisfactory, results. Patients with good results were free from symptoms and led normal social lives. The adults are gainfully employed and some are married. All are perfectly continent.

Trigonosigmoidostomy is an acceptable compromise for patients with bladder exstrophy. The results seem to be more favorable than those obtained with a conventional ureterosigmoidostomy as far as clinical status, renal function and infection are concerned. Three fourths of the present patients had excellent results after a single operation.

▶ [If the bladder is of reasonable size, we prefer to attempt a primary closure as early in life as possible with a secondary operation for continence as described by Jeffs, and Fisher and Retik. However if this treatment fails and diversion is necessary either trigonosigmoidostomy or the Boyce-Vest procedure described at our institution and recently reviewed by Boyce produces very satisfactory results, probably because of the preservation of the ureterovesical junction.–S.S.H.] ◀

Psychiatric Aspects of Recurrent Cystitis in Women. It has long been recognized that a number of

(2) Br. J. Urol. 50:90–94, April, 1978.

women presenting with recurrent cystitis have psychiatric symptoms. D. L. P. Rees and N. Farhoumand[3] (London) studied 207 women urologically for recurrent attacks of dysuria and increased frequency of micturition, after excluding subjects with major urographic abnormalities. Of the 207 patients, 50 were successive unselected admissions; these patients also underwent detailed psychiatric assessment and were the subject of this study. The mean patient age was 34.5 years. The tests included the Eysenck Personality Questionnaire, the Morbid Anxiety Inventory and the Middlesex Hospital Questionnaire. Bladder instability was demonstrated in 7 patients, and 8 others had end-filling pressures of 15 cm water or more without uninhibited detrusor contractions. Eleven patients had inhibited micturition, 3 had bladder outlet obstruction and 10 had a low detrusor voiding pressure. Bacteriuria was established in 14 patients. Twenty-two patients reported dyspareunia.

The study patients exhibited more anxiety, obsessionality and somatization than normal subjects at significant levels but did not differ significantly in depression or neuroticism. Anxiety was even greater in patients with bladder instability. Patients with low detrusor voiding pressure had significantly less anxiety than the other subgroups. Scores for hysterical traits and obsessionality were increased in the group with dyspareunia. Neuroticism scores were high in patients with bladder outlet obstruction and in those with dyspareunia. Interviews indicated that about a third of the patients had had anxiety and/or depression before the onset of micturitional symptoms. Only one fourth of patients were free from psychiatric symptoms at all times.

The most striking finding in this study is the high prevalence of anxiety in women with recurrent cystitis. The findings suggest a direct link between anxiety and voiding pressure. Recognition of the psychologic and psychiatric factors present in women with recurrent cystitis will permit a more balanced, sympathetic and fruitful approach to be made to these patients.

▶ [Since many women with the "urethral syndrome" are included in this study, it is hardly surprising that these patients exhibited more anxiety and somatization than normal subjects. It is interesting that they were not de-

(3) Br. J. Urol. 49:651–658, 1977.

pressed or neurotic. This suggests that reassurance and other treatment aimed at relieving anxiety will benefit these women and that excessive diagnostic studies and treatment measures may increase their anxiety and thus perpetuate the disease.–S.S.H.] ◄

Interstitial Cystitis: Early Diagnosis, Pathology and Treatment. Edward M. Messing and Thomas A. Stamey[4] (Stanford Univ.) reviewed the findings in 52 patients seen in the past 12 years with interstitial cystitis who had cystoscopy with anesthesia. Twenty-eight patients had early lesions on the basis of bladder capacity and 24 had classic lesions. Thirty-eight patients had bladder biopsy with a resectoscope and bladder tissue from 7 patients and 3 controls was evaluated by immunofluorescence methods.

The classic symptoms of interstitial cystitis are continual frequency, urgency and suprapubic pain. Cystoscopy shows a reduced bladder capacity and a Hunner's ulcer. It is not clear, however, whether reduced bladder capacity is essential. Most patients do not have a Hunner's ulcer. Pinpoint petechial hemorrhages are seen throughout the vesical mucosa on the second distention of the bladder. They are generally most prominent on the dome, posterior wall and side walls of the bladder, rarely on the trigone. These lesions rarely occur in patients with normal bladders. The irrigating fluid is clear when emptied after the first distention but becomes blood-tinged in its terminal 50–100 ml. Urinalysis and tests of immune function are of little diagnostic value and the histologic findings are not significantly helpful. Nonspecific submucosal edema and vasodilatation and "pancystitis" are inconsistent findings, even in bladders with classic cystoscopic findings.

Impressive results have been obtained with use of 0.4% oxychlorosene sodium (Clorpactin WCS-90), given in a dose of 1 L at repeated instillations. Full anesthesia is necessary at first. Surgery is indicated only after conservative measures have been exhausted. Over two thirds of patients have become symptom free or nearly so for at least 6 months after the final instillation. One third of successes required only one instillation of oxychlorosene sodium. However, some of the benefits of the therapy must be attributed to hydraulic distention. Severe irritative symptoms may occur for up to 48 hours after instillations. The

(4) Urology 12:381–392, October, 1978.

presently preferred surgical procedure is cecocystoplasty with supratrigonal cystectomy but is not always successful. The only certain method for total relief is supravesical urinary diversion, with or without cystectomy.

▶ [This review points out that one of the problems in understanding interstitial cystitis is that we lack definitive diagnostic criteria. Various published series obviously include different types of patients. Nevertheless, the authors' encouraging results with Clorpactin WCS-90 suggest that this compound may benefit some of these patients.–S.S.H.] ◀

Dimethyl Sulfoxide in Treatment of Inflammatory Genitourinary Disorders. Symptomatic relief has been reported with intravesical dimethyl sulfoxide (DMSO) therapy in about two thirds of patients with classic interstitial cystitis. Sheridan W. Shirley, Bruce H. Stewart and Simon Mirelman[5] reviewed the findings in 213 patients in whom intravesical DMSO was used to treat various inflammatory states of the lower genitourinary tract. A 50-cc volume of 50% DMSO was instilled into the bladder under local urethral lubricant analgesia in the office. A small catheter was used in most instances. Treatments were repeated as needed to control symptoms. Patients with chronic prostatitis had the solution instilled directly into the prostatic urethra and then into the bladder. Intravesical DMSO therapy was used in 100 women with classic chronic interstitial cystitis refractory to conventional therapy; 31 women with intractable bladder irritative symptoms; 14 men with chronic interstitial cystitis; 12 patients with radiation cystitis; and 35 with atypical chronic prostatitis.

The results in women with chronic interstitial cystitis are given in the table. Good to excellent clinical results were obtained in over half the patients, and objective endoscopic improvement was noted in about 85% of all patients. Nine of 14 male patients with chronic interstitial cystitis had good to excellent symptomatic relief and continued on therapy. Five of 12 patients with radiation cystitis gained significant relief. Symptomatic relief was substantial in 75% of male patients with chronic prostatitis. Seventy-four percent of women with atypical chronic cystitis had good to excellent symptomatic relief and remain on therapy. Two of 3 other male patients with atypical in-

(5) Urology 11:215–220, March, 1978.

CHRONIC INTERSTITIAL CYSTITIS—FEMALE:
SYMPTOMATIC RESPONSE TO INTRAVESICAL DMSO*

Type of Response	Ohio	Number Alabama	Total	Percentage	
Excellent	7	14	21	27	54
Good	12	9	21	27	
Fair	3	2	5	6	35
Poor	9	14	23	29	
Relapse	3	6	9	11	11

*Seventy-nine patients treated: 34 in Ohio and 45 in Alabama.

flammation of the bladder had a good response to DMSO therapy. Three female children with chronic inflammatory changes in the trigone and proximal urethra had good results from intermittent intravesical DMSO therapy.

Intravesical DMSO therapy has given significant symptomatic relief in most patients with troublesome genitourinary disorders. No systemic or local toxicity has been observed. This treatment is recommended for patients who have failed to respond to conventional therapy or who present with severe symptoms secondary to chronic inflammatory conditions.

Use of Dimethyl Sulfoxide (DMSO) in Treatment of Interstitial Cystitis. Interstitial cystitis is an uncommon but extremely troublesome condition characterized by intense suprapubic pain and urgency relieved only temporarily by voiding. A. Ek, A. Engberg, L. Frödin and G. Jönsson[6] evaluated dimethyl sulfoxide treatment in 16 women and 1 man aged 30–80 years who had had interstitial cystitis for a mean of 7.5 years. Most of the patients had responded poorly to other conservative treatments. Mean bladder capacity was 189 ml. Instillations generally were done as outpatient procedures with a small-caliber ureteral catheter. A volume of 50 ml of a sterile 50% DMSO solution in water was instilled for 15 minutes into the empty bladder and followed by voiding. Treatment was repeated on alternate weeks; an average of four treatments was given. There were no serious adverse effects.

(6) Scand. J. Urol. Nephrol. 12:129–131, 1978.

On follow-up for $1^{1}/_{2}$–4 years, 5 patients failed to respond and underwent cystolysis or cystoplasty. Twelve reported nearly dramatic improvement after the second DMSO treatment. Pain ceased and micturition frequency was drastically reduced. Three patients had another course of treatments, and 3 underwent cystolysis after having improved 4–7 months after the first treatment. Two other patients responded for 2–4 months and then underwent cystolysis; 1 had only modest improvement after a further course and 1 had ocular symptoms. The cystoscopic findings did not change despite definite subjective improvement. Bladder capacity increased moderately in 2 patients.

Symptoms of interstitial cystitis were controlled by DMSO instillations in two thirds of these patients, but repeated treatment was necessary. Therapy with DMSO is worth trying; in some cases it has a dramatic and lasting effect. Instillations should particularly be considered in older patients and when other conservative treatments fail. Cataract is an absolute contraindication. Patients should avoid alcoholic beverages for 2 days after an instillation.

▶ [These reports support a trial of DMSO in patients with interstitial cystitis. In some patients, DMSO seems to relieve pain associated with bladder distension which in turn allows capacity to increase. Bladders that are contracted due to fibrosis do not enlarge. Worth and Warwick, who described the operation, feel that cystolysis is effective in sensory but not motor vesical disorders (Proc. Am. Assoc. Genitourin. Surg., in press).–S.S.H.] ◀

Interstitial Cystitis, Treated by Prolonged Bladder Distension. The cause of interstitial cystitis remains unknown. Many major operative procedures carrying significant morbidity have been described, and the overall results are disappointing. The benefit from vesical distension has been short-lived. M. Dunn, P. D. Ramsden, J. B. M. Roberts, J. C. Smith and P. J. B. Smith[7] evaluated prolonged bladder distension under epidural anesthesia in 25 patients (22 women and 3 men, with a mean age of 65.5 years) with severe frequency, nocturia and suprapubic pain, a sterile urine and normal urogram and small hemorrhagic patches and linear ulcers with a small bladder capacity at cystoscopy. The mean duration of symptoms was 5 years. Conventional treatment had failed in all patients. The bladder was distended to the systolic blood pressure

(7) Br. J. Urol. 49:641–645, 1977.

| | PAIN AND URGENCY | |
	Before prolonged bladder distension	After prolonged bladder distension
Pain		
Suprapubic	22	6
Urethral	17	5
Urgency		
None	11	22
Moderate	14	3

level with an 18 Ch Latex catheter for 1–3 hours. Distension lasted 3 hours in most patients.

The mean initial bladder capacity was 151 ml, and the mean capacity at the end of distension was 450 ml. The mean capacity at cystometry done 3–6 months later was 278 ml. Changes in symptoms are shown in the table. Sixteen patients were free from symptoms at most recent follow-up, a mean of 14 months after the procedure. Five had had at least one previous prolonged bladder distension. Six patients were symptomatically improved, and 1 of these patients had had a previous distension. Three patients did not improve. Two patients had bladder rupture during prolonged distension and underwent urethral catheter drainage for 10 days. Both these patients have done well.

Prolonged bladder distension appears to be useful in the management of patients with interstitial cystitis. It is a relatively simple procedure with few complications. Since bladder carcinoma may present with the same symptoms and similar cystoscopic changes, biopsy examination of the affected areas is vital in each patient to exclude multifocal submucosal carcinoma.

▶ [Prolonged distension is yet another method to treat this difficult problem. In addition to the treatments outlined in the preceding articles we have used nerve blocks, alcohol injection of the trigone and systemic steroids. Although all treatments improved some patients, none of them is a panacea. The severe problems may still require cystoplasty or diversion.–S.S.H.] ◀

Follow-up of Abdominal Neourethra. Jack Lapides[8] (Univ. of Michigan) has found abdominal neourethrostomy

(8) J. Urol. 119:219–222, February, 1978.

to be a highly satisfactory urinary diversion procedure for patients with irreparable urethral stricture or destruction.

TECHNIQUE.—A 5×5-cm bladder flap is created through a transverse abdominal incision, with the base 1–2 cm wider than the apex in the region of the bladder dome. The flap edges are joined to each other to form a tube, and a 1.5-cm spatulated end is left for later incorporation of a skin flap. The site for the skin flap and stoma of the neourethra should be in an area free of scar and folds, and the stoma should be placed as high as possible on the abdominal wall without tension being present. The skin flap measures 1.5×1.5 cm. The stoma can be placed in the midline or laterally. The skin flap is sutured to the spatulated end of the neourethra with moderately fine chromic gut. A de Pezzer catheter is placed in the bladder through a stab wound before the bladder is closed. The perivesical space is drained. Cystostomy drainage is continued for 2–3 weeks.

Seven patients were followed for 8 years or more after this procedure. The 5 men and 2 women were aged 15–40 years at the time of surgery. Four men had severe posterior urethral strictures from pelvic and urethral trauma, and 1 had a large atonic bladder of unknown etiology. The women had total incontinence after multiple operations. All the patients can now maintain continence for 2–4 hours during the day and throughout the night. Incontinence occurs only when the bladder is permitted to overdistend. When no device is used, the patient can void while sitting or standing, holding tissue under the stoma to prevent soiling. No pyelonephritis has occurred despite episodes of bacteriuria and pyuria in each case. Renal function has remained normal. One patient required revision of the stoma, and in 1 a perivesical abscess and vesicocutaneous fistula developed in the retropubic area. All surviving men are employed and married, and the women are housewives with families.

Abdominal neourethrostomy is worthy of serious consideration as a means of urinary diversion, particularly in patients with a normally functioning bladder who have lost use of the urethra. Creation of a larger skin flap will help avoid too narrow a meatus.

▶ [The author's excellent long-term results including day and night continence suggest that this procedure might be useful in selected patients. In our experience with cutaneous vesicostomy and anterior transposition of the urethra, renal function is well preserved because the ureterovesical junctions are intact. However, our patients have been incontinent which may be related to differences in surgical technique.–S.S.H.] ◀

Clinical Significance of Cystitis Cystica in Girls: Results of a Prospective Study. About 10% of patients with lower urinary tract infection have endoscopic changes of cystitis cystica. A. Barry Belman[9] (Northwestern Univ.) evaluated girls with otherwise normal urinary tracts when cystoscopy showed evidence of cystitis cystica. Alternate children were treated with 25–50 mg nitrofurantoin and 0.5–1 gm sulfisoxazole 3 times daily. Three patients with mild bladder changes were placed on 6 months of continuous treatment, while 19 with more marked changes were assigned to 1 year of treatment. Nineteen patients completed all phases of the study.

Only 3 of 9 patients with significant daytime wetting before urine sterilization became dry with treatment. Cystitis cystica persisted in 5 cases (24%) despite a year of continuous treatment, but marked improvement was noted in all cases. Persistent cystitis was not noted in any mild case. Control of recurrent bacteriuria and pyuria was excellent. Eight patients who were clear endoscopically at follow-up were reinfected within 1 year, most of them within 3 months of discontinuance of treatment. Similar results were obtained with nitrofurantoin and sulfisoxazole therapy. Abdominal discomfort resolved completely in nearly all affected patients.

Early diagnosis of urinary tract infection by culture in infancy may be the only means of preventing bladder changes. The kidneys do not appear to be threatened by this problem; urinary control and abdominal discomfort are the chief clinical problems. Treatment will resolve the discomfort, but wetting is best managed by bladder retraining. The use of an anticholinergic often is needed in addition to a regulated voiding schedule. If urinary infection is recognized in infancy, prevention of all these problems may be possible.

▶ [This study suggests that cystitis cystica responds to long-term antibacterial therapy although lesions may persist in severe cases. Unfortunately, since there was no untreated control group, it is not possible to determine whether the same results would have been obtained if the patients had been treated only for acute infections.–S.S.H.] ◀

(9)   J. Urol. 119:661–663, May, 1978.

The following review articles are recommended to the reader:

Bartholomew, T. H., and Gonzales, E. T.: Urologic management in cloacal dysgenesis, Urology 11:549, 1978.

Bradley, W. E.: Autonomic neuropathy and genitourinary system, J. Urol. 119:299, 1978.

Fletcher, T. F., and Bradley, W. E.: Neuroanatomy of the bladder-urethra, J. Urol. 119:153, 1978.

Pers, M.: The closure of urinary-vaginal fistulas, Scand. J. Plast. Reconstr. Surg. 11:147, 1977.

The Prostate

CARCINOMA

Cohort Mortality for Prostatic Cancer among United States Nonwhites is discussed by Virginia L. Ernster, Steve Selvin and Warren Winkelstein, Jr.[1] (Univ. of California, Berkeley). The occurrence of prostatic cancer in blacks is substantially higher than in whites in the United States, without relation to readily identifiable factors associated with socioeconomic status. Age-adjusted incidence and mortality rates have increased dramatically for blacks in the United States over the past few decades (Fig 54). The relative increase in rates for nonwhites and the decrease in rates for whites since 1940 have been essentially constant. Analysis of mortality rates in men aged

Fig 54.—Annual age-adjusted prostatic cancer mortality rates per 100,000 United States male patients aged 45–84 years. The data are separated for whites and nonwhites, and a computed rate is shown for nonwhites. The rates are shown at 5-year intervals from 1930 to 1970 and are adjusted to the 1950 United States male population aged 45–84 years. (Courtesy of Ernster, V. L., et al.: Science 200:1165–1166, June 9, 1978.)

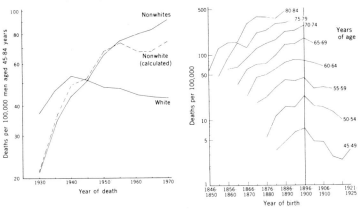

(1)   Science 200:1165–1166, June 9, 1978.

45–84 years from 1846 to 1925 showed a consistent increase in rates for all age groups in cohorts born before 1896–1900 and a fairly consistent decline for those born after this time. Analysis of variance indicated that the cohort effect was nonrandom. No such generational pattern is evident in analyzing mortality data for whites.

These findings presage an arrest and reversal of the time trend in mortality rates as more recent nonwhite cohorts reach the ages of maximal risk. Research into the historical experience of the 1896–1900 and earlier nonwhite birth cohorts might provide clues to agents associated with prostatic cancer, although the amount of time will make the task a difficult one.

Solid Phase Radioimmunoassay for Prostatic Acid Phosphatase. J. Fenimore Cooper, Andras Foti, Harvey H. Herschman and William Finkle[2] compared the sensitivity of a recently developed solid phase radioimmunoassay for human prostatic acid phosphatase with that of an enzymatic method with the use of p-nitrophenylphosphate as substrate. The assays were compared in 109 patients with histologically verified, untreated stages I–IV prostatic cancer and 200 men without such cancer. Forty-four patients had stage I or II intraprostatic carcinomas, and 65 had stage III or IV extraprostatic carcinomas. Serums from 53 elderly men with benign prostatic hyperplasia were also evaluated. Antiserum was produced in rabbits with puri-

FREQUENCY OF CORRECT CLASSIFICATION OF CANCER AND STATISTICAL ASSESSMENT OF DIFFERENCES

	No. Pts.	Correct Classification		Assessment of Differences
		Radioimmuno-assay Test No. (%)	Enzymatic Test No. (%)	p Value
Prostatic cancers	109	80 (73.3)	34 (31.1)	$<10^{-6}$
Stages I–II	44	19 (43.1)	4 (9.1)	$<10^{-3}$
Stages III–IV	65	61 (93.8)	30 (46.1)	$<10^{-6}$
Non-prostatic Ca	90	85 (94.4)	66 (73.3)	$<10^{-4}$
Normal male sera	200	189 (94.4)	193 (96.5)	—

(2) J. Urol. 119:388–391, March, 1978.

fied prostatic acid phosphatase from healthy men and complete adjuvant for use in the assay.

The results are given in the table. The radioimmunoassay was substantially more sensitive and specific than the enzymatic technique. The radioimmunoassay method correctly classified 73% of the prostatic malignancies, compared with 31% for the enzymatic technique. The respective figures for stages I and II cancers were 43 and 9.1% and for the stages III and IV cancers, 94 and 46%. False positive results were obtained in 5.6% of 200 male controls with the radioimmunoassay and in 3.5% with the enzyme assay. Of 90 nonprostatic human cancer serums, 94.5% were classed as negative by the radioimmunoassay, and 73% by the enzymatic method. No false positive values were obtained with the enzymatic assay in the group of patients with prostatic hyperplasia, whereas the radioimmunoassay gave one marginal elevation.

The radioimmunochemical approach to determining human serum prostatic acid phosphatase appears to have distinct biochemical and clinical advantages over a standard enzymatic technique, particularly in detecting early stages I and II prostatic cancers. A prospective study of the utility of the radioimmunoassay for prostatic acid phosphatase in clinical diagnosis is being carried out.

Bone Marrow Acid Phosphatase in Staging of Prostatic Cancer: How Reliable Is It? J. Edson Pontes, B. K. Choe, N. R. Rose and J. M. Pierce, Jr.[3] (Wayne State Univ.) evaluated the reliability of bone marrow acid phosphatase in the staging of prostatic carcinoma by analyzing 50 marrow samples collected at random from a hematology service. The samples were assayed by a colorimetric method using sodium thymolphthalein monophosphate as substrate and by two immunochemical assays, counterimmunoelectrophoresis and radioimmunoassay. The authors' indirect immunofluorescence (IF) technique used a rabbit antibody to prostatic acid phosphatase and a second antibody produced in a chicken against rabbit IgG. The double-antibody technique of radioimmunoassay was used.

The 36 males and 14 females studied had a variety of hematologic disorders. Fourteen had prostatic carcinoma.

(3) J. Urol. 119:772–776, June, 1978.

The colorimetric assay gave significant elevations of marrow acid phosphatase activity in 61% of all patients. All but 1 of the positive results in patients without prostatic disease were negative by counterimmunoelectrophoresis assay; 1 lung cancer patient had a positive result. Five of the patients with prostatic carcinoma had positive colorimetric results. Eight patients, including 2 with localized prostatic cancer and negative counterimmunoelectrophoresis test results, had positive radioimmunoassay results. Three of 5 patients with positive immunologic reactions had positive marrow smears by enzymologic and IF techniques. All patients with advanced prostatic carcinoma had positive assays by all methods. The colorimetric method most consistently showed abnormality in patients with localized disease.

Immunologic methods are reliable in determining prostatic acid phosphatase levels. Determination of marrow acid phosphatase has a place among other urologic tests for the detection of metastasis in patients with prostatic carcinoma, but the methods used at present in hospitals are not specific for prostatic acid phosphatase, and spread of disease should not be assumed from the results of this test alone.

Radioimmunochemical Measurement of Bone Marrow Prostatic Acid Phosphatase. John Fenimore Cooper, Andras Gabor Foti and Paul W. Shank[4] (Kaiser Permanente Med. Center, Los Angeles) report a sensitive immunochemical method for specific measurement of prostatic acid phosphatase in bone marrow as an alternative to the unreliable standard spectrophotometric enzymatic techniques. Twenty-seven men aged 52–81 years with histologic and clinical evidence of stages A-D prostatic cancer were evaluated. Serum prostatic acid phosphatase was measured by the p-nitrophenylphosphate method and the current solid phase radioimmunoassay for bone marrow prostatic acid phosphatase. Bone marrow and serum samples from 19 men with benign prostatic hypertrophy were also evaluated. Bone marrow samples were obtained from the iliac crest or sacral prominence by needle aspiration.

Homogenized bone marrow clots and whole blood clots in

(4) J. Urol. 119:392–395, March, 1978.

TABLE 1.—Benign Prostatic Hyperplasia—19 Cases

	No. Pts.	Enzymatic-p-nitrophen-ylphosphate	Radioimmunoassay-Prostatic Acid Phosphatase
		Range (mean)	Range (mean)
Blood serum	19	0.06–0.17 units (0.10±0.05)	2.3–6.0 ng. (4.3±1.3)
Bone marrow	19	0.08–0.27 units (0.20±0.05)	4.7–15.5 ng. (9.0±3.4)
Normal male serum	200	0.05–0.20 units/ml. (0.12±0.04)	0.5–7.0 ng./0.1 ml. (4.88±0.8)

patients with benign prostatic hyperplasia demonstrated 10-fold higher levels of prostatic acid phosphatase with the enzymatic method than did bone marrow and whole blood serums. The radioimmunoassay results showed no evidence of cross-reactivity between existing prostatic acid phosphatases in the serum and the nonprostatic acid phosphatases in the whole blood cell mass. The results in benign prostatic hyperplasia are given in Table 1 and those in prostatic cancer in Table 2. The serum mean values for each method were significantly elevated in the cancer patients when compared with normal serum. The mean bone marrow levels for prostatic acid phosphatase by both assay methods were 2–3 times more elevated than the concentrations of the enzyme noted in the serum samples. A similar observation was recorded in the group of benign prostatic hyperplasia patients.

The radioimmunoassay for prostatic acid phosphatase in bone marrow and serum holds promise. The method can

TABLE 2.—Prostatic Cancer, Stages B, C and D—25 Cases

	No. Pts.	Enzymatic-p-Nitrophen-ylphosphate	Radioimmunoassay-Prostatic Acid Phosphatase
		Range (mean)	Range (mean)
Blood serum	25	0.01–14.3 units (0.75±0.15)	23–135.0 ng. (21.2±2.3)
Bone marrow	25	0.09–17.4 units (1.9±0.37)	6.0–251.0 ng. (56.3±17.6)
Normal male serum	200	0.05–0.20 units/ml. (0.12±0.04)	0.5–7.0 ng./0.1 ml. (4.88±0.5)

correctly reproducibly classify and support the clinical diagnosis of cancer in samples of bone marrow and serum in suspected patients. The immunochemical assay appears to be technically superior to the enzymatic method in analyzing bone marrow and serum samples. Disruption and hemolysis of the bone marrow cell population during sternal or iliac biopsy procedures may be responsible for the spurious results reported in the recent literature.

▶ [The three previous articles report on the use of bone marrow acid phosphatase to stage prostatic cancer. To be of value to the clinician the test must be reliable, reproducible and well controlled. The incidence of false positives and false negatives must be known. The tests must define sensitivity (probability that it is positive in patients with the disease) and specificity (probability that it is negative in patients without the disease). The chemical tests we now have are sensitive enough to detect serum levels but do not measure only prostatic acid phosphatase so false positives are seen in the bone marrow aspirates. Studies are needed to see if the additional sensitivity of the immunochemical methods will also be more specific in detecting early prostatic cancer or bone marrow metastases.

Obviously more studies are needed before, as one manufacturer suggests, "Immunochemical analysis of acid phosphatase is the equivalent in the male of the PAP test in the female."–J.Y.G.] ◀

Early-Stage Prostatic Cancer Investigated by Pelvic Lymph Node Biopsy and Bone Marrow Acid Phosphatase. Ronald W. Sadlowski[5] (Northwestern Univ.) evaluated 47 patients with early-stage prostatic cancer prospectively by pelvic adenectomy and bone marrow acid phosphatase determinations. Patients seen in 1973–76 with biopsy-proved B1, B2 or C prostatic adenocarcinoma were entered into the study. Marrow biopsies or aspirates and marrow blood for chemical analysis were generally taken from the posterior superior iliac spine.

Nodes positive for tumor were found in 5 of 21 patients with B1 lesions, 3 of 8 with B2 lesions and 5 of 18 with C lesions. There were 17 well-differentiated, 22 moderately well-differentiated and 8 poorly differentiated tumors in the series. Seven of the poorly differentiated tumors were in patients with stage C lesions. The internal iliac nodes were involved most often by metastasis. In no case was the marrow acid phosphatase level above normal, and in no case was the marrow biopsy or aspirate positive for tumor cells. The lactic dehydrogenase (LDH) V:I isoenzyme ratio in the marrow and venous blood was less than 1 in all 6

(5) J. Urol. 119:89–93, January, 1978.

patients studied. Serum and marrow calcium levels were similar in all 12 patients studied, 4 of whom had positive pelvic nodes. No consistent pattern of LDH and alkaline phosphatase in venous and bone marrow sera was observed.

Apparently, pelvic lymphadenectomy has a well-defined role in the diagnostic study of early-stage prostatic cancer, while bone marrow acid phosphatase determination is of no value. Using this protocol, excepting the bone marrow and marrow acid phosphatase aspect, one can make a more rational decision in individual patients with early-stage prostatic cancer as to whether surgery or radiotherapy is preferable.

None of the patients in this study had evidence of bone metastasis. In no case was the bone survey more sensitive than the bone scan in detecting suspicious bone lesions.

▶ [For better management of prostatic cancer it is essential to diagnose and stage it accurately. More prospective studies such as this one are needed.—J.Y.G.] ◀

Plasma Testosterone in Patients Receiving Diethylstilbestrol. Controversy over the proper dose of diethylstilbestrol (DES) to use in treating prostatic carcinoma arose when cardiovascular complications were recognized with higher doses. Phillip H. Beck, Jack W. McAninch, James L. Goebel and Ray E. Stutzman[6] (San Francisco) monitored plasma testosterone levels in patients with prostatic carcinoma given 1 mg DES daily as their only hormonal therapy and in patients receiving the same dose after orchiectomy. Sixteen patients with prostatic adenocarcinoma were studied before and after starting DES therapy. Most of these patients had previously had prostatectomy, radiotherapy, or both. In all patients the diagnosis was proved histologically. Plasma testosterone was measured by radioimmunoassay.

Normal men and carcinoma patients had similar plasma testosterone levels initially. Patients above and below age 60 also had similar levels. Patients on DES and castrated patients showed a marked depression of plasma testosterone (Fig 55). Patients treated for less than 6 months had a mean plasma testosterone level of 69 ng/dl, compared with 80 ng/dl for those studied after 6–12 months of therapy.

(6) Urology 11:157–160, February, 1978.

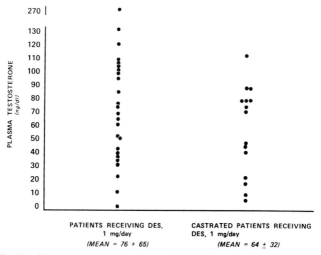

Fig 55.—Plasma testosterone in patients on DES and in castrated patients on DES. There is wide variation in plasma testosterone values, especially in castrated patients. One patient on DES had much higher plasma testosterone than others. (Courtesy of Beck, P. H., et al.: Urology 11:157–160, February, 1978.)

Three of the 16 patients studied had plasma testosterone levels well above the castrate range during DES therapy. Fourteen patients had levels well into the castrate range. Four patients showed objective responses to DES therapy, whereas 1 showed progression of disease on bone scanning while receiving DES. Deep thrombophlebitis developed in 1 patient.

The levels of circulating plasma testosterone in patients receiving 1 mg DES daily are variable, but most patients who take the drug reliably can be expected to show a fall in the plasma testosterone level to the castrate range. The plasma testosterone assay can show whether a patient is taking DES, whether adrenal testosterone is being produced at an accelerated rate or whether carcinoma is progressing despite very low testosterone levels, thus making further hormonal manipulation ineffective.

▶ [If the goal in using estrogen is to produce plasma testosterone levels as low as possible, then when 1 mg/day of diethylstilbestrol is used, it will be necessary to monitor the levels as 3 of 16 patients in this study responded with levels in the castrate range. We use a dose of 2 or 3 mg/day of diethylstilbestrol since all patients with 3 mg/day have plasma testosterone levels in the castrate range (Br. Med. J. 4:391, 1971). As these authors pointed out, orchiectomy solves the dilemma of which estrogen dose to use.–J.Y.G.] ◄

Treatment of Advanced Prostatic Carcinoma with Estramustine Phosphate (Estracyt).

Estracyt is a nitrogen mustard derivative of estradiol-17β, designed to utilize the cellular specificity of steroids because of the presence of hormone receptors in some malignant cells. It has marked antiandrogenic and antigonadotropic activities but low estrogenic activity. Gösta Jönsson, Bertil Högberg and Torgny Nilsson[7] used Estracyt to treat 154 patients with stage IV prostatic carcinoma, all followed for over a year after the start of treatment. Sixty-three patients received Estracyt from the outset, whereas 91 had received other endocrine therapy for an average of 4.5 years. Most of the latter patients were in the very poor condition and had a life expectancy of less than 6 months. Most of the tumors were poorly or moderately differentiated. Estracyt was given intravenously in a dose of 150–600 mg daily for about 3–4 weeks; a dose of 300 mg was commonly used. If the response was good, 300 mg were given twice weekly for a varying period. The oral dose of Estracyt was 8–12 mg/kg daily.

The results are summarized in Table 1. The acid phosphatase fell by at least 50% during treatment in 71 patients and in 47 it became normal; 9 patients however showed no change in general condition. Re-elevation of the acid phosphatase was usually associated with new deterioration. The cancers exhibited cellular pyknosis, vacuolization, cell membrane rupture and squamous epithelial

TABLE 1.—RESULTS

Response

	Objective	Subjective only	None
Primary treatment group (63 patients)	46 (73%)	12 (19%)	5 (8%)
Secondary treatment group (91 patients)	28 (30.7%)	24 (26.4%)	39 (42.9%)
Total	74 (48%)	36 (23.4%)	44 (28.6%)

(7)   Scand. J. Urol. Nephrol. 11:231–238, 1977.

TABLE 2.—MEDIAN SURVIVAL FROM START OF
ESTRACYT THERAPY TO DEATH

		No.	Median survival (months)	
Objective responders	p	24	24.6	
	s	21 } 45	24.3 } 24.5	
Subjective responders	p	4	23.0	
	s	18 } 22	10.1 } 12.4	
Non-responders	p	4	8.8	
	s	37 } 41	10.0 } 9.7	

metaplasia. Survival is shown in Table 2. Most deaths
were due to the basic disease and its complications. The
most conspicuous side effects of Estracyt were nausea and
vomiting. Six patients had jaundice and increased trans-
aminases but 2 of them had progressive liver metastases.
Of the 63 patients given Estracyt as primary therapy, 13
(20.6%) had mild gynecomastia.

Objective partial remissions occurred with Estracyt in
30% of patients in this series who no longer responded to
conventional endocrine therapy and objective responders
who died survived over 2 years. Estracyt is a valuable supplement to the treatment of prostatic carcinoma.

▶ [As the authors state, management of advanced prostatic carcinoma which
is refractory to conventional endocrine therapy is a difficult problem. One
problem in evaluating Estracyt has been separating the endocrine from the
chemotherapeutic effects. The objective response in 30% of patients who no
longer responded to conventional endocrine therapy, although not great,
suggests that Estracyt should be considered.–J.Y.G.] ◀

**Biopsy and Clinical Course after Cryosurgery for
Prostatic Cancer.** David S. Petersen, Leo A. Milleman,
Earl F. Rose, William W. Bonney, Joseph D. Schmidt,
Charles E. Hawtrey and David A. Culp[8] (Iowa City, Iowa)
obtained postcryosurgery biopsies of the prostate in 39 of
154 consecutive prostatic cancer patients who underwent
open perineal cryosurgical prostatectomy. In 2 of these patients prostatic tissue was removed at autopsy. In every
other patient, there was a clinical indication for biopsy,
either voiding difficulty or a nodule on rectal examination.

(8) J. Urol. 120:308–311, September, 1978.

TABLE 1.—Tumor Stage, Survival and Carcinoma in
Postcryosurgical Biopsy

Initial Stage	Ca Present*	Ca Absent*	Totals*
B	0	1/2	1/2
C	9/15	5/5	14/20
D	4/10	4/5	8/15
All stages	13/25	10/12	23/37

*Number of patients surviving/number of patients having biopsy examination.

A total of 42 procedures were carried out, 28 of them 10 days to 3 months postoperatively, and 14 after 4–43 months. Transurethral resection was done in 31 patients. All patients were followed for at least 18 months after cryosurgery.

Fourteen patients have died, 12 of carcinoma (Tables 1 and 2). Ten of 15 survivors with stage B and C disease are free from cancer. Initial tumor stage did not correlate with survival rates. Carcinoma was found at biopsy in 25 of 37 patients. Negative biopsies correlated with good survival in patients with all stages of disease. The tissue reactions observed after cryosurgery are shown in Table 3. Acute necrosis was seen in the first 3 months and fibrosis during this period and later. Inflammation was mainly confined to the first 3 months. Squamous metaplasia was seen both early and late. Inflammatory infiltrates correlated with superior survival rates and with the absence of cancer in postcryosurgical biopsies. Lymphocytic and plasma cell infiltrates occurred mainly in patients not given estrogen.

TABLE 2.—Initial Histologic Grade, Survival and Carcinoma in
Postcryosurgical Biopsy*

Grade	Ca Present†	Ca Absent†	Total†
Well differentiated and moderately well differentiated	9/12	8/10	17/22
Poorly differentiated and anaplastic	1/9	1/1	2/10
Cribriform	2/2	1/1	3/3
All grades	12/23	10/12	22/35

*Patients with available pretreatment biopsy slides.
†Number of patients surviving/number of patients having biopsy examination.

TABLE 3.—Prostatic Tissue Reaction after Cryosurgery

Histology	Mos. After Cryosurgery	No. Pts.	Ca Present
Acute necrosis	0–3	10*	7
Eosinophilic infiltration	0–3	7†	3
Lymphocytic and plasmacytic infiltration	0–3	15‡	8
Granuloma	1	1	0
Fibrosis	1–31	13	8
Squamous metaplasia	1–43	5§	3
Tissue unchanged from pre-cryosurgery	1–22	8	7

*Including one biopsy at 12 months.
†Two patients with orchiectomy plus estrogen and 2 with orchiectomy alone. Survival 6 of 7 patients.
‡Including two biopsies that showed minimal infiltration at 17 and 43 months. Survival: 11 of 15 patients.
§All had orchiectomy and 4 on estrogen.

Local recurrence followed all positive biopsies obtained 4 weeks or more after cryosurgery, but earlier positive biopsies did not correlate with local recurrences.

Cryosurgery of the prostate by the open perineal approach has been highly effective in eradicating the local lesion. Its possible role in stimulating an immunologic response warrants further investigation.

▶ [The authors' conclusions that cryosurgery by the open perineal approach controls the local lesions and that positive biopsies after 1 month correlate with local recurrences seem justified.–J.Y.G.] ◀

Carcinoma of the Prostate: Treatment with External Radiotherapy. Leon Harisiadis, Ralph J. Veenema, John J. Senyszyn, Peter J. Puchner, Patricia Tretter, Nicholas A. Romas, Chu H. Chang, John K. Lattimer and Myron Tannenbaum[9] (Columbia-Presbyterian Med. Center, New York) report the results of curative radiotherapy in 146 patients with prostatic carcinoma not extending beyond the pelvis. Six patients lost to follow-up were counted as dead at the date of last follow-up. Thirteen patients had stage A disease; 21 stage B patients had palpable nodules suggestive of cancer; and 112 patients had locally advanced, stage C disease. The mean age was 65.6 years.

(9) Cancer 41:2131–2142, June, 1978.

Well to moderately well differentiated adenocarcinoma was present in 116 cases and poorly differentiated carcinoma in 16. Twelve patients had carcinoma of periurethral prostatic duct origin. Hormonal manipulation before radiotherapy consisted of both bilateral orchiectomy and estrogen therapy in 59 patients. All patients received megavoltage x-ray or gamma-ray therapy. Only 8% received a tumor dose less than 6,000 rads, and about 38% received a dose greater than 6,500 rads. The present policy is the delivery of a tumor dose of 6,800 rads in 7 weeks.

The actuarial 5- and 10-year survival rates for stage C patients were 58 and 35%, respectively (Fig 56). The 5-year rates for patients with stages A and B were 88.2 and 86.8% respectively, and the overall 5- and 10-year rates were 64.1 and 40.5%. Age did not significantly influence survival, and acid phosphatase was not a significant factor. Obstructive changes on pyelography was an adverse prognostic factor. An increased tumor dose was associated with a higher survival rate. An increase in irradiated volume was not associated with improved survival for either early or advanced disease. Twelve patients (8.2%) had complications of radiotherapy. Nine patients had second primary tumors. The treatment failure rate was 19%.

These results are encouraging. The combination of radiotherapy with hormonal therapy for prostatic carcinoma re-

Fig 56.—The effect of stage on prognosis observed among 146 patients treated with radiotherapy. The difference between stages A and B vs. stage C was statistically significant (P = 0.017). (Courtesy of Harisiadis, L., et al.: Cancer 41:2131–2142, June, 1978.)

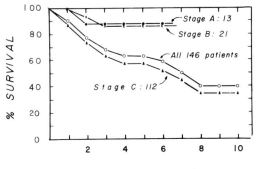

mains controversial. External radiotherapy offers several advantages over interstitial brachytherapy. The present results show how misleading the impression of "radioresistance" or "unresponsiveness" can be when the initial response rate is used as a measure of the efficacy of radiotherapy.

▶ [Such studies are needed to provide information regarding morbidity and long-term care.–J.Y.G.] ◀

Latent Residual Tumor Following External Radiotherapy for Prostate Adenocarcinoma. Little is known about biopsy evidence of residual tumor more than 2 years after radiotherapy for prostatic carcinoma. Daniel A. Nachtsheim, Jr., Jack W. McAninch, Ray E. Stutzman and James L. Goebel[1] (San Francisco) reviewed the findings in 50 patients with prostatic adenocarcinoma who received external supervoltage radiotherapy and underwent needle biopsies at timed intervals after the completion of treatment. About 6,500 rads were delivered to the prostatic bed, and 4,500 rads to the pelvic lymph node drainage. A masitron 2000 machine was used. Biopsies were not done within 6 months after completion of therapy. Individual patients had biopsy examinations up to 48 months after treatment.

Six of 17 patients with stages A and B cancer had residual tumor present, as did 15 of 33 with stage C disease. Eight of the latter patients progressed to stage D, all had residual tumor present in posttreatment biopsies. No earlier lesions progressed to stage C. No metastasis was identified in stages A and B patients. The results are summarized in Tables 1 and 2. Most negative biopsy specimens

TABLE 1.—STAGE OF TUMORS

Tumor Stage	No. Pts.	Residual Tumor No. (%)
A	5	1 (20)
B	12	5 (45)
C	33	15 (45)
Totals	50	21 (42)

(1)   J. Urol. 120:312–314, September, 1978.

TABLE 2.—Biopsies Based on Timed Interval

Timed Interval Biopsies (mos.)	No. Pts.	Residual Tumor
		No. (%)
Before 18	21	6 (29)
18 and beyond	29	15 (52)
36 and beyond	17	10 (59)

showed a large amount of fibrous tissue with little residual adenomatous tissue present. Virtually no radiation effect was found in many positive biopsy specimens.

Patients with residual prostatic adenocarcinoma 18 months after radiotherapy probably will not have resolution of the tumor at a future time and represent treatment failures. Residual tumor in stage C patients may be the result of bulk tumor at the time of initial radiotherapy, whereas stages A and B tumors may be more responsive to therapy. Estrogen therapy has been instituted in selected patients only after positive biopsy material was obtained.

▶ [The persistence of tumor in 15 of 29 patients at 18 months after external radiation is worrisome. More information is needed to determine if the disease progresses in patients with positive biopsies.–J.Y.G.] ◀

Defense of Radical Perineal Prostatectomy. Harry S. Pond, Charles L. Rutherford, Jr., William H. Cooner, B. R. Mosley and Jeff H. Beard[2] (Mobile, Ala.) performed radical perineal prostatectomy on 31 patients for localized prostatic cancer in the past 6 years. They tolerated the procedure with no mortality and little morbidity, and only 1 has subsequently died of the disease. Age range was 54–72 years. Eleven patients had open perineal biopsy at definitive surgery. Six patients were temporarily incontinent after operation and 1 patient had permanent incontinence. Only 1 had rectal injury. Two required removal of a Vest suture. No patient had recognized postoperative infections or complications referable to other organ systems. None had serious systemic complications. All are impotent, but none elected to receive a penile implant. Seven patients developed strictures that responded satisfactorily to dilations. Castration or estrogen, or both, was used in 8 un-

(2) South. Med. J. 71:541–542, May, 1978.

derstaged patients. Two of 3 patients with undifferentiated cancer are without local symptoms at present.

The data support continued use of radical perineal prostatectomy as the optimal way to remove localized prostatic cancer. Further long-term follow-up is needed to determine whether pelvic node dissection improves long-term patient survival. Extirpative surgery would not be withheld even if tumor were known to be present in regional nodes, since in patients so affected quality of life can be improved after removal of the local bulk of their tumors.

▶ [Disagreement continues about the management of localized prostatic carcinoma because of inadequate data to make a sound clinical judgment. Recently (February 8, 1979) Richard Chopp and Willit Whitmore presented a paper on delayed management of prostatic carcinoma. They noted progression of the cancer for 2 years or longer in 4 of 17 stage A, 15 of 39 stage B (most a nodule), and 3 of 4 stage C. They concluded that these results justified conservative management. Others, including myself, feel that the results justify a more aggressive approach.

Aggressive therapy options include hormones, castration, interstitial and external radiation with or without node dissection, and radical prostatectomy with or without node dissection. I still favor a radical perineal prostatectomy in the cancerous nodule. We stage larger tumors with lymphadenectomy and do a radical retropubic prostatectomy or interstitial gold supplemented by external radiation. I hope our future residents do not complete training without learning how to operate in the perineum. We have had a similar experience of very low morbidity (except impotence) with radical perineal prostatectomy.–J.Y.G.] ◀

MISCELLANEOUS

Use of Prophylactic Low-Dose Heparin in Transurethral Prostatectomy. Evan J. Kass, Paul Sonda, Charles Gershon and C. Peter Fischer[3] (Univ. of Michigan) evaluated the safety of low-dose heparin prophylaxis in patients being considered for transurethral prostatectomy. A dose of 5,000 units of sodium heparin was given subcutaneously 2 hours before surgery and then every 12 hours for about 4 days. All patients treated had normal coagulation factors preoperatively.

Thirty heparin-treated patients were compared to 31 patients randomly selected from patients having had prostatectomy a year before. The use of heparin did not increase operative blood loss or postoperative recovery time. Pro-

(3)   J. Urol. 120:186–187, August, 1978.

longed hematuria was not observed in either group. Catheters were removed by 2–3 days after operation in all cases. Transfusion was more frequent in the heparin-treated group, but the difference was not significant. Twenty-five heparin-treated patients had spinal anesthesia without complications.

Heparin prophylaxis should not be used in patients having transurethral surgery when conventional heparin therapy would be excluded. Aspirin should not be given concomitantly. At present, the use of warfarin seems unjustified in transurethral prostatectomy, but low-dose heparin must be considered for high-risk patients. Postoperative pulmonary emboli frequently seem to occur in patients who are hospitalized for a number of days before surgery. Therefore, subcutaneous heparin often is begun at admission if a delay before surgery is expected or significant predisposing factors are identified. Heparin prophylaxis should continue throughout the postoperative hospitalization.

▶ [Unfortunately, the authors give no data as to whether the heparin actually prevented deep vein thrombosis. Transurethral prostatectomy is reported to have only a 10% incidence of deep vein thrombosis by fibrinogen testing (Hedlund, P.O., Scand. J. Urol. Nephrol. 1:100, 1975). The incidence of pulmonary emboli after transurethral prostatectomy is reported to be 0.3 to 2.2% (Valk et al., Urol. Clin. North Am. 2:85, 1975 and Antila et al., Acta Chir. Scand. 357:95, 1966).–J.Y.G.] ◀

Prophylactic Use—or Misuse—of Antibiotics in Transurethral Prostatectomy. Controversy continues as to the value of prophylactic antibiotics in elective transurethral prostatectomy. Robert P. Gibbons, Roger A. Stark, Roy J. Correa, Jr., Kenneth B. Cummings and J. Tate Mason[4] conducted a prospective randomized study of kanamycin in patients with negative urine cultures undergoing elective transurethral prostatectomy. None had required a catheter preoperatively or had received antibiotics in the preceding month. Fifty patients received 500 mg kanamycin intramuscularly an hour before operation and every 8 hours afterward until the catheter was removed. The total dose did not exceed 7.5 gm. A control group of 50 patients were not treated unless symptomatic urinary tract infection occurred postoperatively. Irrigation was with a

(4) J. Urol. 119:381–383, March, 1978.

EFFECT OF KANAMYCIN PROPHYLAXIS ON POSTOPERATIVE INFECTION*

	24 Hrs. After Catheter Removal	2 Wks. After Discharge	6 Wks. After Discharge	Totals No. Pts. (%)
Kanamycin (50 pts.):				
Infected at each interval	3	5	0	
Previously uninfected	3	4	0	7 (14)
7 (14)				
Symptomatic	1	5	0	
Control, non-risk (45 pts.):				
Infected at each interval	2	2	1	
Previously uninfected	2	2	1	5 (11)
Symptomatic	1	2	1	
Control, at risk (5 pts.):				
Infected at each interval	4	4	0	
Previously uninfected	4	1	0	5 (100)
Symptomatic	2	4	0	

*Bacteriuria > 10,000 colonies per ml.

closed system of 1.5% glycine. The catheter most often was removed 2 days postoperatively.

Seven study and 10 control patients had more than 10,000 colonies per ml in urine cultures within 6 weeks after operation (table). The overall infection rate was 11% in the control patients not a risk of infection and 14% in the study group. One study patient had a symptomatic infection from kanamycin-resistant *Pseudomonas aeruginosa*. All patients with bacteriuria at 2 weeks were symptomatic and required antibiotic therapy.

Biologically, inert catheters, sterile closed irrigation and catheter drainage systems and early catheter removal contribute to the decrease of the incidence of postprostatectomy urinary tract infection. With the use of currently available technical refinements, there appears to be no advantage in the use of routine prophylactic kanamycin in uninfected, nonrisk patients undergoing elective transurethral prostatectomy.

► [Our policy has been to use antibiotics only if the cultures are positive before or after operation.–J.Y.G.] ◄

Androgen Receptor Content of Normal and Hyperplastic Canine Prostate. Current concepts of steroid hormone regulation of cell function envision a process whereby effector steroid initially interacts with cytoplasmic receptor proteins. The capacity of the prostate to accumulate specifically 5α-dihydrotestosterone (effector steroid) would be expected to be related to the tissue content of cytoplasmic and nuclear androgen receptor. Sydney A.

Shain and Robert W. Boesel[5] (Southwest Found. for Research and Education, San Antonio, Texas) quantitated the androgen receptor content of the normal and hyperplastic prostates obtained from young (2.5 or 4.6 years old) and aged 12.5 years old) beagles and from mongrel dogs of indeterminate age in an attempt to study age-associated changes in steroid hormone regulation of target tissue function. The protocol utilized exchange saturation analysis at 15 C with the use of the synthetic androgen R1881 as the ligand probe and quantitatively detected total cytoplasmic androgen receptor. This protocol was used in conjunction with a tissue mince saturation analysis procedure (for quantitation of nuclear androgen receptor) to quantitate total androgen receptor content of the normal and hyperplastic prostates.

The total cytoplasmic androgen receptor content of hyperplastic prostates was 4.6 times greater than that of normal prostates. The total nuclear androgen receptor content of hyperplastic prostates was fivefold greater than that of normal prostates in 4.6-year-old dogs and 7.8 times greater in 2.5-year-old dogs. Androgen receptor content per cell was identical in hyperplastic and normal prostates, except for a reduction in nuclear androgen receptor in prostates from 2.5-year-old dogs. The cell content per gram dry weight was identical in hyperplastic and normal prostates.

Canine prostatic hyperplasia is characterized by coordinate proliferation of androgen receptor-positive and androgen receptor-negative cells and is not a consequence of increased accumulation of 5α-dihydrotestosterone due to proliferation of androgen receptors per prostate cell. The high rate of prostatic hyperplasia and low rate of adenocarcinoma in the aging canine prostate, compared with the absence of hyperplasia and high incidence of adenocarcinoma of the ventral prostate of the aging AXC rat, may be related to altered hormonal regulation of cell function, which is reflected in the different relationships between aging and prostatic androgen receptor content of these two species.

▶ [We hope that more data on effects of hormones on the prostate will enable us to better understand prostatic hyperplasia and cancer. Conclusions depend upon the reliability and accuracy of the assay techniques. These authors

(5) J. Clin. Invest. 61:654–660, March, 1978.

seem to have a reliable one. Their studies showing opposite results in dogs with hyperplasia and the ventral prostate of the aging AXC rat with a high incidence of adenocarcinoma are very interesting.–J.Y.G.] ◄

Studies on Mechanism of 3α-Androstanediol-Induced Growth of the Dog Prostate. Administration of 3α-androstanediol in pharmacologic amounts induces prostatic growth in the castrate dog comparable to that seen in spontaneous canine prostatic hypertrophy, and 17β-estradiol exerts a synergistic effect. Günther H. Jacobi, Ronald J. Moore and Jean D. Wilson[6] (Univ. of Texas, Dallas) investigated the mechanism by which 3α-androstanediol induces prostatic growth in animals in which the prostate was initially either normal or large in size. Pharmacologic treatment was begun 2 weeks after castration and continued for 4 weeks or else was given immediately after castration. The total weekly dosage was 75 mg of androgen and 0.75 mg of 17β-estradiol. The 3α-hydroxysteroid dehydrogenase assay utilized [1,2³H] dihydrotestosterone.

When androgen replacement was begun immediately after castration of dogs with preexisting prostatic hypertrophy, dihydrotestosterone was as effective as 3α-androstanediol in maintaining prostatic weight. Under all other conditions, only 3α-androstanediol induced significant prostatic growth. The maximal effect of 3α-androstanediol was observed in 12 weeks. Estrogen administration enhanced with growth-promoting action of 3α-androstanediol but did not affect the action of dihydrotestosterone or alter 3α-hydroxysteroid dehydrogenase activity in prostate.

The synergistic effect of 17β-estradiol and 3α-androstanediol seems to be independent of any effect on the interconversion of the two androgens. The activity of 3-hydroxysteroid dehydrogenase in the dog prostate appears to be under androgenic control. Conceivably, the natural equilibrium is toward dihydrotestosterone formation. If so, the net effect of an increase in enzyme content would be to enhance the dihydrotestosterone concentration in the tissue. Identification of the effective intracellular mediator of prostatic growth will require a means of measuring androgens attached to the critical intracellular receptors.

► [Such studies are needed if we are to understand the etiology of prostatic hypertrophy.–J.Y.G.] ◄

(6) Endocrinology 102:1748–1755, June, 1978.

Partial Inhibition of Castration-Induced Ventral Prostate Regression with Actinomycin D and Cycloheximide. Castration-induced regression of the rat ventral prostate is associated with an increased rate of ^{3}H-uridine incorporation into prostatic RNA in vitro, whereas such parameters as protein and DNA synthesis decline after castration. Thomas Stanisic, Ronald Sadlowski, Chung Lee and John T. Grayhack[7] (Northwestern Univ.) used actinomycin D and cycloheximide to determine whether an enhanced rate of RNA synthesis is essential to the regressive process. Sprague-Dawley rats were castrated and given subcutaneous injections of 50 µg actinomycin D in saline. Treatment was repeated daily for 4 subsequent days, and the rats were killed 24 hours after the last dose. A similar experiment was performed with 5 days of daily subcutaneous injections of cycloheximide in a dose of 100 mg/100 gm body weight.

Castration reduced prostatic wet weight to 25% of control in 5 days. When actinomycin D was given, prostatic wet weight was maintained at 43% of control. The difference in weights between actinomycin-treated and saline-treated rats was significant. Actinomycin-treated rats lost 22% of their body weight. Testosterone concentrations fell rapidly in both actinomycin-treated and saline-treated rats. Serum corticosteroid levels were similar in treated and untreated castrated rats. Prostatic acini were less atrophic in actinomycin D-treated rats. The effects of cycloheximide were similar to those of actinomycin D. Prostatic weight loss after castration was significantly less in cycloheximide-treated than in control rats.

Tissue regression appears to be an active metabolic process, requiring enhanced RNA synthesis, but the evidence supporting this hypothesis is only indirect. Studies correlating the presence of specific RNA species with the amounts of hydrolytic enzymes present during regression might provide insight into the basic mechanism of the process. Understanding of the mechanism of tissue regression ultimately may afford a basis for manipulation of regression in benign and malignant growth of the prostate.

▶ [These results support the concept that the regression is an active meta-

(7) Invest. Urol. 16:19–22, July, 1978.

bolic process rather than a passive atrophy. A better understanding of prostatic regression should give us more insight into the management of benign hypertrophy and prostatic cancer.—J.Y.G.] ◄

The following review articles are recommended to the reader:

Catalona, W. J., and Scott, W. W.: Carcinoma of the prostate, J. Urol. 119:1, 1978.

Shain, S. A., and Boesel, R. W.: State of the Art: Human prostate steroid hormone receptor quantitation: Current methodology and Possible utility as a clinical discriminant in carcinoma, Invest. Urol. 16:169, 1978.

The Genitalia

PENIS AND POTENCY

Frequency of Sexual Dysfunction in "Normal" Couples. Relatively little attention has been paid to the prevalence of sexual dysfunction in couples not seeking treatment for sexual problems. Ellen Frank, Carol Anderson and Debra Rubinstein[8] (Univ. of Pittsburgh) analyzed the responses of 100 predominantly white, Christian, well-educated, happily married couples to a self-report questionnaire covering many aspects of marriage, including sexual activities. Reported sexual problems are summarized in the table. The predominant functional complaint by men was premature ejaculation. The frequency of sexual dysfunction was much higher in women, and women also reported a high frequency of sexual difficulties. Wives' perceptions of their husbands' dysfunction and the husbands' own reports were similar, but the men tended to underestimate the occurrence of sexual dysfunction in their wives. Only 15% of

FREQUENCY OF SELF-REPORTED SEXUAL PROBLEMS			
PROBLEM	WOMEN (%)	MEN (%)	P*
Sexual dysfunctions — women:			
Difficulty getting excited	48		
Difficulty maintaining excitement	33		
Reaching orgasm too quickly	11		
Difficulty in reaching orgasm	46		
Inability to have an orgasm	15		
Sexual dysfunctions — men:			
Difficulty getting an erection		7	
Difficulty maintaining an erection		9	
Ejaculating too quickly		36	
Difficulty in ejaculating		4	
Inability to ejaculate		0	

*Significance of t test comparing men and women; NS, not significant.

(8) N. Engl. J. Med. 299:111–115, July 20, 1978.

subjects considered their sexual relations less than moderately satisfying. There was a strong relation between the number of difficulties experienced by men and the number experienced by their wives. About half the couples reported having intercourse more than once a week.

These are self-reported data from volunteer subjects who believe that their marriages are working. Forty percent of the men reported erectile or ejaculatory dysfunction, and 63% of the women reported arousal or orgasmic dysfunction. Half the men and about three-fourths of the women reported difficulty that was not dysfunctional in nature, such as lack of interest or inability to relax. The number of "difficulties" was more strongly and consistently related to overall sexual dissatisfaction than the number of "dysfunctions." Couples from the upper portion of the socioeconomic spectrum are not immune to sexual problems. The couples are apparently able to tolerate a relatively high level of specific sexual dysfunctions and difficulties while still feeling very positive about their sexual relations and their marriages. The sexual difficulties probably reflect interpersonal problems to which both the husband and wife contribute. It is not the quality of sexual performance but the affective tone of the marriage that determines how most couples perceive the quality of their sexual relations.

▶ [This report provides information regarding sexual function in normal middle class married couples. The authors emphasize that 40% of the men had sexual problems although only 15% reported problems with erection.–S.S.H.]

Prolactin-Secreting Tumors and Hypogonadism in 22 Men. Reproductive dysfunction is one of the most common clinical findings in women with elevated prolactin concentrations. John N. Carter, John E. Tyson, George Tolis, Stuart Van Vliet, Charles Faiman and Henry G. Friesen[9] studied 22 men with prolactin-secreting pituitary tumors. Mean age was 37.8 years. Seventeen tumors were confirmed histologically; 16 were chromophobe adenomas and 1 was an eosinophilic adenoma.

Twenty patients reported decreased libido and potency. Nine had visual impairment. Only 6 had headaches. Three had galactorrhea, gynecomastia or both. The median pretreatment serum prolactin concentration was 880 ng/ml. Concentrations remained elevated in all 17 men studied

(9) N. Engl. J. Med. 299:847–852, Oct. 19, 1978.

after operation or radiotherapy. Eleven patients showed major reductions in prolactin concentrations and improved potency after treatment with bromocriptine. Plasma testosterone concentrations increased in these patients. Testosterone therapy alone failed to correct impotence in 4 patients. Basal serum LH concentrations were low-normal or low in these patients. Only 2 had marginally elevated baseline FSH concentrations. Gonadotropin responses to LH releasing hormone were in the normal range in all 9 patients tested. Administration of human chorionic gonadotropin produced a normal rise in testosterone concentrations in all 10 patients studied. Two patients who failed to respond to testosterone alone responded to bromocriptine therapy with a return of potency.

Dramatic responses of hyperprolactinemic men to bromocriptine therapy were confirmed in this study. Decreased libido and impotence may be explained by a defect in conversion of testosterone by 5α-reductase to dihydrotestosterone in hyperprolactinemic states. Alternatively, impotence may result from a direct effect of prolactin on the central nervous system. Bromocriptine therapy is ineffective in men with sexual impotence but no endocrine abnormalities.

▶ [This series confirms the findings of several other investigators. Actually most of these patients are quite ill and complain of malaise and decreased libido rather than impotency. We have recently studied a group of 30 impotent men and found that none of them had an elevated serum prolactin. Thus, except for individuals with pituitary tumors, hyperprolactemia rarely, if ever, is found in impotent men.–S.S.H.] ◀

Sexual Dysfunction Following Proctocolectomy is supposed to be rare in women, but opinions still differ regarding this complication in men. S. Fasth, S. Filipsson, R. Hellberg, L. Hultén, J. Lindhagen and S. Nordgren[1] (Univ. of Göteborg, Sweden) evaluated the occurrence of permanent impairment of sexual function in proctocolectomy patients. Sixty-six men and 56 women were interviewed regarding postoperative change in sexual function. The procedure was performed electively in most patients. Twenty-five patients had a two-stage procedure. Two-thirds of the ileostomy patients were married at the time of surgery, and more than half of these had children.

---

(1) Ann. Chir. Gynaecol. 67:8–12, 1978.

Sexual dysfunction was reported by 29% of the men. Potency was affected in 12 men, but only 5 had true impotence, and all these were more than age 40 years. Only 2 men less than age 40 had "partial" impotence. Ejaculation was reported completely abolished in 6 of the male patients. Seven women (12%) considered their sexual function impaired, with dyspareunia and/or inability to achieve orgasm.

Gross sexual disorder occurred in 17% of men in this series after proctocolectomy. Sexual dysfunction appears to be less frequent in female patients. It appears most unlikely that the ileostomy alone would cause sexual disturbances in these patients. Impotence might be improved by medical information and encouragement. Such management is also indicated for female patients. It is highly doubtful if the rectum should be spared in order to preserve sexual function in male patients. Several serious complications might result, including perirectal inflammation and fibrosis.

▶ [The type and degree of sexual dysfunction after proctocolectomy depend on the psychologic status of the patient and the surgical technique employed. Nevertheless, this series documents that postoperatively approximately 9% lose the ability to ejaculate, 7.5% are totally impotent and 10.5% are partially impotent.–S.S.H.] ◀

Preservation of Erectile Function after Aortoiliac Reconstruction. An organic pattern of erectile dysfunction after aortic reconstruction may be due to surgical interruption of autonomic fibers supplying the genital system. Ralph G. DePalma, Stephen B. Levine and Stewart Feldman[2] (Case Western Reserve Univ.) compared the results of a nerve-sparing dissection with those of conventional dissection in 30 nondiabetic men aged 43–67 years who underwent aortoiliac reconstructions in 1973–76. In the 11 operations done urgently conventional dissection and vascular control techniques were used. In the 19 elective cases the anterior aortic and superior hypogastric plexus and sympathetic nerve trunks were preserved. For both occlusive disease and aneurysm, the dissection limits mobilization of vessels and spares the longitudinal course of the autonomic nerve fibers. The aorta is exposed proximally by a longitudinal incision over its right lateral as-

(2) Arch. Surg. 113:958–962, August, 1978.

pect. The technique of aortic division is shown in Figures 57 and 58. The iliac arteries are controlled, where necessary, by limited dissection and passage of elastic vessel loops.

All 11 patients requiring conventional dissections were preoperatively and postoperatively impotent, as were 4 of the 19 in whom nerve-sparing dissection was performed. Seven of the latter 19 maintained preoperative potency after operation. Eight patients had improved or restored potency after operation. Two patients with advanced internal iliac atherosclerosis recovered potency after nerve-sparing dissections. Various predisposing factors were present in the patients who were impotent after nerve-sparing dissections, including long-standing internal iliac artery occlusion, embolization and extensive aneurysmal involvement of the common and internal iliac arteries.

Fig 57 (top).—Dissection of infrarenal artery to spare nerve fibers supplying genitals.

Fig 58 (bottom).—Complete aortic division after limited dissection to spare nerve fibers. Closure of distal aorta to prevent embolization of atherosclerotic debris.

(Courtesy of DePalma, R. G., et al.: Arch. Surg. 113:958–962, August, 1978; copyright 1978, American Medical Association.)

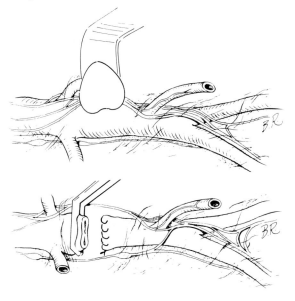

Erectile function is most likely to be preserved when elective operation is done at an early stage of aortic disease. Nerve-sparing aortic dissection increases the probability of normal function. Revascularization of the corpora cavernosa may be of use in persistently dysfunctional patients, provided nerve function is intact after proximal reconstruction.

▶ [The authors found that 11 of 11 men remained impotent after "conventional" dissection whereas 8 of 12 regained potency after "nerve-sparing" dissection.

In apparent disagreement with these findings is the fact that impotency does not occur after extensive node dissection which is certainly not "nerve-sparing." The critical factor may be the extent of the vascular compromise rather than the neurologic status.–S.S.H.] ◀

Phalloarteriography in Diagnosis of Erectile Impotence. V. Michal and J. Pospíchal[3] (Prague) devised an angiographic method for visualization of the arteries supplying the cavernous bodies of the penis, the internal iliac and internal pudendal arteries and the penile artery and its dorsal, deep and bulbocavernosus branches. Thirty patients were studied; 12 had diabetes but 14 had no associated disease. Four controls with obvious psychogenic impotence were also evaluated. A plastic cannula was placed dorsally into the cavernous body through the preputial insertion under general anesthesia, and saline with heparin was infused at an increasing rate until erection was achieved and then decreased to determine the threshold value that would maintain erection. Seldinger catheters were placed in the internal iliac arteries, and 30 ml contrast was injected at a rate of 2 ml per second. In 5 patients 1 mg acetylcholine was injected before contrast medium, followed by 40 ml contrast injected at a rate of 5 ml per second. Retrograde arteriography was necessary in 1 patient.

Erection was attained at infusion rates of 45–160 ml per minute (mean, 90), depending on the size of the penis. The maintenance infusion rate was about 60% of the initial erectile rate. Pulsation of the dorsal artery was lacking during erection in 7 patients. Peyronie's disease was seen during erection in 7 patients. No patient had normal penile vessels on angiography. All showed varying degrees of nar-

(3) World J. Surg. 2:239–248, March, 1978.

rowing and obliteration of the prudendal or penile arteries or their branches. Collateral vessels, usually from the region of the internal obturator or caudal vesical arteries, partially bypassed stenoses of the internal pudendal and penile arteries. Controls required average flows of 95 ml per minute to produce erection and 62 ml per minute to maintain erection. All had normal angiographic findings.

Most impotence is the functional result of arterial disease. Phalloarteriography permits precise anatomical diagnosis and can suggest surgical correction.

▶ [Although the success rate of vascular surgery to correct impotence has thus far been very disappointing, there is no doubt that impotence can be secondary to vascular insufficiency. Studies such as this may lead to improved—perhaps microsurgical—techniques to reverse impotence in selected men. However, the vascular physiology is complicated and poorly understood. Newman et al. (Invest. Urol. 1:350, 1964) found that in cadavers erections could be initiated and maintained at much lower infusion rates than reported in this study. The difference probably relates to important factors of corporal elasticity and outflow resistance.–S.S.H.] ◀

Current Status of Inflatable Penile Prosthesis in Management of Impotence: Mayo Clinic Experience Updated. William L. Furlow[4] (Mayo Clinic and Found., Rochester, Minn.) reviewed experience with the inflatable penile prosthesis in 63 consecutive patients treated in a 2-year period and followed for at least 6 months. Another 37 patients have had implantation during the past 5 months. Evidence is now accumulating that supports implantation in the psychologically impotent male subject. Diabetic patients and those with postprostatectomy impotence have been treated (Table 1).

Mechanical complications occurred in 27% of the 63 patients evaluated (Table 2); all were correctable. The most difficult mechanical problem was disturbance in cylinder symmetry associated with ballooning of the cylinder. More emphasis must be placed on technique if the rate of mechanical complications is to be reduced to an acceptable level. Cylinder problems have decreased with time and have not occurred in the last 20 patients who have undergone implantation. Sixty patients have satisfactory erections, and 59 have had satisfactory intercourse with the device. Three failures resulted from infection around the

(4)   J. Urol. 119:363–364, March, 1978.

TABLE 1.—Causes of Impotence in 63 Patients with
Inflatable Penile Prosthesis

	No. Pts.
Post-prostatectomy	22
Post-adenectomy	1
Post-cystectomy	2
Diabetes	18
Peripheral vascular disease	1
Abdominoperineal resection	1
Neurologic dysfunction:	9
Spinal cord injury, 6	
Multiple sclerosis, 2	
Imperforate anus, 1	
Perineal trauma	7
Physiologic	2
Total	63

prosthesis. The longevity of the device remains uncertain. Nine patients have used the device actively for more than 18 months and 24 for more than a year without difficulty.

Implantation of the penile prosthesis produces a near physiologic mechanical response and an efficient change from penile rigidity to flaccidity and vice versa. Disadvantages include infection leading to failure and physician dependence. An expandable prosthesis maintains a near normal physiologic state that will safely permit cystoscopy in the diabetic patient with neurogenic vesical dysfunction.

TABLE 2.—Mechanical Complications Associated with
Inflatable Penile Prosthesis*

	No. Cases	Disposition†
Cylinder kink	4	Replaced
Cylinder ballooning	4	Replaced
Cylinder leak	1	Replaced
Cylinder rupture	1	Replaced
Cylinder recession	2	Replaced (1)
Reservoir leak	1	Replaced
System leak	2	Replaced
Defective pump	1	Replaced
Pump malposition	1	Repositioned
Tubing kink	3	Repaired

*Of the 63 patients, 17 had twenty complications, 3 having two mechanical complications each.
†Normal function in all.

Small-Carrion Penile Prosthesis: Report on 160 Cases and Review of the Literature. Michael P. Small[5] (Univ. of Miami) evaluated the Small-Carrion penile prosthesis in 160 patients, aged 19–77 years, seen during 1973–76. This prosthesis is available in thirteen lengths and two diameters, as well as in custom sizes. Usually the 17- or 18-cm prosthesis with a 1.1-cm diameter is required. Tobramycin is given intramuscularly to prevent wound infection, and doxycycline is given intravenously at operation. The prosthesis is soaked in polymyxin B-neomycin solution after autoclaving, and the corpora and wound are irrigated with the solution. Dilation of the corpora is performed entirely under the glans penis so that the glans will not flex over the prosthesis.

Complications have been minimal after the adoption of antibiotic coverage (table). The overall rate has been less than 0.5%. Most patients had no pain at discharge, but some had pain or discomfort in the penis and perineum for 4–6 weeks. A water-soluble lubricant is recommended the first few times intercourse is performed to minimize discomfort in the glans. Another 100 patients have had implantation more recently, for a total of 260 patients. The

COMPLICATIONS

	No. Pts.
*20 patients who did not receive antibiotic coverage**	
Urinary retention (temporary)	2
Severe wound infection with extrusion of prosthesis	2
Incorrect placement of prosthesis	1
Superficial wound infection, without sequelae	3
Inability to insert prosthesis because of extensive corporeal scarring (post-priapism)	1
140 patients who received antibiotic therapy†	
Inability to insert prosthesis because of extensive scarring in corpora (post-priapism)	1
Septicemia requiring removal of prosthesis, incision and drainage of perineum and abscess of corpora (diabetic)	1
Urinary retention (diabetic)	1
Paraphimosis – treated with dorsal relaxing incision	1
Surgical perforation of glans (scleroderma)	1

*Three serious complications.
†Two serious complications.

(5) J. Urol. 119:365–368, March, 1978.

only additional complication was severe postoperative infection in a diabetic patient, necessitating removal of the prosthesis.

Bilateral intracorporeal placement of the Small-Carrion penile prosthesis produces a normal state of erection that is adequate for intercourse. The phallus is inconspicuous under various types of shorts in the normal position or against the abdominal wall. If a prostatectomy or bladder neck operation is necessary, it should be done before the prosthesis is inserted. Recently, the Rosen incontinence device has been combined with the Small-Carrion penile prosthesis in patients with impotence and incontinence, with encouraging results.

▶ [Our experience is similar to Dr. Small's. We feel that surgery for impotence is a proved modality and a very useful addition to the urologist's armamentarium. Surgeons doing the procedure for the first time should be certain to cut deeply enough into the crura and avoid the temptation to use too small a prosthesis. We offer our patients the option of the inflatable penile prosthesis but because of the higher complication rate mentioned by Furlow and the greater expense, most opt for the noninflatable prosthesis.–S.S.H.] ◀

Experience with the Horton-Devine Dermal Graft in the Treatment of Peyronie's Disease. Efforts at ameliorating Peyronie's disease have had less than satisfactory results. Chester C. Hicks, David P. O'Brien, III, John Bostwick, III and Kenneth N. Walton[6] (Emory Univ.) used the dermal graft technique of Horton and Devine in 15 patients seen since 1974 with severe or refractory Peyronie's disease. All had had progressive symptoms for over 6 months, the average period being 1 year. Ten had been on vitamin E therapy for over 6 months. The average age was 54 years. Five patients had Dupuytren's contracture of the palmar fascia. All patients had dorsal penile plaques; only 1 had multiple areas of plaque formation.

TECHNIQUE.—The plaque is dissected sharply and excised after complete circumcision, and a dermal graft is then taken from a hairless area in the lower flank or abdominal wall, the epidermis excised and the dermis, with a thin layer of fat, sutured to the tunica albuginea in the penile defect with the fat side toward the skin. Permanent sutures of 4–0 Tevdek are used. Saline instillation is used to induce an erection as a check for residual chordee. Cephalosporin is used routinely.

(6) J. Urol. 119:504–506, April, 1978.

Only minimal pain and local edema followed the operation. In time the graft was indistinguishable from the surrounding penile tissue. Twelve patients had normal sexual function without pain or residual chordee on follow-up an average of 1 year postoperatively. The patient with multiple plaques was a surgical failure. One patient had an acceptable surgical result but could not have erections, probably on a psychogenic basis. One man without residual chordee continued to have painful erections postoperatively.

A surgical approach to Peyronie's disease should be reserved for severe cases or patients with significant progression despite vitamin E therapy. The dermal graft technique holds the best potential for cure of this frequently incapacitating condition. It should be considered the surgical procedure of choice for intractable Peyronie's disease.

▶ [This work confirms the reports of successful treatment of Peyronie's disease with the dermal graft technique. Nevertheless it is wise to deal cautiously with this disease since spontaneous remissions often occur and dermal grafting has been complicated by impotence. We usually inject steroids into the plaque before advising surgery.–S.S.H.] ◀

Synergistic Gangrene of the Scrotum and Penis Secondary to Colorectal Disease. Robert C. Flanigan, Elroy D. Kursh, W. Scott McDougal and Lester Persky[7] (Case Western Reserve Univ.) recently encountered 5 patients with synergistic gangrene of the genitalia secondary to colorectal disease. This number of cases suggests that there may be an increasing incidence of this entity. Three patients had diabetes, and 2 had neurologic deficits in the involved areas. *Pseudomonas* was one of the organisms cultured in all cases. Six cases of synergistic gangrene of the genitalia arising from a gastrointestinal source have previously been reported. Some cases of spontaneous Fournier's gangrene may have been initiated by a colorectal source that was overlooked. An ischiorectal abscess was responsible in 3 of the present cases, and perforated diverticulitis and a perforated rectal carcinoma in 1 case each. Microaerophilic *Streptococcus* and *S. aureus* are usually isolated in patients with synergistic gangrene when the primary source is other than the colon or rectum. Subcu-

---

(7) J. Urol. 119:369–371, March, 1978.

taneous necrosis with obliterative endarteritis has been proposed as the mechanism of injury.

When synergistic gangrene is suspected, immediate aggressive treatment with broad-spectrum antibiotics is indicated. Surgery must be done as soon as possible, since a delay of only a few hours may be fatal. Three of the present patients died. Early, repeated radical debridement into normal tissue is recommended whenever a gastrointestinal source is discovered, and the colorectal disease must be dealt with. A diverting colostomy is often necessary. Intra- and extra-abdominal abscess cavities must be drained. The role of suprapubic cystostomy is unclear. Eventually the testes may be implanted into the thigh or abdomen if necessary. Early application of split-thickness skin grafts is helpful in obtaining coverage. The lower gastrointestinal tract should be considered as a possible cause of infection in all cases of synergistic gangrene of the scrotum and penis.

Dextran Polymer Particles (Debrisan) in Treatment of Penile Ulcers. Genital ulcers, especially those of the glans penis, pose a frequent diagnostic problem and also a problem in treatment. Systemic antibiotic therapy is often ineffective, and the results of local therapy are usually poor. Recently, a very hydrophilic dextran polymer, dextranomer, has been reported to be highly effective in the treatment of burns, infected wounds and leg ulcers. A. Lassus, J. Karvonen and T. Juvakoski[8] (Univ. of Helsinki, Finland) evaluated the effects of dextranomer on nonvenereal penile ulcers in 25 patients (mean age 26 years) seen during 1975–76 with ulcers on the glans and/or preputium. Herpes genitalis was diagnosed in 14 patients, dequalinum necrosis in 3 and nonspecific ulceration in 8. Dry dextranomer beads were applied twice daily to the ulcers to fill the cavity.

The ulcers of genital herpes healed more rapidly than those in the other patients. Six patients without signs of secondary infection were completely cured in 3–4 days, and 6 others were cured in 2 weeks. The patients with dequalinum chloride ulcerations had clean sores with granulation after 1 week of treatment, and 2 had complete heal-

---

(8) Acta Derm. Venereol. (Stockh.) 57:361–363, 1977.

ing within 3 weeks. Two patients without a specific diagnosis were cured after 2 weeks, and the others after 3–4 weeks of treatment. No side effects were observed in any of the 25 patients. Pain was almost immediately relieved after treatment was instituted.

The use of dextranomer beads to treat penile ulcers is very efficient and convenient, even in very therapy-resistant cases. No mucosal irritation was noted, and the rapid relief of pain was encouraging. Occlusion is not necessary in treating penile ulcers. It may be concluded that dextranomer is highly effective in the treatment of penile ulcers.

▶ [If the treatment is as effective as the authors claim, it will become the therapy of choice for genital ulcers.–S.S.H.] ◀

URETHRA

Posterior Urethral Valves in Infants: Therapeutic Approach is presented by Zygmunt Kaliciński, Jerzy Kansy, Barbara Kotarbińska and Wlodzimierz Joszt[9] (Military Med. Academy, Warsaw). Posterior urethral valves are one of the chief causes of congenital lower urinary tract obstruction and one of the most difficult problems in pediatric urology. Both newborn-infant-type valves, with serious symptoms such as failure to thrive and severe renal insufficiency, and later-age-group micturition difficulty and incontinence are observed. Treatment depends on the severity of the symptoms. The authors' technique is described.

TECHNIQUE.—A Foley catheter is inserted under ketamine anesthesia, and the balloon is filled with 1–1.5 ml of contrast medium. The filled balloon is pulled down in the urethra under x-ray control. The catheter is then reinserted, and the balloon is filled with 1.5–2 ml of contrast and rapidly pulled down to rupture the valves. The catheter is kept in place for 2–3 days.

Nine children have had this procedure in the past 4 years. Three had severe changes in the entire urinary tract, and 1 had large vesical diverticula. All newborns and infants showed proper micturition and no urinary retention after the procedure. Voiding cystourethrography showed considerable recovery of the urethra after 3–6

(9) Eur. Urol. 4:182–184, 1978.

months. Vesicoureteric reflux disappeared in 4 cases. Only 1 of the 3 children with severe changes has grown properly, however.

Urinary flow obstruction in the urethra due to posterior urethral valves in newborns and infants can be removed by rupturing the valves with the balloon of a Foley catheter. The procedure is simple and can be done in the first days of life without open operation. No stress incontinence has been observed in these children, in contrast to infants having endourethral incision. Removal of posterior urethral valves should be done as early as possible in the newborn period to prevent progressive renal damage.

▶ [The method described in this report is similar in concept to use of a Fogarty catheter or a hooked electrode both described by Mr. D. I. Williams et al. (Br. J. Urol. 45:200, 1973). We still prefer to fulgurate valves endoscopically under direct vision.–S.S.H.] ◀

Evaluation and Treatment of Patients with Failed Hypospadias Repair. Charles J. Devine, Jr., John P. Franz and Charles E. Horton[1] (Eastern Virginia Med. School) have performed primary repair of hypospadias and chordee in about 500 cases in the past 22 years, using a variety of one-stage procedures, and in the past 15 years have done surgical corrections in more than 75 patients with failures of primary repair and complications severe enough to require more than a simple procedure.

Nine personal cases and 61 referred patients were reviewed. The average number of previous procedures was 5.5. No common factor in the failures was identified. In most cases, several techniques were used in the same session to correct various deformities. Two operations on the average were necessary to complete the repair. Nineteen patients required only 1 operation; the maximum was 5. Several patients had planned multistaged procedures. The commonest complications were fistula, stricture, chordee, retracted meatus, flap necrosis and urethral diverticulum.

Inadequate resection of chordee was the most frequent major problem in referred patients with previous treatment failure. Artificial erection to evaluate the completeness of release of chordee could prevent these failures. When a satisfactory urethra is present with residual chordee, the urethra is not sacrificed. Urethral stenosis often

(1) J. Urol. 119:223–226, February, 1978.

occurs distal to a urethral fistula and the adequacy of the entire channel must be demonstrated preoperatively. A voiding urethrogram shows the functional capacity of the urethra. Urethral fistulas are closed after mobilizing the skin widely. The urethra is closed by inverting the edges, with a trapdoor flap of skin or by a free full-thickness patch graft. Flaps used to cover the penis must have adequate blood supply. Penile skin is the best substitute for the urethra. When a fistula develops, a catheter should be reinserted and left indwelling for 10 days. Definitive reconstruction is not begun until 4–6 months after inflammation and edema have resolved.

▶ [This article summarizes the authors' extensive experience in the correction of failed hypospadias repair and contains several helpful suggestions such as the use of intravenous fluorescein dye and ultraviolet light to evaluate the blood supply to tenuous skin flaps.—S.S.H.] ◀

Pull-Through Intraurethral Bladder Flap. Continence is a result of resistance of the opposed walls of the male posterior urethra to fluid pressure. Manuel Neto[2] (VA Center, Leavenworth, Kan.) describes a new technique for correcting postprostatectomy incontinence in which a tube constructed from a bladder flap is used to restore the damaged internal sphincter mechanism.

TECHNIQUE.—The bulbous urethra is exposed by a vertical perineal urethrostomy and a Foley catheter placed. The bladder is exposed suprapubically, and a rectangular flap is made from its anterior wall with the pedicle toward the dome (Fig 59, A). A tube is made of the 2.5×4.5-cm flap around a no 18 catheter, 4–0 plain gut sutures being used for the uroepithelium and interrupted no. 3 chromic sutures for the seromuscular layers (B). The catheters are removed, the membranous urethra is calibrated with metal sounds, and a bladder incision is made for suprapubic urinary drainage. A no. 18 Foley catheter is placed through the tube and sutures at the apex of the tube are tied around it (C). The tube is drawn down to the level of the perineal urethrostomy (D) and fixed to the bulbous urethra, and the base of the bladder flap is approximated to the bladder neck (E). The perineal urethrostomy can be left open. The urethral stent is removed after 10–14 days and the suprapubic catheter after successful voiding.

Four patients who had been incontinent for 11 months to 7 years 4 months after various operations on the prostate underwent this operation. One was improved. The 3 who

(2) J. Urol. 119:699–701, May, 1978.

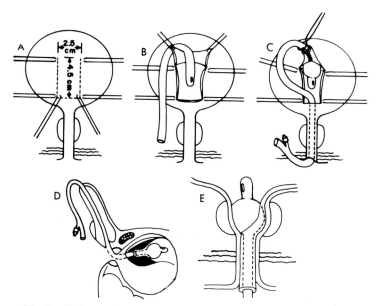

Fig 59.—Technique for construction of pull-through intraurethral bladder flap. (Courtesy of Neto, M.: J. Urol. 119:699–701, May, 1978.)

had had unsuccessful Kaufman prostheses were cured during follow-up for 3–10 months postoperatively, with gradual improvement in voiding from increase in bladder capacity.

This procedure appears to offer better results than any other. It can be used in all situations of postprostatectomy incontinence in patients with bladders of relatively good capacity.

▶ [This procedure is similar to that described by Tanagho and Smith (Trans. Am. Assoc. Genitourin. Surg. 63:103, 1971) except that Neto pulls the tube through the bladder neck. Although the preliminary results are encouraging, the value of the operation will depend on its long-term success rate in the hands of other surgeons.–S.S.H.] ◀

The Sloughed Urethra Syndrome. Extensive or complete sloughing of the urethra usually leads to total urinary incontinence, the treatment of which is a challenge. The success of constructing a new urethra from the vaginal wall has been limited, and some patients must then require a urinary diversion. J. E. Morgan, G. A. Farrow and

R. H. Sims[3] (Univ. of Toronto, Canada) describe an operative approach that has successfully rebuilt the urethra and bladder neck and restored satisfactory bladder function in 8 of 9 patients who presented with a destroyed urethra.

PROCEDURE.—The urethra is reconstructed from a widely mobilized flap of vaginal mucosa. Blood supply and support to the bladder neck and new urethra are ensured by a Martius bulbocavernosus graft. A Marlex sling is usually also used. (A split labial graft was necessary in 2 patients to re-epithelialize the vagina.) A wide U-shaped incision is made in the anterior vaginal wall (Fig 60), and thick flaps of vaginal mucosa are dissected free (Fig 61). The edges are closed over a silicone rubber catheter (Fig 62). After the abdominal team has freed the bladder and anterior urethra from the pubic symphysis and vaginal periurethral tunnels have been formed, the Martius bulbocavernosus fat pad graft from the labia is placed across the new urethra at the blad-

Fig 60 (left).—Only the superior portion of the urethra is preserved. The flaps of vaginal mucosa fashioned from the upper portion of the U-shaped incision *(broken line)* will be rolled in to form the lateral walls of the new urethra. The flap from the lower portion of the incision *(solid line)* will be brought forward to form the floor of the new urethra.

Fig 61 (right).—Closure of the vaginal flaps is commenced at the vault.

(Courtesy of Morgan, J. E., et al.: Am. J. Obstet. Gynecol. 130:521–524, Mar. 1, 1978.)

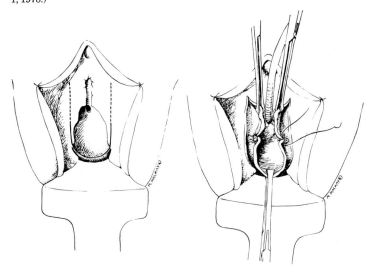

(3) Am. J. Obstet. Gynecol. 130:521–524, Mar. 1, 1978.

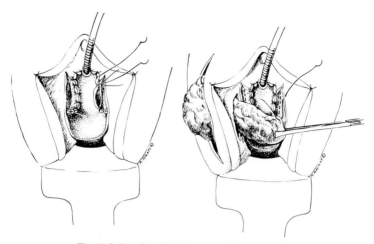

Fig 62 (left).—Completed closure of the new urethra.
   Fig 63 (right).—Vascular graft on a posterior pedicle from the right labia majora is placed across the new urethra.
   (Courtesy of Morgan, J. E., et al.: Am. J. Obstet. Gynecol. 130:521–524, Mar. 1, 1978.)

   Fig 64 (left).—The strip of Marlex mesh at the junction of the bladder and new urethra with the ends of the strip passed through periurethral tunnels.
   Fig 65 (right).—The pedicle graft at the bladder neck lies between the new urethra and the Marlex mesh. The urethrovesical junction is pulled into a retropubic position and held there by suturing the mesh to Cooper's ligaments (cl).
   (Courtesy of Morgan, J. E., et al.: Am. J. Obstet. Gynecol. 130:521–524, Mar. 1, 1978.)

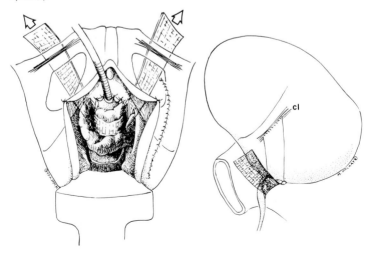

der neck (Fig 63). A strip of Marlex mesh is then placed under the graft, the ends are passed through the tunnels (Fig 64) and the mesh is anchored to Cooper's ligament (Fig 65). The bladder is drained with a suprapubic cystostomy tube. The rubber catheter is removed in 3 weeks.

No immediate surgical or medical complications resulted. Four patients had acute cystitis that responded to antibiotics. Chronic cystitis ensued in one instance. One patient had urethral stenosis requiring dilatation under anesthesia. No fistulas occurred. On follow-up for 6 months to 5 years, 5 patients were totally continent and fully active and 3 improved. Two of the latter did not have a Marlex sling procedure. One patient remained incontinent due to radiation cystitis.

This combined procedure is indicated for patients who present with a sloughed urethra. The safety of the procedure depends on the two-team approach.

Loss of the Urethra: Report on 50 Patients. Loss of the urethral floor with total urinary incontinence is a difficult problem. Richard E. Symmonds and Lyndon M. Hill[4] (Mayo Clinic and Found., Rochester, Minn.) reviewed the results of treatment of 50 patients presenting with total incontinence due to traumatic loss of much or all of the urethral floor and bladder neck. They had previously undergone 94 unsuccessful operations. Surgical reconstruction was accomplished by creating a small-caliber urethra from the contractile tissues that had retracted into the urethral roof. The anterior vaginal wall was replaced by a labial skin flap that included the bulbocavernosus muscle or a simple fibrofatty-bulbocavernosus muscle flap of the Martius type. When necessary, a delayed retropubic urethrovesical suspension was done to provide complete urinary continence. The mean patient age was 44.1 years. The causes of urethral destruction are given in Table 1. The operative technique is illustrated in Figures 66 and 67.

The results of surgery are given in Table 2. All patients were followed for at least a year. Thirty-seven patients (75%) have been completely continent of urine for 1–17 years after operation. Four others consider the operation to have been successful despite some continuing incontinence.

---

(4) Am. J. Obstet. Gynecol. 130:130–138, Jan. 15, 1978.

TABLE 1.—CAUSES OF URETHRAL DESTRUCTION (1959–75)

Cause	No. of cases	
Congenital	4	
Hypospadias		1
Epispadias		2
Short urethra		1
Obstetric trauma	4	
Trauma (automobile accident)	1	
Irradiation injury	1	
Surgical	40	
Anterior colporrhaphy with and without vaginal hysterectomy		27
Repair of urethral diverticulum		11
Transurethral bladder neck resection or cautery		2
Total	50	

Fig 66.—Technique of mobilization of tissue. **A,** incision adjacent to margin of defect. B and C, vaginal flaps widely dissected but urethral "roof" undermined only enough to allow a tension-free closure. (Courtesy of Symmonds, R. E., and Hill, L. M.: Am. J. Obstet. Gynecol. 130:130–138, Jan. 15, 1978; from Symmonds, R. E.: Am. J. Obstet. Gynecol. 103:665, 1969.)

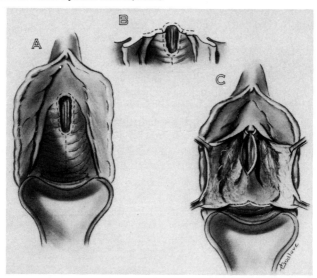

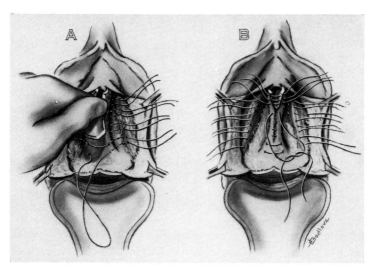

Fig 67.—Technique of closure of urethra. Technique of urethral reconstruction; finger inserted into bladder for accurate placement of plicating sutures at bladder neck. Initial pairs of sutures are placed in supporting tissues and held laterally **(A)**, while small-caliber urethra is reconstructed **(B)**. (Courtesy of Symmonds, R. E., and Hill, L. M.: Am. J. Obstet. Gynecol. 130:130–138, Jan. 15, 1978; from Symmonds, R. E.: Am. J. Obstet. Gynecol. 103:665, 1969.)

Three additional patients had estimated improvement of 50–75%. Four of 6 patients without significant benefit had incomplete operations. Twenty patients required a retropubic suspension. Six required a repeat urethral reconstruction. Complications have been relatively minor. Only 1 of 6 patients with separation of the urethral repair had had a labial skin flap used in the repair.

TABLE 2.—RESULTS IN 50 CASES OF URETHRAL RECONSTRUCTION (1959–75)

| | Years after operation | | | | Total | |
Result	1-5	6-10	11-15	>15	No.	%
Cured	20	7	9	1	37	74.0
Improved 75 to 90%	1	1	1	1	4	8.0
Improved 50 to 75%	2	1	0	0	3	6.0
Unchanged	2	1	3	0	6	12.0
Total	25	10	13	2	50	100.0

After a follow-up period of 5–15 years, 37 of the 50 patients (74%) were cured, and an additional 4 patients were greatly improved. Unfortunately it is not possible to determine the quantity or quality of smooth muscle that may still be present. In some cases a "second-stage" retropubic suspension may be necessary to increase urethral support and resistance and provide better urinary continence.

▶ [Loss of urethra and subsequent total urinary incontinence is a devastating problem for any woman but is particularly tragic when it occurs during childbirth in a young woman. Urologists have usually attempted to repair this injury using the Leadbetter modification of the Young-Dees procedure. Unfortunately this technique is not always successful. The preceding two reports from the gynecologic literature offer an interesting alternative approach.–S.S.H.] ◄

Rectourethral Fistula: Treatment by Abdominoperineal Pull-Through Resection of the Rectum. Rectourethral fistula is a rare condition that is secondary to trauma, inflammation, neoplasia, pelvic or perineal surgery, irradiation or congenital malformations. Large fistulas may be very difficult to handle. Kjell J. Tveter and Willy Mathisen[5] (Natl. Hosp. of Norway, Oslo) treated 4 difficult cases by abdominoperineal pull-through resection of the rectum and obtained very satisfactory results, with primary closure of the fistula in all cases. All the fistulas had been present for several years. Three patients had been operated on several times and had abundant scar and fibrous tissue. Closure of the urethral side of the fistula with absorbable suture material is recommended after transection, unless the fistula is small.

Boy, 5, had a rectourethral fistula caused by sitting on a piece of glass. He was operated on at least 12 times from the perineum without closure of the fistula. Laparotomy was done once, with transection and suture of the fistula and interposition of greater omentum between the bowel and prostate, but the fistula recurred. At age 15 a fistula was present between the urethra and rectum at the level of the prostate. An abdominoperineal pull-through resection of the rectum was carried out, with removal of scar tissue and suture of the urethral side of the fistula with chromic gut. The rectum was sutured to the anus and external sphincter. The fistula closed primarily. The cystostomy catheter was removed after 2 months, and the transversostomy was closed 3 months later. The patient is well 7 years after the operation. Urethrography shows no signs of communication with the rectum.

(5) Eur. Urol. 4:303–305, 1978.

Abdominoperineal pull-through resection of the rectum should be added to the list of surgical alternatives for the management of difficult rectourethral fistulas.

▶ [Recently, we had the opportunity to see a patient who had a prostatic urethroperineal fistula after an abdominal perineal operation for colitis. He had had multiple previous failures. The large defect was easily and successfully closed using the gracilis muscle as a pedicled patch.–J.Y.G.] ◀

Direct Vision Urethrotomy in Management of Urethral Strictures. H. Lipsky and G. Hubmer[6] (Univ. of Graz, Austria) performed direct vision urethrotomy in 32 patients (average age 43 years) with urethral strictures. Ten strictures were inflammatory; 8, traumatic; 6, iatrogenic; and 3, congenital. The penile urethra was involved in 10 patients, the bulbar segment in 18 and the membranous urethra in 4. No patient had urinary infection at the time of operation, but 60% had had urinary infection previously. Eight had had intermittent dilatation for several years. General anesthesia was used in 30 patients and local anesthesia in 2. A ureteric catheter was passed at urethroscopy before the cutting of the stricture at 12 o'clock along the catheter. Irrigation was carried out with isotonic solution. A 22 F catheter was inserted after urethrotomy. All patients received antibacterial therapy. Catheters were left in place for 5–14 days, and patients practiced "hydraulic self dilatation" for 6 months. Ten patients had weekly instillations of steroid jelly.

In 2 patients in whom a ureteric catheter could not be passed, the urethrotomy resulted in a false passage with massive extravasation of irrigation fluid, and the first stage of a conventional urethroplasty was carried out. Both patients had an uneventful course. No patient had fever, serious bleeding or epididymitis. Twenty patients had good results at follow-up, which varied from 9 months to 3 years, with flow rates of 15 ml/second or more and a normal urethrogram. Five patients were improved, and 5 had bad results. Nine patients required a second procedure (table). All recurrences were evident within 3 months.

Direct vision urethrotomy can be performed easily and without major risk in all patients with urethral stricture. At many centers, it is done on an outpatient basis under local anesthesia. The results compare favorably with those

(6) Br. J. Urol. 49:725–728, 1977.

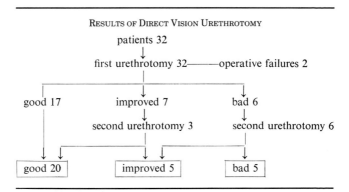

RESULTS OF DIRECT VISION URETHROTOMY

patients 32
↓
first urethrotomy 32————operative failures 2

good 17   improved 7   bad 6
                       ↓   ↓
              second urethrotomy 3   second urethrotomy 6

good 20   improved 5   bad 5

of open surgery. If restenosis occurs, urethrotomy can be repeated without appreciable risk to the patient or the local situation. Conventional urethroplasty can always be done at a later time. A stricture longer than 3 cm is likely to recur in a short time. Traumatic strictures with dense scar tissue also tend to recur. The ideal indication is a short stricture without inflammatory changes, which has never been dilated.

▶ [This report serves to emphasize that in spite of recent enthusiasm for patch graft urethroplasties and transpubic surgery, many patients with urethral strictures can be treated by more traditional methods. It is difficult to know whether the use of "hydraulic self dilation" and/or steroid jelly contributed to the good results.–S.S.H.] ◀

Radiation Treatment of Primary Carcinoma of the Female Urethra. Primary carcinoma of the female urethra is rare. Thongbliew Prempree, Morris J. Wizenberg and Ralph M. Scott[7] reviewed experience with 16 women seen in 1961–76 with histologically diagnosed urethral carcinomas who received radiotherapy. Ten were treated definitively and the other 6 palliatively from the outset. The 10 patients with disease in stages I–III were treated by radium implantation (Fig 68) alone or with external whole pelvis irradiation plus interstitial therapy in more advanced cases. Only a small-volume radium implant was used where disease was limited to the distal half of the urethra or involvement of periurethral tissues was minimal. Cobalt or 4-Mev supervoltage therapy was used when

———
(7)   Cancer 42:1177–1184, September, 1978.

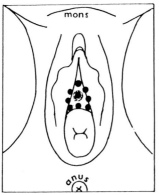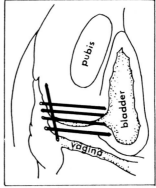

Fig 68.—Radium implant for stage I urethral carcinoma. Three-cm active length, half-intensity radium needles are used. Crossing needles are usually 3 cm in active length and full intensity. (Courtesy of Prempree, T., et al.: Cancer 42:1177–1184, September, 1978.)

the entire urethra was involved, with interstitial radium. When the vulva or vagina was involved, whole pelvis irradiation was followed by radium implantation. Direction of external therapy included the lymphatic drainage.

Excellent control was obtained without complications in all 3 cases of anterior urethral disease. Two of 3 cases involving the entire urethra were controlled. Disease in 3 patients with involvement of the vulva, vagina or both was controlled, but 1 had a urethral stricture. A patient with bladder neck involvement represented local failure and died of disease. Four of the 6 patients treated palliatively obtained a partial symptomatic response, but all 6 died of disease within 6–12 months.

Interstitial radium therapy alone is adequate treatment for cancer limited to the distal female urethra. A dose of 5,500–6,000 rad is delivered in 4 or 5 days. Patients with more advanced disease are given both external and interstitial therapy in a total dose of 6,000–6,500 rads in 6 to 7 weeks. Involvement of the bladder neck, parametrial tissues or inguinal nodes carries a poor prognosis. Palliative irradiation offers only a short-term symptomatic response. Complications from radiotherapy are infrequent and self-limited.

▶ [We, and others, agree that early distal urethral carcinoma is well treated with interstitial radiation and that disease in stage IV has a grave prognosis.

These authors' results with intermediate stages are better than most (Bracken et al., J. Urol. 116:118, 1976). Although this is encouraging it may be related to the small number of cases and clinical upstaging rather than the treatment. We feel that many of these lesions are best treated with preoperative radiotherapy and surgery.–S.S.H.] ◀

TESTES

The Testes after Torsion. Many testes that undergo torsion are "saved," but the quality of these testes and the contralateral companions over the long-term is not known. Torben Krarup[8] (Univ. of Copenhagen, Denmark) attempted to determine whether testes "saved" by detorsion really survive, whether external manual rotation is as safe as surgery and whether prophylactic fixation of the contralateral testis is necessary. Seventy-four patients were treated for torsion during 1961–1974, and 48 volunteered for follow-up in 1974. The mean age at torsion was 16 years. The mean interval between torsion and follow-up was $4^{1}/_{2}$ years. Ten patients had surgical detorsion with, and 13 without, contralateral fixation; 5 had external manual detorsion; 9 had orchiectomy with, and 7 without, contralateral fixation; and 4 had surgical fixation for chronic torsion.

Only 9 of 28 "saved" testes were of normal size. Surgery within 4 hours of torsion did not assure the survival of a full-sized testis. One patient who had been treated by manipulation only had lost his testis by a misdiagnosed recurrent torsion 1 year later, and 2 other patients had intermittent swelling and pain in the testis. All prophylactically fixed contralateral testes were normal, but 8 of the others were painful and 2 patients had required fixation. Semen quality was doubtful in 6 of 19 patients, pathologic in 3 and severely pathologic in 9. Even patients with high sperm concentrations had many dead or abnormal sperms. Sperm numbers appeared to be lowest in patients who had had a testis removed, but the group differences were insignificant.

The duration of testicular torsion is clearly correlated with the degree of subsequent testicular atrophy. The findings confirm the importance of fixing the contralateral tes-

_____

(8) Br. J. Urol. 50:43–46, February, 1978.

tis prophylactically. Sperm count data do not offer any argument against prophylactic fixation. Patients operated on for unilateral testicular torsion appear to have bilateral testicular abnormality. Studies are in progress to elucidate the bilateral testicular disease in patients with torsion.

▶ [The authors document a very high incidence of late atrophy (68%) after "successful" surgical correction of testis torsion. They also show that control fixation does not have obvious deleterious effects on the normal testis. Their semen analysis data are difficult to interpret in the absence of control data but suggest that some patients may have decreased fertility.–S.S.H.] ◀

Endocrine Tests in Phenotypic Children with Bilateral Impalpable Testes Can Reliably Predict "Congenital" Anorchism. The normal phenotypic male with impalpable gonads poses a serious clinical dilemma. The term anorchism implies a distinct clinical entity. Surgical exploration has not proved completely reliable in differentiating anorchism from nonfunctioning cryptorchid testes. A test that could reliably identify functioning testicular tissue would be of value in planning the extent of exploration. Selwyn B. Levitt, Edna H. Sobel, Stanley J. Kogan, Robin H. Mortimer, Keith M. Schneider, Rainer M. E. Engel and Jerrold M. Becker[9] report the endocrine findings in 11 anorchic males, 10 of whom had "congenital" anorchism.

Baseline plasma testosterone levels were measured by immunoassay before and the day after intramuscular injection of 4,500 IU of human chorionic gonadotropin (hCG). Extensive testing has shown hCG can stimulate Leydig cells to secrete testosterone over basal levels even in immature testes (positive test). No rise over basal levels indicates absence of testicular tissue (negative test).

Basal plasma gonadotropin (FSH and LH) levels were measured before a single bolus injection of 100 μg of luteinizing hormone releasing factor (LHRF) and at 15-minute intervals for 2 hours after. Plasma FSH levels are strikingly elevated in presence of primary gonadal failure; LH levels are less so. Peak gonadotropin levels after LHRF stimulation correlated directly with basal levels. Functioning testicular tissue was reliably excluded in all but 1 patient, who had had an infarcted testis within an incarcerated left inguinal hernia and absent right testicular tissue.

In a normal phenotypic male child with a 46 XY kary-

(9) Urology 11:11–17, January, 1978.

otype and no müllerian structures palpable at rectal examination, a negative hCG test indicates no rise in gonadotropins and congenital anorchism. This precludes the need for surgical confirmation. In contrast, a positive hCG test appears to mandate thorough and extensive surgical exploration. Exploration is also necessary with a negative hCG response in a boy with ambiguous external genitalia, karotype abnormality or suspected müllerian duct structures on rectal examination. Children with acquired loss of a testis postnatally could conceivably harbor a nonfunctioning dysgenetic testis despite a normal male phenotype and a 46 XY karyotype. Caution is needed in extrapolating these recommendations to adults, since beyond age 35–40 abnormally retained testes may undergo premature failure of androgen function.

▶ [We agree that boys with nonpalpable gonads should have an hCG stimulation test and measurement of the serum gonadotropins. Postive tests indicate functioning gonadal tissue. However, negative tests may require expert interpretation. Certainly a negative hCG stimulation test by itself is inconclusive. Although it may be correct, we feel it is premature to endorse the authors' recommendation that some of these patients do not need exploration because very few of these patients have been operated on to document anorchia. Also we could find no basis for the statement that testicular function changes at age 35 to 40.–S.S.H.] ◀

Orchiopexy in the Prune Belly Syndrome. The prune belly syndrome is characterized by deficient abdominal musculature, undescended (intra-abdominal) testes and dilatation of the urinary collecting system. The early mortality has exceeded 50%. Reports of successful orchiopexy in these patients have been rare. The major technical problem in orchiopexy has been insufficient length of the spermatic vessels. John R. Woodard and Thomas S. Parrott[1] (Emory Univ.) have taken an aggressive approach to these infants, performing orchiopexy in the first 6 months of life, in conjunction with major urinary reconstructions.

Sixteen new patients have been treated since 1969. Ten, aged 1 day to 6 years on admission, had severe uropathy but sufficient renal parenchyma to permit total urinary reconstructive procedures. Seven of 8 neonates in the 10 had reconstructive surgery in the first 6 months of life, with orchiopexy done at the same time. Two other patients had bilateral transabdominal orchiopexy at age 5 and 7 years,

---

(1) Br. J. Urol. 50:348–351, August, 1978.

respectively. One patient had a loop cutaneous ureterostomy and later unilateral orchiopexy during urinary
reconstruction.

In the 10 patients, orchiopexy was performed on 17
testes. Six testes never reached the scrotum completely or
retracted into the groin. Two 2d-stage procedures have succeeded. Fourteen testes now are in the scrotum and without atrophy. At least 1 scrotal testis without atrophy was
achieved at one operation in all cases in which orchiopexy
was combined with neonatal or early infantile urinary reconstruction. Only 1 of 3 children having delayed orchiopexy had a good result with a single operation. The only
testis biopsy showed immature testicular tissue and immature but structurally preserved tubules.

These results support the view that orchiopexy in the
neonate or young infant with prune belly syndrome offers
the best chance of obtaining viable testes in the scrotum.
Orthiopexy done during ureteric straightening in young infants easily allows for sufficient cord length without division of the testicular vessels and without atrophy.

▶ [This is a very significant observation. It is clear that such patients should
have orchiopexy early in life. For those who come later to medical attention,
microvascular autotransplant should be considered.–S.S.H.] ◀

**Diagnosis and Management of Testes in Superficial
Inguinal Pouch.** In general, testes away from the low
scrotal position may be arrested, deviated or retractile.
Testes that retract readily to the external ring do not require operation, but the status of those that persistently
lie lateral to the external ring and can be coaxed passively
some way into the scrotum, but will not stay there, is less
certain. In the literature there is a lack of clear distinction
between testes at the external ring and those lateral to it.
E. C. Ashby[2] (Chichester, West Sussex, England) reviewed the findings in boys less than age 14 years who presented during 1971–75 with abnormalities of testicular position. With testes at the external ring, tensing the
muscles by straight-leg raising to 45 degrees tended to
drive deviated testes laterally, whereas retractile testes
either stayed in the same position or moved toward the
scrotum. The prominent factor in the malposition of the
testes is given in the table.

(2) Lancet 1:468–470, Mar. 4, 1978.

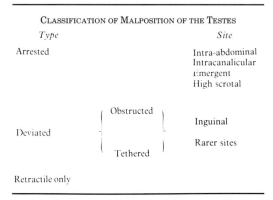

CLASSIFICATION OF MALPOSITION OF THE TESTES

Type	Site
Arrested	Intra-abdominal Intracanalicular Emergent High scrotal
Deviated { Obstructed Tethered }	Inguinal Rarer sites
Retractile only	

In this study, 111 orchiopexies were performed on 86 boys. Three testes found at times lateral to the external ring subsequently came to rest spontaneously well down in the scrotum at age 12 years, but all had at presentation been noted by boy and parent to have been occasionally in the scrotum. Deviated obstructed testes were invariably associated with marked fibrosis at the neck of the scrotum, whereas tethered testes were not. Retroperitoneal dissection was performed in 60% of the patients. Failure to reach the normal low position could not be attributed to cremasteric contraction alone in a majority of tethered, deviated testes.

Tensing the abdominal muscles by straight-leg raising facilitates palpation of deviating testes and helps demonstrate lateral deviation. The cord was too short in over half of nonobstructed deviated testes in this series. With testes in abnormal sites, errors of omission are potentially more damaging than errors of commission, and a well-executed orchiopexy is remarkably free from complications. In 3 of the present patients with deviated testes, a transcutaneous transfixing suture at the bottom of the scrotum left in place for 10 days resulted in permanent adoption of a low position.

▶ [Ashby feels that certain testes classified as retractile actually lie lateral to the external ring and will not descend spontaneously. If this observation can be confirmed by others it will explain the observations of Scorer (Arch. Dis. Child. 39:605, 1964) and most clinicians that some "retractile" testes do not end up in the scrotum and will thus alter the treatment of such patients.—S.S.H.] ◀

Regional Lymph Nodes in Infants with Embryonal Carcinoma of Testis. Regional nodes draining the testis are the most common site of early metastasis of germ cell tumors of the testis other than choriocarcinoma in adults, but in infants with embryonal carcinoma of the testis hematogenous spread is far more common. R. B. Bracken, D. E. Johnson, A. Cangir and A. Ayala[3] (Univ. of Texas, Houston) evaluated the potential role of retroperitoneal lymphadenectomy in 16 children with embryonal carcinoma of the testis. The patients, seen in 1951–77, were all under age 4 years; the median age at diagnosis was 16.6 months. All presented with painless scrotal enlargement; 3 had an associated hydrocele. All patients had had the primary tumor removed. Three patients had unilateral and 9 had bilateral retroperitoneal lymphadenectomy; 5 who had had scrotal orchiectomy had partial scrotectomy with removal of the remaining spermatic cord. The regional nodes were clinically involved in 1 of the 15 evaluable patients.

Adenectomy was negative for metastasis in the 12 patients with disease clinically limited to the testis. One stage I patient who had had radiotherapy did not have adenectomy. Another was referred after pulmonary metastases were evident. The patient with clinical node disease had unresectable retroperitoneal metastases proved at laparotomy. One patient who was not adequately staged at diagnosis had evidence of retroperitoneal node disease on referral a year later. Eleven of the 14 clinical stage I patients are alive without evidence of disease 1 month to 17 years after treatment; 2 had lung metastases and died of disease and 1 referred with metastases died without evidence of retroperitoneal disease at autopsy. The clinical stage II patient had unresectable retroperitoneal disease at laparotomy and died despite aggressive chemotherapy. The inadequately staged patient died with inoperable retroperitoneal disease. The lymphangiographic findings were confirmed surgically in 10 patients. Pyelography was normal in the stage I patient in whom it was performed and showed ureteral displacement in the stage II patient.

Lymphangiography is indicated when embryonal carcinoma of the testis is confirmed by inguinal orchiectomy. If

(3) Urology 11:376–379, April, 1978.

the findings are normal, a bilateral retroperitoneal adenectomy is done. Patients presenting with regional disease are given radiotherapy before adenectomy and chemotherapy afterward.

▶ [From the authors' data and that in the literature it is clear that clinical stage I embryonal carcinoma in infants rarely involves the regional lymphatics. Nevertheless the literature suggests (see the following article and Sabio et al., Cancer 34:2118, 1974, and Matsumoto et al., J. Urol. 104:778, 1970) but does not prove in a controlled fashion that lymph node dissection and/or radiotherapy increases survival. Perhaps this is why the authors recommend lymphadenectomy despite the fact that their findings suggest it is not rational.–S.S.H.] ◀

Management of Testicular Tumors in Children remains controversial. Timothy B. Hopkins, Norman Jaffe, Arnold Colodny, J. Robert Cassady and Robert M. Filler[4] (Harvard Med. School) reviewed the records of 43 children aged less than 16 who were discharged in 1930–75 with a diagnosis of testicular tumor. All patients with malignancy were followed for at least 20 months and all but 2 for at least 3 years or to death. Thirty tumors were of germinal origin. There also were 7 sarcomas and 2 interstitial cell tumors.

Twenty patients had embryonal cell carcinoma. The mean age at diagnosis was 18 months, and the average duration of symptoms was 3.2 months. All 3 patients presenting with metastases before 1957 have died. Five of 9 having only orchiectomy died within 3–18 months. All 11 patients having retroperitoneal adenectomy were found to have stage A disease, and all survived. Ten children received actinomycin D, and 1 received Thiotepa. Nine received irradiation in addition. Two of 3 children with teratocarcinoma have survived. One with choriocarcinoma has died. All 6 children with benign teratoma have done well. Both patients with interstitial cell tumors have survived. Two of 5 patients with rhabdomyosarcoma of the testicular tunics had only orchiectomy and died of metastases.

Any solid scrotal mass in an infant must be considered malignant until proved otherwise. All patients in this series who received combination therapy for embryonal cell carcinoma have survived. Radical inguinal orchiectomy, extended unilateral retroperitoneal lymphadenectomy and adjuvant chemotherapy are recommended at present. Che-

(4) J. Urol. 120:96–102, July, 1978.

motherapy consists of actinomycin D, vincristine and cyclophosphamide, given in repeated courses for 2 years. Radiotherapy is withheld if the removed nodal tissue is negative for tumor.

Cryptorchidism and Testicular Neoplasia. The risk of malignancy in the undescended testis is 35 times that in the scrotal testis, and the abdominal testis is at 4 times greater risk than is the inguinal. The contralateral eutopic testis is affected in 20% of unilateral cryptorchid patients who develop testis tumors. Rufus Green, H. Herr, M. Scott, M. Cosgrove, H. Schwarz and D. Martin[5] reviewed 20 cases of cryptorchid testis seen in 1966–76 in which testicular neoplasia subsequently developed.

Seminoma accounted for 64% of cases. Average age at presentation was 35 years. Most cases were stage 1. Over 60% of the intra-abdominal tumors were seminomas. Seven patients had had orchiopexy, 6 after age 10 years. There were 2 cases of male pseudohermaphroditism in the series. The most common symptom was pain at the tumor site. A mass was present in about two thirds of intra-abdominal cases. Average delay in diagnosis was 7.7 months. Patients with stage 1 and stage 2 seminomas were treated by radical orchiectomy or resection; adjuvant chemotherapy was used in stage 3 cases. Adenectomy was performed for nonseminomatous stage 1 and stage 2 tumors, and chemotherapy was added if nodes were involved. Two patients with stage 3 lesions died before operation, and another died a year after operation and radiotherapy with multiple metastases. All patients with stage 1 lesions and two thirds of those with stage 2 tumors were without disease at 3 years. Half the patients with stage 3 disease were alive at 1 year on chemotherapy. Survival was inversely related to stage of disease. All stage 3 deaths were in patients with nonseminomatous tumors.

An aggressive approach is indicated in the evaluation and management of postpuberal cryptorchid males. Intra-abdominal exploration is indicated if inguinal and retroperitoneal search is nonrevelatory. The patient seen after puberty with a unilateral intra-abdominal undescended testis should undergo orchiectomy. Orchiectomy is also recommended for the postpuberal patient under age 50 who is

(5) J. Natl. Med. Assoc.'70:659–664, September, 1978.

seen with a unilateral undescended testis in the inguinal region.

▶ [Although the precise incidence of cancer in abdominal and inguinal cryptorchid testis is unknown because of inadequate data, the figures given in this review are reasonable. We agree with the recommendation that cryptorchid testes be removed in postpuberal patients younger than 45 to 50.–S.S.H.] ◀

Lymphangiography in Patients with Malignancy in a Nondescended Testicle. The undescended testis is at increased risk of developing malignant change. K. Jonsson, S. Wallace, B. S. Jing, L. E. Boyle and D. E. Johnson[6] (M. D. Anderson Hosp., Houston) report experience with lymphangiography in 23 patients with malignancy in an undescended testis. The mean age of the patients was 36 years. Eight patients had had orchiopexy at age 4–35 years, with failure in 3 of them. The histologic diagnosis was seminoma in 14 patients, embryonal cell carcinoma in 6, mixed tumors in 2 and teratoma in 1. Bilateral pedal lymphangiography was performed on all patients.

Lymphangiography was normal in 15 patients. The other 8 showed evidence of node metastases: in the lumbar region in 3, the external iliac nodes in 1 and the lumbar and iliac nodes in 4 (Fig 69). Two orchiopexy patients had lumbar and iliac node metastases, and 1 had lumbar node metastases. Metastases were in continuity between the iliac and lumbar areas in all but 1 of the patients operated on.

The lymphangiographic findings were confirmed by node dissection or biopsy in 10 patients. Microscopic foci of disease were found in lumbar nodes in 2 patients with normal lymphangiograms. The 1 patient with epididymal involvement had a normal lymphangiogram. Follow-up of 11 patients showed survival times of 1.5–13 years. Three patients died of metastatic disease 1.5–4 years after diagnosis; these had lumbar node metastases at initial lymphangiography.

Iliac or lumbar metastases may occur alone or in combination, independent of previous orchiopexy, in patients with malignancy in an undescended testis. Node metastases in these cases are not necessarily the same as in malignancy in a normally descended testis. The iliac nodes may be the only site of metastasis. Surgeons and radiother-

(6) J. Urol. 119:614–617, May, 1978.

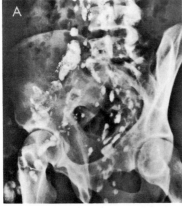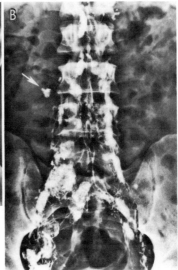

Fig 69.—Lymphangiograms of man, aged 35, with seminoma in right undescended testis, showing metastasis in **(A)** right external and common iliac region and **(B)** right lumbar node *(arrow)*.
(Courtesy of Jonsson, K., et al.: J. Urol. 119:614–617, May, 1978.)

apists must be aware of this possibility so that the node dissection may be extended to the ipsilateral iliac region or the nodes may be included in the treatment portal.

▶ [The fact that malignancies in cryptorchid testes metastasize more frequently to iliac lymph nodes than do tumors in normally descended testes is of obvious clinical significance to surgeons and radiotherapists. However this report should be interpreted somewhat cautiously since in only 2 patients with iliac metastasis were the lymphangiographic findings histologically confirmed. –S.S.H.] ◀

Sandwich Therapy in Testis Tumor: Current Experience. Donald F. Lynch, Jr., Larry P. McCord, Thomas C. Nicholson, Jerome P. Richie and C. Rolland Sargents[7] (Naval Regional Med. Center, San Diego, Calif.) evaluated sandwich therapy, that is, lymphadenectomy preceded and followed by irradiation, in 13 patients with stage A and B nonseminomatous testis tumors, treated during 1970–73 and followed for 3–6 years. All cases were considered resectable. An average of 2,000 rad was given

(7) J. Urol. 119:612–613, May, 1978.

to the entire abdomen over 28 days after orchiectomy, and bilateral retroperitoneal lymphadenectomy was done within a week. An average of 2,500 rad was delivered through a restricted port excluding the kidneys about 3 weeks postoperatively. An average of 4,200 rad was delivered to the mediastinum and supraclavicular areas several weeks after the completion of abdominal radiotherapy.

Eleven patients (84%) have survived at least 3 years without recurrent disease. One stage B patient died of metastatic disease, and 1 died of peritonitis after lymphadenectomy. One patient died of complications of thrombocytopenic purpura 3 years after treatment, without evidence of tumor at autopsy. In 1 patient, a scrotal abscess developed during postoperative radiotherapy, and 1 had chylous ascites that persisted several months postoperatively. Forty-eight patients have now received sandwich therapy, and 83% of them survived at least 3 years (table). Eight have died of metastases or as a direct result of treatment complications. Serious complications required the discontinuance of therapy in at least 5 patients. Commonly encountered complications have included ejaculatory impotence, bone marrow depression, prolonged ileus, superficial wound infections and weight loss.

Sandwich therapy of stage A and B nonseminomatous testis tumors has been superseded by more effective approaches that give equal if not superior survival results with fewer potential serious side effects. A new protocol, based on thorough retroperitoneal lymphadenectomy in conjunction with chemotherapy, is being designed, with

THREE-YEAR SURVIVAL RATES—TOTAL SERIES (1958–74)

Pathologic Stage

	A	B	Total No. Pts. (%)
	No. Pts. (%)	No. Pts. (%)	
Teratoca.	15/16 (93)	6*/9 (67)	
Embryonal cell Ca	15/18 (83)	4/5 (80)	
	30/34 (88)	10*/14 (71)	40/48 (83)

*Includes 1 operative death.

radiotherapy reserved for the adjunctive treatment of recurrent tumor or unresectable retroperitoneal metastases.

▶ [The fact that the original proponents of "sandwich therapy" are now abandoning the technique speaks for itself. We prefer modified bilateral retroperitoneal lymph node dissection with adjuvant chemotherapy in patients with positive nodes. We do not always use chemotherapy, as has been recently recommended, when the nodes are negative.–S.S.H.] ◀

Evolution of Mature Teratoma from Malignant Testicular Tumors. Evolution of a purely mature teratoma in a patient with a previously diagnosed fully malignant testicular cancer appears to be increasing in frequency. Waun Ki Hong, Robert E. Wittes, Steven T. Hajdu, Esteban Cvitkovic, Willet F. Whitmore and Robert B. Golbey[8] (Mem'l Sloan-Kettering Cancer Center, New York) reviewed the case reports of 12 patients with malignant germ cell tumor of the testis seen during 1969–1976 in whom metastases composed of fully mature teratoma subsequently developed. In 4 patients, biopsy specimens showed the existence of malignant tumor at the same site at which mature teratoma was found months or years later. The patients had a variety of primary germ cell tumors in the testis and received radiotherapy and/or chemotherapy, as well as surgical treatment. The teratomas most often contained cartilage, ciliated respiratory-type epithelium, enteric epithelium and neurogenic tissue. Only 1 patient has died with known persistent cancer.

Treatment may selectively kill the malignant cells in these cases, leaving the differentiated component behind to appear later as a fully mature teratoma. Alternately, treatment may directly induce the evolution of malignant cells into highly differentiated, benign-appearing tissues, or benign evolution may be an inherent property of the malignant cell. The latter hypothesis is supported by much experimental evidence in the murine teratocarcinoma system. These various possibilities are not mutually exclusive, and two or more might be operative in a given patient. Although the appearance of mature teratoma does not imply certain cure, it seems to be a favorable prognostic sign. Eleven living patients have been at risk for a median of 25 months from the time of diagnosis of cancer and 16 patients from the initial diagnosis of mature teratoma.

(8)   Cancer 40:2987–2992, December, 1977.

Continued therapy has been recommended for most patients in whom mature teratoma has developed.

▶ [It is interesting that in 3 patients the mature teratomas were enlarging before excision. Theoretically, if the cellular physiology of the evolution of a teratoma from a germ cell cancer can be determined, the principles could be used to treat many forms of malignancy.–S.S.H.] ◀

Direct Inhibitory Effect of Estrogen on Leydig Cell Function of Hypophysectomized Rats. The testes both produce and bind sex steroids, and an intratesticular short-loop regulation of testicular function by these hormones is possible. A. J. W. Hsueh, M. L. Dufau and K. J. Catt[9] (Natl. Inst. of Health) examined the influence of estrogen on various parameters of testicular function under controlled conditions of gonadotropin stimulation in the rat. Hypophysectomized rats treated with FSH were used as a model of stable, known gonadotropin input. Follicle-stimulating hormone reduces the regression in testicular function that follows hypophysectomy and enhances LH-induced testosterone production in hypophysectomized rats. Immature hypophysectomized rats received 50 µg FSH for 7 days, with or without diethylstilbestrol (DES). The increase in testis weight produced by FSH injections was inhibited by concomitant DES treatment.

Follicle-stimulating hormone induced an increase in testicular LH-human chorionic gonadotropin (hCG) receptor content. The increase in ^{125}I-iodo-hCG binding was unaffected by daily injections of 0.01–0.2 µg DES, but it was prevented by treatment with 5 and 20 µg. No significant change in ^{125}I-iodo-FSH binding capacity was observed in any group. Both basal production and hCG-stimulated testosterone production by the decapsulated testis were increased markedly by daily FSH treatments. Diethylstilbestrol caused reductions in testosterone production, with or without concomitant FSH. The inhibitory effect of DES was dose dependent. A decrease in cyclic adenosine monophosphate production was seen in FSH-treated rats. The inhibitory action of FSH was not affected by DES.

A direct inhibitory effect of estrogen on steroidogenic responses has been demonstrated in the Leydig cells of hypophysectomized immature rats. It is accompanied by a decrease in testis weight and is partially correlated with a

(9) Endocrinology 103:1096–1102, October, 1978.

decrease in LH-hCG receptor content. It may be hypothe-
sized that when LH induces an increase in intratesticular
concentration of testosterone, the FSH-inducible aromatiz-
ing enzymes in Sertoli cells convert androgens to estrogens, which then diffuse outside the tubule compartment
into Leydig cells to inhibit further testosterone production
by the Leydig cells. This intratesticular short-loop feedback system may be important in maintenance of normal
testicular function.

▶ [The confirmation of a direct nonpituitary inhibitory effect of estrogen on
testosterone production by Leydig cells and the previous discovery of estrogen receptors in the Leydig cells suggest that estrogens may have a direct
testicular effect in men with prostatic cancer. Indeed it has been shown in
such men that testicular androgen production decreases before serum LH
falls (Dorner et al., Endokrinologie 66:221, 1975).–S.S.H.] ◀

FERTILITY AND STERILITY

Low-Dose Cortisone for Male Infertility. Low-dosage
cortisone is a popular treatment for men with idiopathic
infertility. David T. Uehling[1] (Univ. of Wisconsin) compared the effectiveness of low-dosage cortisone therapy
with that of low-dosage thyroid therapy in 38 men seen in
1970–75 with a primary complaint of infertility. The wives
lacked irremediable factors for failure to conceive, and
there had been no pregnancies after 2 years of unprotected
intercourse. The sperm count was below 40 million per ml.
Patients received 2.5 mg cortisone 4 times daily or 1 grain
thyroid USP daily. Most patients received both treatments.
Ten patients subsequently received 5 mg cortisone acetate
for 6 months.

Pregnancy followed thyroid therapy in 4 of 30 courses
and cortisone therapy in 7 of 33. Pretreatment and posttreatment mean sperm counts did not differ significantly
(table). Differences in motility before and after treatment
also were insignificant. The 11 patients whose wives conceived had a higher mean pretreatment count, but no
higher pretreatment motility, than those whose wives did
not become pregnant. No pregnancies occurred in the wives
of 10 patients given 5 mg cortisone, and mean counts and
motility were unchanged in this group.

(1) Fertil. Steril. 29:220–221, February, 1978.

	Pretreatment	After cortisone treatment	After thyroid treatment
RESULTS OF TREATMENT WITH LOW-DOSAGE CORTISONE OR THYROID*			
Mean count (million/ml)	12 ± 8	13 ± 7	11 ± 9
Mean motility (%)	45 ± 2	43 ± 2	44 ± 2

*Values are means ± SD.

It is difficult to select empirical therapy for idiopathic infertility. Progress in treatment will most likely result from narrowing the idiopathic group by delineating specific endocrine abnormalities.

▶ [This is one of the few controlled studies of the effect of treatment on idiopathic male infertility. It clearly shows that low-dose cortisone treatment is not effective therapy for this condition. The results are not surprising since there is no good scientific rationale for this approach.–S.S.H.] ◀

Quantitative Evaluation of Testicular Biopsies before and after Operation for Varicocele. Testicular biopsies in patients with varicocele have shown bilaterally decreased spermatogenesis, desquamation of germ cells and increased numbers of Leydig cells. Svend G. Johnsen and Peter Agger[2] (Copenhagen) obtained testicular biopsy specimens before and about 1 year after operation for varicocele from 39 men, 15 operated on for scrotal symptoms (group A) and 24 treated for infertility, which had been present for a mean of 4 years (group B). Respective mean ages were 22 and 33 years. Varicocele had disappeared in all patients but 2 at follow-up, and in these it was considerably smaller than before operation. Mean follow-up was 14 months.

There were 2 cases of Del Castillo syndrome (Sertoli cell-only syndrome) in group B. All the other patients initially showed desquamation of immature germ cells in the tubular lumen, disorganized spermatogenesis, Leydig cell hyperplasia and various degrees of hyalinization of the basement membranes. Only 3 patients had mean biopsy scores in the normal range, compared with 6 after operation. Scores were highest in group A. The overall mean score

(2)   Fertil. Steril. 29:58–63, January, 1978.

increased significantly after varicocelectomy; nearly all the increase was in group B. Total sperm counts and numbers of abnormal head forms decreased to about the same extent in the two groups after operation. The wives of 4 group B patients became pregnant during follow-up. These patients did not differ from the others before or after operation.

The most marked change after varicocelectomy is found in sperm motility, and varicocele may have an effect on the function of the epididymis and ductus deferens. These organs share the vascular supply of the testis. Few testes in this series became perfectly normal after operation for varicocele. The duration and size of the varicocele appear to have little effect on the state of the testicular tissue or the changes in it after operation.

Varicocele: Review of Radiologic and Anatomical Features in Relation to Surgical Treatment is presented by J. T. Hill and N. Alan Green[3] (Norwich, England). A variety of radiologic procedures has been used to evaluate venous drainage of the testis and scrotum in patients with varicocele, including left renal venography, and at the time of operation by ascending venography and retrograde contrast injection into prominent varicosities. Left renal venography was performed in 26 patients by percutaneous femoral vein puncture. Operative venography was performed at the time of definitive surgery through the scrotum into the most prominent vein or veins. Retrograde injection of contrast medium into the cremasteric vein was often difficult or impossible. Crosscommunication with veins on the right side of the pelvis through retropubic or sacral veins was a constant finding at operative venography.

A total of 48 patients with a mean age of 30.1 years were studied. Of these, 26 were subfertile. Only 2 had bilateral varicoceles. Eleven of 22 patients classified by operative venography had cremasteric varicocele. Only 3 of 14 patients having left renal venography as well had the pure cremasteric vein type of varicocele. Twelve patients had all the studies; only 1 patient had a pure cremasteric varicocele with conclusive evidence of cremasteric valve incompetence. Five patients were unclassified (Table 1). The re-

(3) Br. J. Surg. 64:747–752, October, 1977.

TABLE 1.—Overall Classification of 48 Varicoceles

Type of varicocele	No. of cases
Internal spermatic	18
Cremasteric	15
Mixed	10
Unclassified	5
Total	48

sults of left renal venography are summarized in Table 2. Representative results of retrograde cremasteric venography are shown in Figures 70 and 71. Of 24 patients followed for 5 years or more after surgery, 83% were completely cured of their varicocele. Seven of 13 subfertile patients had an improved sperm count and satisfactory motility after surgery, and the wives of 6 of these patients have conceived. No patient had complications of radiologic study or surgery apart from temporary hematoma formation.

Cremasteric varicoceles appear to be less common than has been thought. The surgical treatment of varicocele should be tailored to the etiology in each case. If incompetence is found in the cremasteric vein, it seems logical to ligate these radicals both in the scrotum and at the junction of the definitive vein with the inferior epigastric vein. Incompetence of the internal spermatic vein calls for ligation at the level of the deep inguinal ring. In subfertile patients, those with gross internal spermatic vein reflux and those with evidence of contralateral venous communi-

TABLE 2.—Results of Left Renal Venograms

No. of cases	Retrograde filling of internal spermatic vein
5	None
6	Slight
10	Free
5	Gross
Total 26	Significant reflux 15/26

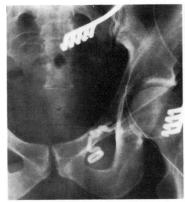

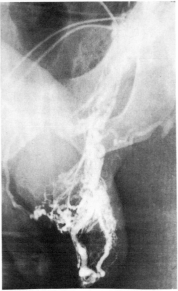

Fig 70 (above).—Retrograde cremasteric venogram showing valvular competence.

Fig 71 (right).—Retrograde cremasteric venogram showing valvular incompetence and free flow into the scrotum.

(Courtesy of Hill, J. T., and Green, N. A.: Br. J. Surg. 64:747–752, October, 1977.)

cation in the abdomen, a case can be made for ligation at the entry of the vein into the left renal vein.

▶ [It is encouraging to see two serious studies of this common clinical problem. *If* there was no bias in patient selection *and* the scoring of the biopsies was done in a blind fashion, the Johnsen and Agger study is extremely important because it objectively documents that varicocele repair has a favorable effect on the germinal epithelium.

Hill and Green state that varicocele may be due to either cremasteric or internal spermatic vein pathology and recommend that treatment be individualized. We feel this work is interesting but still use high ligation of the internal spermatic vein in all cases because: (1) It seems to work well; (2) the studies used by the authors are too cumbersome for routine practice; and, (3) it is difficult to interpret their data because many patients had "mixed" lesions and all subjects did not undergo the same studies.–S.S.H.] ◀

Prolactin and Testosterone Levels in Plasma of Fertile and Infertile Men. Male infertility has proved difficult to treat, although some success has been achieved with gonadotropin and androgen therapy. Prolactin remains something of an enigma in men, although there now is considerable evidence that it can have profound effects both on the testis and on the accessory sex glands of animals. C. G. Pierrepoint, B. M. John, G. V. Groom, D. W. Wilson and J. G. Gow[4] routinely measured the concentrations of testosterone and prolactin in plasma of men attending an infertility clinic. The infertile men studied had been unsuccessful, over a period of at least 2 years, in impregnating their wives in whom no abnormality had been found. The median sperm count for infertile men, excluding azoospermic men, was 6.9×10^6, compared with a figure of 64×10^6 for fertile men. The concentrations of both testosterone and prolactin were significantly lower in infertile than in fertile men.

A reduction in testosterone in oligospermic men was confirmed in this study. The finding of a low level of prolactin is of interest in view of the fact that this hormone has been incriminated in cases of hypogonadism and impotence. Whether the low levels of prolactin and testosterone in infertile men are related is a matter for speculation, although some interesting data from Rubin et al. (1976) strongly suggest that this could be so. It may well be that, in concert with other hormones, a deficiency in prolactin is as detrimental as an excess.

▶ [The documentation of lower than normal concentrations of testosterone in a group of infertile men is neither new nor surprising since some of these men have small abnormal testicles. The claim of a low serum prolactin is intriguing because several authors have reported a high serum prolactin in infertile men. A more detailed analysis of this data might help to determine whether this finding is confined to a small subgroup of infertile men.–S.S.H.] ◀

Vas Deferens Reanastomosis without Splints and without Magnification. Intravasal splints usually have been used in the attempt to reanastomose the vas deferens after bilateral vasectomy, and magnification is sometimes advocated. Sperm cells have returned to the semen in 38–94% of reported cases, with pregnancy rates of 10–60%.

Richard G. Middleton and David Henderson[5] (Univ. of Utah) describe a simple technique of bilateral vas deferens reanastomosis in which no splint or magnification of the operative site is used. The operation is performed with general or spinal anesthesia.

(4) J. Endocrinol. 76:171–172, January, 1978.
(5) J. Urol. 119:763–764, June, 1978.

TECHNIQUE.—Short anterior scrotal incisions are made bilaterally, and all scar tissue is excised at the vasectomy site until healthy, patent segments of the vas deferens are obtained. A short piece of 000 plain gut is inserted into each lumen to guide placement of 6–0 or 7–0 prolene sutures through the edges of the proximal and distal segments of the vas at two points. Usually an additional suture is placed at each 90-degree quadrant, through the muscular edges only (Fig 72). The scrotal incisions are closed with fine chromic gut sutures.

A total of 110 vas reanastomoses were done bilaterally in vasectomy patients during 6¹/₂-years. In the 72 cases available for analysis, there were 28 (39%) pregnancies. Another 25 men (35%) have postoperative sperm counts of over 25 million per cc. Fifteen men have low counts and are not considered hopeful cases. There were 4 total failures, with aspermia present 6 months or more after operation. The outcome does not appear to be related to the interval between vasectomy and vas reanastomosis.

The results of vas reanastomosis appear to have improved with elimination of intravasal splints. Vas reanastomosis performed with regular instruments can be fairly successful. A somewhat optimistic success rate of 74% was obtained in the present series.

▶ [It is most impressive that the author was able to obtain a 95% patency rate without microsurgery. The controversy over surgical technique for vasovasostomy will not be easy to settle. However it is clear that experienced surgeons, regardless of techniques, are not reporting patency rates greater than 80% and pregnancy rates of 40% or more. We prefer a microscopic two-layer anastomosis. There is strong evidence from other investigators that the fertility rate decreases if the interval between vasectomy and reanastomosis is long.–S.S.H.] ◀

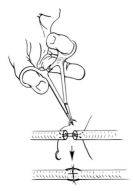

Fig 72.—Technique of vas deferens reanastomosis without splints or magnification of site. (Courtesy of Middleton, R. G., and Henderson, D.: J. Urol. 119:763–764, June, 1978.)

Antigenic Status of Semen from the Viewpoints of the Female and Male. Alan E. Beer and William B. Neaves[6] (Univ. of Texas Health Sciences Center, Dallas) observe that the female reproductive tract is repeatedly inoculated with millions of immunogenetically alien spermatozoa through sexual activity, as well as other cell types including leukocytes and the complex, protein-containing seminal plasma. Much evidence supports the premise that immunologic approaches in experimental animals can reduce fertility, and there is growing suspicion that infertility due to immune responses to seminal antigens may occur in human females and males. However, there is no unequivocal evidence of such an association.

Antibody activity in the serum correlates poorly with activity in reproductive tract secretions. Some subjects exhibit antisperm antibodies in the cervical mucus but not in the blood. Both IgA and IgG are present in cervical mucus; the concentration of IgA is far greater than that in the serum. The complement components necessary for sperm antibody to be cytotoxic for spermatozoa normally are absent from cervical mucus. Semen has potent anticomplement activity and contains substances that are markedly inhibitory to the elicitation and expression of immune responses. Local antibodies could arm macrophages and enhance phagocytic clearing of spermatozoa from the genital tract, be cytotoxic to sperm, prevent sperm from adequately penetrating the cervical mucus, interfere with capacitation or cross-react with components of oocytes and inhibit their development. Local antibodies might, under normal circumstances, play an important role in sperm selection.

Some manifestations of spermatozoal autoimmunity appear to constitute a sufficient cause of otherwise unexplained infertility in men. An example is the presence of sperm-immobilizing antibodies in seminal plasma at levels producing a rapid loss of motility of most ejaculated spermatozoa. Only a minority of infertile men, however, show any evidence of sensitization to spermatozoal autoantigens. This suggests that autoimmunity may be involved in extremely few cases of male infertility. However, it may sim-

(6) Fertil. Steril. 29:3–22, January, 1978.

ply reflect the limited ability of existing tests to detect varied manifestations of functionally significant spermatozoal autoimmunity.

▶ [This is a scholarly review of a controversial topic. We agree that current evidence suggests most male infertility is not immunologic and that in infertile men with serum or semen antibodies, a cause-and-effect relationship has not been established. At this time immunologic testing of infertile men is a research rather than a practical clinical approach.–S.S.H.] ◀

Bipolar Needle for Vasectomy: I. Experience with the First 1,000 Cases. All present techniques of vasectomy are those of open surgery. Stanwood S. Schmidt (Univ. of California, San Francisco) and Michael J. Free[7] (Battelle Northwest Labs., Richland, Wash.) evaluated a battery-powered, bipolar electrocoagulator in over 1,000 vasectomies done since 1973. The instrument destroys only the mucosa and one or two muscle cell layers of the vas, leaving adequate live muscle to serve as a source of fibroblasts to seal off the lumen. The procedure is done under local anesthesia in the office. The vas is exposed high in the scrotum and divided, and the bipolar needle is inserted to a depth of 2 mm on the urethral side and withdrawn as the current is applied over 1 to 2 seconds. The needle is then placed 4 to 5 mm on the testicular side for 3 to 4 seconds of electrocoagulation.

Subjects aged 20–68 years were treated with the bipolar needle. The electrocoagulation-fascial interposition technique has never failed in the senior author's hands. Spermatic granuloma of the vas occurred with equal frequency with use of the bipolar needle and a monopolar electrode. The bipolar needle is an effective instrument for sealing the cut vas without ligatures, clips or other devices. A trial is planned to evaluate a modified needle with a sharpened tip for sealing the undivided vas. Should it prove to be successful, the technique and equipment for percutaneous vasectomy will be available.

Recanalization Rate Following Methods of Vasectomy Using Interposition of Fascial Sheath of Vas Deferens. Many studies have shown recanalization rates ranging from 0 to 3.3% after partial vasectomy by the ligation method (table). Julius O. Esho and Alexander S.

---

(7) Fertil. Steril. 29:676–680, June, 1978.

COMPARISON OF RECANALIZATION RATE WITH METHOD OF VASECTOMY

Reference	No. Pts.	Method	Recanalization No. (%)
Kase and Goldfarb	500	Ligation and fulguration	2 (0.4)
Bennett	500	Double clip ligation	0
Kaplan and Huether	2,197	Ligation	26 (1.2)
Livingstone	3,200	Ligation	4 (0.1)
Leader and associates	2,227	Ligation	6 (0.3)*
	484	Double clip ligation	0 *
Rees	754	Ligation	3 (0.4)
Barnes and associates	929	Ligation	6 (0.6)
Moss	565	Double clip ligation	3 (0.5)
	1,300	Fulguration and fascial sheath interposition	0
Klapproth and Young	800	Ligation	8 (1.0)
	200	Fulguration and fascial sheath interposition	0
Schmidt	150	Ligation	5 (3.3)
	135	Ligation and fascial sheath interposition	0
	1,000	Fulguration and fascial sheath interposition	0
Current study	497	Ligation	6 (1.2)
	820	Fulguration and fascial sheath interposition	0

*Plus 1 with method unknown.

Cass[8] (St. Paul-Ramsey Hosp., St. Paul, Minn.) compared rates with the ligation and the fulguration-fascial sheath interposition methods in 1,527 patients having bilateral partial vasectomy to achieve sterility during 1970–76. The ligation method was used in 564 patients and the fulguration method with fascial sheath interposition in 963. Patients submitted semen specimens for analysis 8 weeks after vasectomy.

The clearance rate of sperm after vasectomy was about the same in the two groups. There was a 1.2% incidence of recanalization with the ligation method, but no proved case of recanalization with the fulguration-fascial sheath method. One of the patients who underwent the latter method had sperm present $8^{1}/_{2}$ months after the procedure and insisted on having a repeat vasectomy. A sperm granuloma was found on one side. Attempts to demonstrate recanalization by contrast injection from one end of the excised vas length failed. Two semen examinations after the repeat vasectomy were negative. A tender mass was present at the vasectomy site in 2.1% of patients after ligation and in 0.5% after fulguration with fascial sheath interposition.

A small but definite recanalization rate follows the vas

(8) J. Urol. 120:178–179, August, 1978.

ligation method of partial vasectomy and is eliminated by
interposing a fascial sheath between the divided ends of
the vas. It is not clear why the vas ligation method without
fascial sheath interposition is still being used.

▶ [A recent survey showed that 50% of the malpractice suits against urologists studied related to vasectomy. Therefore it is important to the physician
as well as the patient that this operation be done properly. Claims and
counterclaims notwithstanding, two principles seem to be emerging. First,
methods that do not necrotize the end of the vasa are advisable and, second, fascial sheath interposition is beneficial.–S.S.H.] ◀

**Evolution of Properties of Semen Immediately Fol-
lowing Vasectomy.** Spermatozoal motility often has not
been considered in the outcome of vasectomy. Pierre
Jouannet and Georges David[9] (Paris) analyzed sperm numbers and motility parameters in 76 men before and after
vasectomy. The men had an average of about 5 spermio-
grams before vasectomy and an average of 2.7 after operation. Semen properties were examined as a function of ejaculation frequency in 68 subjects.

Average semen volumes were 4.03 ml before and 3.37 ml
after vasectomy; the decrease was significant. A decrease
in number of spermatozoa was correlated primarily with
the number of ejaculations. In nearly all cases the total of
spermatozoa in all semen samples obtained after vasectomy was clearly lower than the average in one ejaculation
before operation. Motile spermatozoa were never observed
after the 15th postoperative day. Reappearance of motile
spermatozoa after that time was an almost certain sign of
a defect in the vas block or of recanalization of the vas deferens. Reappearance of motile spermatozoa was observed
in only 1 patient after total asthenospermia had been observed. An incomplete vas block was confirmed by a regular increase in numbers of motile and immotile spermatozoa over three successive examinations. Histologic study
after the second operation showed formation of new canals
within the scar tissue surrounding the vas stumps on one
side.

Biologic control of a vasectomy should be assured by a
spermiogram performed 15–20 days after operation and repeated 1 week later. The absence of motile spermatozoa at
both studies should be sufficient proof of successful opera-

(9) Fertil. Steril. 29:435–441, April, 1978.

tion. An increase in number of spermatozoa and reappearance of motile spermatozoa are almost certain indications of a defect in the block or of recanalization of the vas deferens.

▶ [Although several similar studies have been conducted, this is the most complete and carefully done. The absence of motile sperm after the 15th postoperative day seems to be an indication of successful vasectomy.—S.S.H.] ◀

INTERSEXUALITY

The Phenotypic Expression of Selective Disorders of Male Sexual Differentiation is reviewed by Patrick C. Walsh and Claude J. Migeon[1] (Johns Hopkins Hosp.). Male sexual differentiation can be divided into: 1) an early phase (1st trimester) during which time chromosomal factors direct differentiation of the testes and hormonal factors induce regression of the müllerian ducts and virilization of the wolffian ducts and external genitalia; and 2) a late phase (2nd and 3rd trimesters) during which there is growth of the external genitalia and descent of the testes (table). Any disturbance during embryogenesis may be reflected as a disorder of sexual differentiation. The genetic sex of the individual, established at fertilization, directs differentiation of the gonadal sex and this in turn determines establishment of phenotypic sex in which the mature male or female phenotype is developed.

Chromosomal abnormalities may lead to failure of testicular differentiation, preventing normal male phenotypic development. Complete deletion of the Y chromosome results in a 45×0 complement and bilateral streak ovaries (Turner's syndrome); deletion of the short arm of the Y chromosome will produce the same phenotype.

A defect in any of several enzymes involved in conversion of cholesterol to testosterone may result in inadequate testosterone synthesis in utero and incomplete virilization, with absence of the wolffian ducts and female differentiation of the urogenital sinus and external genitalia. Testicular feminization and 5α-reductase deficiency are two clinical syndromes in which testosterone synthesis is normal

(1) J. Urol. 119:627–629, May, 1978.

SEQUENTIAL STEPS IN MALE SEXUAL DIFFERENTIATION

Event	Determinant	Approximate Time (wks.)
Testicular differentiation	Chromosomal (X,Y,?autosome)	6–9
Müllerian regression	Müllerian-inhibiting substance	9–11
Wolffian duct differentiation	Testosterone	10–11
Virilization of the urogenital sinus and external genitalia	Dihydrotestosterone	10–15
Growth of penis, descent of testes	Androgen (secreted by fetal Leydig cells under pituitary gonadotropin regulation)	23–37

but the target organ response to androgen is defective. A defect in müllerian-inhibiting substance secretion or action results in the persistence of müllerian structures in otherwise normal males. Defective timing of endocrine function of the fetal testes may result in *both* incomplete virilization and inadequate müllerian regression. Patients with a defect in pituitary gonadotropin production may present with microphallus and undescended testes.

Investigation of these patients for accurate diagnosis includes family history; evaluation of genetic sex by nuclear chromatin studies, fluorescent staining of the Y chromosome, karyotyping and, if possible, H-Y antigen; biochemical studies of urine and plasma steroids before and after human chorionic gonadotropin stimulation; x-ray and endoscopic studies of urogenital sinus and internal duct structures; laparotomy and gonadal biopsy; and assessment of androgen action.

▶ [The pathophysiologic mechanisms by which selective disorders of male sexual differentiation may produce specific phenotypes are outlined in this review. However, in many patients the classical findings are not present because the defect is incomplete, thus producing a spectrum of clinical findings. Consequently, one must be cautious in using phenotypic expression as a diagnostic tool.—Patrick C. Walsh] ◀

Endocrine Studies in Male Pseudohermaphroditism in Childhood and Adolescence. M. O. Savage, J. L. Chaussain, D. Evain, M. Roger, P. Canlorbe and J. C.

Job[2] (Paris) reviewed the findings in 50 cases of male pseudohermaphroditism and XY karyotype in subjects aged 6 months to 20 years. Thirty-two subjects were prepuberal, and the other 18, 10 of whom developed gynecomastia, were puberal. There were four pairs of siblings and 3 other children with a family history of deficient masculinization in the series. Male pubic hair ratings alone were used to stage puberal development. Plasma hormone concentrations were determined by radioimmunoassays. The binding capacity of serum testosterone-estradiol binding globulin (TeBG) for tritium-labeled dihydrotestosterone (^{3}H-DHT) was measured by steady-state polyacrylamide gel electrophoresis. The luteinizing hormone releasing hormone (LH-RH) test was done after overnight fast; 0.1 mg LH-RH per sq m was used.

A definite etiology was established in 6 subjects; 4 had mixed gonadal dysgenesis and 2 had defective testosterone biosynthesis. No definite cause was found in 44 subjects. The mean basal plasma testosterone concentration was slightly elevated in stage 1 subjects over age 1 year and markedly elevated in subjects in stages 2–4. The mean basal plasma estrone and estradiol concentrations were elevated in stage 1 subjects. Puberal subjects had elevated serum TeBG binding capacities and markedly elevated basal LH values. The peak FSH concentration was elevated in stage 2 and stage 3 subjects. Dihydrotestosterone concentrations after human chorionic gonadotropin administration were 0.3–1.28 mg/ml in puberal subjects. Prepuberal subjects had plasma androstenedione concentrations of 0.12–0.9 ng/ml.

Deficient testosterone synthesis accounted for only a small proportion of cases of male pseudohermaphroditism in this series. Mixed gonadal dysgenesis associated with a peripheral XY karyotype was present in 8%. In the other cases, a disorder of androgen function at the target areas is suggested. This may involve a defect of conversion in the target cell of testosterone to dihydrotestosterone or a defect of androgen binding to the intracellular receptor protein. Significant testosterone, estradiol, TeBG binding capacity and LH elevations in puberal subjects with male pseudo-

ˑhermaphroditism appear to be characteristic of androgen unresponsiveness. The finding of slight elevations of testosterone and estradiol concentrations before puberty suggests that some of these changes may be present from early childhood.

▶ [Male pseudohermaphroditism is a disorder in which 46 XY individuals with bilateral testes fail to masculinize normally. Because patients with mixed gonadal dysgenesis lack a normal 46 XY karotype, they should not be classified as male pseudohermaphrodites. Thus, a definite diagnosis using endocrine studies was made in only 2 of 46 subjects. However, indirect evidence for androgen resistance at the target organ was provided by the finding of elevated plasma testosterone *and* LH levels in some pre- and postpuberal patients. Assessment of androgen action in cultured fibroblasts is necessary. See the next article.—Patrick C. Walsh] ◀

Studies on Pathogenesis of Incomplete Forms of Androgen Resistance in Man. A variety of disorders has been characterized in which hereditary male pseudohermaphroditism is due to resistance to androgen action at a cellular level. James E. Griffin and Jean D. Wilson[3] (Univ. of Texas Southwestern Med. School, Dallas) assessed the affinity and turnover of the specific dihydrotestosterone binding protein in fibroblasts cultured from genital skin from a variety of control subjects and 4 patients with incomplete hereditary male pseudohermaphroditism due to androgen resistance (incomplete testicular feminization and Reifenstein syndrome). In some studies, the uptakes of both ^{3}H-testosterone and ^{3}H-dihydrotestosterone were determined in parallel.

The amount of dihydrotestosterone binding in the four mutant cell strains was low, but both the affinity of the protein for dihydrotestosterone, assessed by the concentration at which half-maximal binding occurred, and the turnover of the binding protein were within normal limits. No qualitative abnormality was detected.

These findings suggest that the mutations in incomplete testicular feminization and the Reifenstein syndrome affect the synthesis of dihydrotestosterone binding protein. If the interpretation is correct that the mutations in these two disorders involve the regulation (direct or indirect) of the activity and/or synthesis of the binding protein, it can also be inferred that more than one gene is involved in the reg-

(3)   J. Clin. Endocrinol. Metab. 45:1137–1143, December, 1977.

ulatory process. Although it is not certain whether intermediate levels of dihydrotestosterone binding represent primary manifestations of the mutant genes in question, it is likely that at least two genes (allelic or nonallelic) are involved in the regulation of dihydrotestosterone binding.

▶ [Defects in the amount or function of the androgen receptor appear to be responsible for the complete (testicular feminization syndrome) and incomplete (Reifenstein syndrome, incomplete testicular feminization syndrome) forms of androgen resistance. This article suggests that a defect in the synthesis of the receptor may be responsible for the incomplete forms of androgen resistance. However, the factors that normally regulate the synthesis of the receptor are unclear.–Patrick C. Walsh] ◀

Microphallus: Clinical and Endocrinologic Characteristics. Terry D. Allen[4] (Univ. of Texas Health Science Center, Dallas) reviews the findings in 15 males with small, normally formed external genitalia. Nine had simple microphallus alone, while 6 had associated central nervous system defects. The size of the penis was somewhat age related but was always smaller than normal standards. In the 6 patients aged less than 4 years the stretch length never exceeded 2 cm. The testes were invariably small and usually cryptorchid or, in 4 cases, impalpable. Anomalies of the epididymis and vas were seldom observed. Testicular biopsy showed infantile testes regardless of the patient's age. The patients usually were behind the average for their peer group in growth, and retarded bone age was documented in several instances. Pubertal development always was incomplete. The body configuration remained boyish or became gynecoidal, and obesity was a frequent problem. The pubic hair distribution was more female than male. Erections occasionally occurred, but no patient reported ejaculations.

Four patients had identifiable syndromes; 2 had Kallmann's syndrome, and 1 each had Robinow's syndrome and Prader-Willi syndrome. One patient had developmental retardation with inability to vocalize, and 1 had arrested hydrocephalus. The serum testosterone level was low in the face of low serum luteinizing-hormone (LH) and FSH levels. All 6 patients tested responded to infusion of LH-releasing hormone. The serum testosterone level rose on treatment with human chorionic gonadotropin (hCG).

(4) J. Urol. 119:750–753, June, 1978.

The penis exhibited an ability to respond well to testosterone, especially in younger patients, in whom a doubling in size in 3 months was not unusual. A normal penile size could result, but equivalent responses were not seen in previously untreated adults.

Unfortunately, testosterone therapy alone does not promote testicular development in these patients. Long-term gonadotropin therapy might be better, but no overt testicular enlargement has been seen during long-term hCG stimulation tests. Continuous therapy with LH-releasing hormone might be more physiologic. Experience with LH and FSH therapy in hypogonadotropic hypogonadism suggests that endocrine therapy may hold out hope for fertility in some of these patients.

Clinical and Endocrinologic Evaluation of Patients with Congenital Microphallus. Patrick C. Walsh, Jean D. Wilson, Terry D. Allen, James D. Madden, John C. Porter, William B. Neaves, James E. Griffin and Willard E. Goodwin[5] report the findings in 8 prepuberal boys with isolated microphallus. All patients, aged 3–13 years, had a stretched penile length below the 3d percentile. Five had a family history of a similar disorder, and 3 of these had a relative with documented hypogonadotropic hypogonadism. The patients were compared with 6 normal boys, 4 with bilateral cryptorchidism, 1 with anorchia and 1 adult with hypogonadotrophic hypogonadism. Some patients had hormone measurements made before and after administration of human chorionic gonadotropin (hCG).

The testes were incompletely descended in all cases. Five patients had undetectable plasma luteinizing hormone (LH) and a normal plasma testosterone response to hCG. Three of these had maternal relatives with evidence of hypogonadotropic hypogonadism. The other 2 patients were brothers.

Three patients had detectable plasma LH values and no significant rise in plasma testosterone level after hCG treatment. One of these patients had normal plasma gonadotropin values after LH-releasing hormone administration. Plasma cortisol responses to ACTH were normal, and plasma androstenedione values after hCG also were nor-

(5) J. Urol. 120:90–95, July, 1978.

mal. Testicular biopsy in 2 of the 3 patients showed normal immature testes. When tissue removed at circumcision from 2 patients was incubated with radioactive testosterone, dihydrotestosterone formation was normal.

Three and possibly 5 of these 8 patients with microphallus have hypogonadotropic hypogonadism, while the others are sporadic cases. A primary testicular disorder appears to be responsible in the latter cases. Microphallus appears to result from defective testicular function in the 2d and 3d trimesters of gestation as a result of either defective gonadotropin secretion or defective androgen synthesis.

▶ [There appears to be general agreement that microphallus results from defective testicular function in the 2nd and 3rd trimesters of gestation as the result of either defective gonadotropin secretion (most common) or defective androgen synthesis. However, there is still uncertainty about the management of the newborn with microphallus. Although treatment with testosterone in infancy can induce enlargment of the penis, it is unknown whether growth at adulthood will be satisfactory. If a decision is made to rear the patient as male, then treatment with testosterone should be initiated at an early age. However, until long-term follow-up information on these patients is available, the wisdom of this treatment plan is uncertain.–Patrick C. Walsh] ◀

Serum Testosterone during Oral Administration of Testosterone in Hypogonadal Men and Transsexual Women. It is generally thought that oral testosterone is ineffective, but an increase in serum testosterone level and a clinical effect have been observed after the oral administration of testosterone to men (Johnsen et al., 1974), a study which used tablets having a very small crystal size. Marie Fogh, Charles S. Corker, Helen McLean, Ivan Bruunshuus Petersen, John Philip and Niels E. Skakkebaek[6] (Copenhagen, Denmark) studied the effect of oral testosterone on serum testosterone levels in 3 subjects with low androgen production evaluated over a 2-week period. Tablets of 25, 50 and 200 mg of crystal size 2–5 μm were administered at 9 A.M. and 9 P.M. from days 2 to 11 of the study. Seven similar subjects received tablets of crystal size 125–400 μm, and serial blood samples were collected. Serum testosterone levels were measured by radioimmunoassay. Most subjects were hospitalized but ambulatory; all received a normal diet.

In the first study, a significant rise in serum testoster-

(6) Acta Endocrinol. (Kbh.) 87:643–649, March, 1978.

one levels occurred with 25 mg testosterone in small crystal size. Maximal serum levels occurred 2 hours after administration. Repeated administration did not have a cumulative effect on serum levels. In the second study, peak serum testosterone levels of up to 1,200 ng/100 ml occurred 1–5 hours after administration. Five subjects maintained serum levels within the normal male range for 5–8 hours. Two subjects exhibited poorer responses.

It is possible to maintain serum testosterone levels in the normal male range in subjects with low androgen production with orally administered testosterone, but convenience to patients must be balanced against the cost and possible side effects of the large doses required. Androgen-induced hepatomas have been reported with the use of synthetic anabolic steroids, and the possibility of similar effects occurring with large doses of oral testosterone should not be overlooked.

▶ [Following the oral administration of enormous amounts of crystalline testosterone (15 to 30 times the normal daily testicular production rate) plasma testosterone levels remained in the normal range for 5 to 7 hours. However, because the cost of such therapy would probably be unacceptably high and the possibility of inducing liver disease uncertain, it is unlikely that this form of treatment will ever be practical.–Patrick C. Walsh] ◀

Construction of Male Genitalia in the Transsexual, Using a Tubed Groin Flap for the Penis and a Hydraulic Inflation Device.

Penile reconstruction in trauma patients and transsexuals has left much to be desired in both function and appearance. Charles L. Puckett and Joseph E. Montie[7] (Univ. of Missouri) recently used a groin flap and the Scott penile inflation device to construct male genitalia in a transsexual conversion.

Woman, 29, who had been living as a man for about 2 years and had had a complete mastectomy, was considered psychiatrically to be a stable candidate for conversion. A total hysterectomy with salpingo-oophorectomy was performed, with delay of a McGregor groin flap. After construction of a glans, a Brantly-Scott penile inflation device was inserted in the left labium majus. A testicular prosthesis was inserted into the right labium majus. The clitoris was divided and inserted into the base of the penis, and the remaining labia minora were partially resected and sutured to create a scrotal fusion. The seven operations were followed by an inflation regimen. The patient reports erection ad-

(7) Plast. Reconstr. Surg. 61:523–530, April, 1978.

equate for sexual function and consistent orgasm during intercourse, with an actual increase in clitoral sensation.

The groin flap measured about 13 × 27 cm; the extra length was required to avoid the pubic hair. The flap was initially tubed as a delay procedure. When the distal part was inset at the mons pubis, an 8-cm segment was "de-epithelized" and split into two tails and, after dissection of a tunnel into each labium majus, the tails were inserted to simulate the legs of the corpora cavernosa. An arterial delay was done before complete division. Glans "sculpturing" then was undertaken by removal of a series of diamond-shaped sections of skin of unequal length. Two months were allowed for healing before implantation of the prosthesis. At the time of insertion of the Scott prosthesis, only one inflation tube was utilized. Seven to ten pumps have produced satisfactory erections. The seven operations were done over a 9-month period, but scheduling problems resulted in about 3 months' delay. The appearance and function of the constructed genitalia have been quite satisfactory.

► [This article contradicts all of my preconceived concepts. The authors have fashioned a cosmetically acceptable phallus and have wisely avoided constructing a penile urethra. Rather, they have inserted a Brantley-Scott prosthesis and have relocated the clitoris to the undershaft of the penis to provide erotic stimulation. It will be interesting to determine whether excellent functional results will be obtained in other patients.–Patrick C. Walsh] ◄

Male Transsexualism: Review of Genital Surgical Reconstruction is presented by U. G. Turner III, Richard F. Edlich and Milton T. Edgerton[8] (Univ. of Virginia). Transsexuals represent one variety of gender dysphoria, presenting with normal genitalia and a chronic, intense desire for change to the opposite sex. The condition is 4 times more frequent in men. Patients should be at least 18 years old and must have substantital living experience in the cross-gender role before surgery is planned. True self-reliance in living as a woman should be demonstrated. Hormone therapy is begun before castration. The use of penile skin as a pedicle flap to line the vagina eliminates the disadvantages of free skin grafting. Rish has used an inverted penile tube pedicle to form both vagina and external genitalia in a single operation. The authors now use a V-Y monsplasty to minimize avascular necrosis of the penile tube vaginal lining.

Fifty-three male transsexuals have had primary genital surgery at the authors' institution since 1971. All 47 fol-

(8) Am. J. Obstet. Gynecol. 132:119–133, Sept. 15, 1978.

lowed at 1 year felt positive about the conversion and reported relief from anxiety and improved social adjustment. Psychologic testing has substantiated these claims. No patient has regretted the change in gender, and no psychotic breakdowns or suicides have occurred. Many patients required secondary corrective surgery for postoperative complications, but the primary operative results have improved with experience. The most common late complication is vaginal vault stenosis. Nineteen patients have had secondary operations for vaginal stenosis and shortening. Meatoplasty can easily correct stenosis of the urethral meatus. Nonsurgical complications can potentially result from long-term hormone therapy. Further attention should be given to sexual function and response after genital surgery for transsexualism.

MISCELLANEOUS

Therapy of Gonorrhea: Comparison of Trimethoprim-Sulfamethoxazole and Ampicillin. The sudden emergence of penicillinase-producing organisms throughout the world in 1975 and 1976 mandated a search for new, nonpenicillin drugs for treatment of gonococcal infections. Fred R. Sattler and Joel Ruskin[9] (Kaiser-Permanente Med. Center, Los Angeles) treated 89 men who had gonococcal urethritis with either 320 mg trimethoprim (TMP) plus 1,600 mg sulfamethoxazole (SMX) twice daily for 2 days or 3.5 gm ampicillin plus 1 gm probenecid in a single dose. Forty-three patients received TMP-SMX and 42 received ampicillin. The patient group was representative of the younger members of a health plan population. Patient compliance with both regimens appeared to be excellent.

Forty-one of 43 patients treated with TMP-SMX were cured; the 2 in whom treatment failed responded to retreatment with ampicillin. All but 1 of the 42 patients given ampicillin were cured. The exception was successfully retreated with TMP-SMX. Adverse side effects of the drugs were minimal and their frequency was similar in the two treatment groups. Postgonococcal urethritis occurred

(9) J.A.M.A. 240:2267–2270, Nov. 17, 1978.

in 2.3% of the TMP-SMX group and 9.5% of the ampicillin group, not a significant difference. All isolates studied were considered to be susceptible to TMP-SMX. The only clearly ampicillin-resistant isolate produced penicillinase; the patient had received TMP-SMX and had been cured. Lack of response could not be related to higher pretreatment minimum inhibitory concentrations (MICs). The MICs of TMP-SMX showed no strict correlation with those of ampicillin.

Trimethoprim-sulfamethoxazole in a dosage of 4 tablets twice daily for 2 days was comparable with single-dose ampicillin therapy in treatment of gonococcal urethritis in men in this study. The drug was well tolerated and patient compliance was excellent. Trimethoprim-sulfamethoxazole is effective in treatment of pharyngeal infection, and because of its activity against *Chlamydia trachomatis* in vitro, it should also be capable of reducing the incidence of chlamydia-associated postgonococcal urethritis.

▶ [Since the authors found that treatment of gonorrhea with trimethoprim-sulfamethoxazole is rather effective, it seems reasonable to use this combination to treat patients who are allergic to penicillin.–S.S.H.] ◀

Corpus Cavernosum-Corpus Spongiosum Shunts have become an accepted means of correcting idiopathic priapism to minimize thrombosis of the corpora and eventual impotence. Nonoperative methods rarely resolve true idiopathic priapism. Corpus cavernosum-saphenous vein shunts are difficult to perform and to keep open. William Graham Guerriero[1] (Baylor College of Medicine, Houston) reviewed 22 corpus cavernosum-corpus spongiosum shunts performed in the past 8 years. These shunts are technically much simpler to perform and tend to remain open long enough for the acute process to resolve. The anastomosis can be placed anywhere in the penis but should not be placed too far posteriorly; a site in the region of the distal deep bulb of the urethra is probably best.

PROCEDURE.—The patient is placed in the lithotomy position, and a vertical incision is made in the midline over the corpus spongiosum. The corpus spongiosum and corpus cavernosum are mobilized in such a manner that the anastomosis between the corpus cavernosum and corpus spongiosum can be made as far dorsal on the corpus cavernosum and corpus spongiosum as is pos-

(1) Surg. Gynecol. Obstet. 146:792–794, May, 1978.

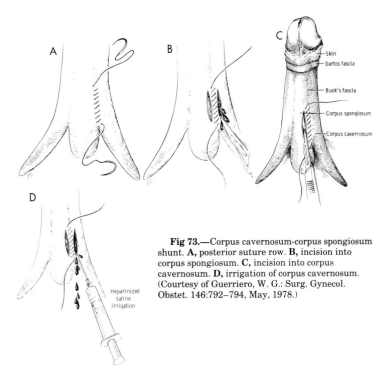

Fig 73.—Corpus cavernosum-corpus spongiosum shunt. **A,** posterior suture row. **B,** incision into corpus spongiosum. **C,** incision into corpus cavernosum. **D,** irrigation of corpus cavernosum. (Courtesy of Guerriero, W. G.: Surg. Gynecol. Obstet. 146:792–794, May, 1978.)

sible. A posterior row of sutures is placed in the corpus cavernosum and corpus spongiosum (Fig 73); a double-armed 3–0 or 4–0 suture is used. A linear incision 4–6 cm long is then made in the corpus spongiosum, not penetrating into the urethra, followed by a parallel incision on the other side of the suture row in the corpus cavernosum. The corpus cavernosum is irrigated with heparinized saline solution. The upper and then the lower half of the ventral portion of the shunt is then sutured. If light compression does not easily produce detumescence, the other side is incised and a second shunt created. Suprapubic cystostomy is useful in those patients who require penile compression as compression over a firm catheter may result in necrosis of the skin or urethritis.

If this procedure is followed in the creation of a corpus cavernosum-corpus spongiosum shunt, the patient is usually able to ambulate rapidly and be discharged from hospital after several days.

▶ [We initially use the Winter's procedure in all priapism patients except those with sickle cell disease in whom it does not work. Corpus cavernosum-corpus spongiosum shunting which is nicely described by the author is attempted if the glans-corpus cavernosum shunt fails.–S.S.H.] ◄

5-Fluorouracil Urethral Suppositories for the Eradication of Condyloma Acuminata. Condylomata acuminata of the urethra and urethral meatus are difficult to eradicate. Podophyllin is irritating and cytotoxic to intraurethral mucosal surfaces, and surgical methods can result in stricture. Dretler and Klein (1975) reported the successful use of 5-fluorouracil (5-FU) cream in treating intraurethral condylomata. George W. Weimar, Leo A. Milleman, Thomas L. Reiland and David A. Culp[2] (Univ. of Iowa) devised a method of forming a 5-FU intraurethral suppository that can be inserted to a predetermined depth into the urethra. The suppositories are made from fluoracil powder incorporated in a polyethylene glycol base, which is poured into a mold, lubricated with mineral oil and refrigerated. Suppositories are inserted twice daily for 7–10 days.

Twelve patients of both sexes were treated successfully with 5-FU suppositories. No significant complications have occurred on follow-up for 4 months to 3 years. Spillage has caused superficial scrotal ulcerations, but this has not been a problem. No urethral strictures or systemic side effects have occurred. There have been no changes in blood cell or platelet counts during or after treatment. Meatal skin irritation is minimized by wearing an athletic support with gauze over the meatus and washing the meatus 15 minutes after insertion of the suppository. Denuded mucosa heals spontaneously after sloughing of condyloma lesions. Panendoscopy is not advised until 3–4 weeks after treatment.

The action of 5-FU on rapidly metabolizing cells makes it ideal for use in patients with condyloma acuminata. The use of 5-FU in intraurethral suppositories has effected good patient compliance and more accurate dosing. Both males and females may be treated in this way.

► [This and Wallin's report (Br. J. Vener. Dis. 54:240, 1977) confirm the original observation of Dretler and Klein that 5-FU cream is effective treatment for condylomata acuminata. The suppository devised by the authors may facilitate drug delivery to the urethra. However we still prefer to use podophyllin as the initial treatment modality.–S.S.H.] ◄

(2) J. Urol. 120:174–175, August, 1978.

Prostatic Maldevelopment in the Prune Belly Syndrome: Defect in Prostatic Stromal-Epithelial Interaction. The prune belly syndrome consists of deficient abdominal wall musculature, cryptorchidism and urinary tract anomalies. Lack of development of the epithelial elements of the prostate is a recognized but poorly described feature of the syndrome. D. P. Deklerk and W. W. Scott[3] (Johns Hopkins Hosp., Baltimore) reviewed the findings from autopsy in 8 patients with well-documented prune belly syndrome, 3 with posterior urethral valves, 4 with isolated bilateral undescended testes after full-term pregnancy and 2 with so-called pseudo-prune belly syndrome.

Prostatic epithelial elements were absent in 5 of 8 patients with prune belly syndrome and glands were sparse in another patient; in 1 patient no prostatic tissue was demonstrated at autopsy. The prostatic utricle was markedly dilated and showed squamous metaplasia in 3 of 5 patients, where it was clearly identified. In 2 cases the membranous urethra was completely obstructed; 3 patients had membranous urethral stenosis, 1 had mid-penile urethral stenosis and 1 had prostatic urethral stenosis. One patient had associated megalourethra. One patient with pseudo-prune belly syndrome had hypoplastic prostatic epithelial elements and 1 had membranous urethral stenosis and a prominent posterior urethral squamous cyst, probably originating from the prostatic utricle. Prostatic glandular elements were compressed and dilated but otherwise normal in the patients with posterior urethral valves. In cases of cryptorchidism the prostate was normally developed.

The etiology of prune belly syndrome remains obscure. Primary mesenchymal developmental arrest, presumably of the lateral and possibly of the intermediate mesoderm, at 5–10 weeks' gestation seems likely. Lack of induction of prostatic epithelium by the urogenital sinus mesenchyme may be a result of this poor mesenchymal development. The lack of development is not attributable to a testicular defect or to compression from massive posterior urethral distention. Whether the mesenchymal induction defect in prune belly syndrome has a hormonal component is conjectural.

▶ [The lack of development of the prostatic epithelial elements may account

(3) J. Urol. 120:341–344, September, 1978.

for the typical radiographic picture of a funneled posterior urethra seen in this syndrome and may also in part account for voiding abnormalities. We have found that α-adrenergic blockade improves the voiding flow rate in such boys.—S.S.H.] ◄

Paratesticular Rhabdomyosarcoma in Childhood. Paratesticular rhabdomyosarcoma is one of the most common nongerminal neoplasms affecting the scrotal contents of children and adolescents. Inguinal lymph node metastases are unusual because the scrotal skin is only occasionally infiltrated by tumor; spread to para-aortic and renal hilar nodes is more likely. R. Beverly Raney, Jr., Daniel M. Hays, Walter Lawrence, Jr., Edward H. Soule, Melvin Tefft and Milton H. Donaldson[4] (Intergroup Rhabdomyosarcoma Study Committee) reviewed the findings in 20 children with paratesticular rhabdomyosarcoma entered in the Intergroup Rhabdomyosarcoma Study. Patients with completely resected tumors and no regional lymph node involvement (group I) generally received similar combination chemotherapy, and half received local radiotherapy as well. Patients with local residual and/or regional nodal tumor (group II) and those with gross residual tumor or distant metastases received similar radiotherapy but differing chemotherapy, as did patients with gross residual tumor (group III) or distant metastases (group IV). Radiotherapy consisted of at least 4,000 rad in 4 weeks. Chemotherapy was continued for 1–2 years or until relapse.

The average age at diagnosis was 9 years. Radical orchiectomy was done initially in 19 patients, and 15 patients had retroperitoneal exploration. Twelve of these had a retroperitoneal node dissection. One of six lymphangiograms was falsely negative. Retroperitoneal nodal tumor was found in 6 patients. Thirteen patients had localized, clinically completely resected tumors after surgery. Only three primary tumor specimens showed evidence of venous invasion. Sixteen of 18 evaluable patients were free from disease a median of 23 months after treatment was begun. Both patients who died of tumor had distant metastases as the initial sign of relapse. All evaluable patients with completely resected tumor were free from disease at a median of 24 months.

(4) Cancer 42:729–736, August, 1978.

Nodal Metastasis in Childhood Paratesticular Rhabdomyosarcoma

Source	Number of patients	Number with retroperitoneal node dissection or biopsy	Number positive	Number with inguinal node biopsy	Number positive
References 4,7,9,11,13,14,16,19–21, 25,35,36,40,42	58	31	14 (45%)	8	2 (25%)
Current Series	20	15	6 (40%)	5	0
Total	78	46	20 (43.5%)	13	2 (15.4%)

There is a high likelihood of retroperitoneal nodal involvement in patients with paratesticular rhabdomyosarcoma (table). It is not clear whether a unilateral or bilateral retroperitoneal adenectomy should be performed, but at least any suspicious contralateral nodes should be evaluated by frozen section study. Doses of radiation on the order of 4,000–5,000 rad in 4–5 weeks may be necessary to prevent local recurrence despite concomitant systemic chemotherapy when residual microscopic disease is present. Temporary transplantation of the other testis in the thigh before scrotal radiotherapy should be considered.

► [Aggressive multimodality therapy has dramatically improved survival rates in children with rhabdomyosarcoma. Pediatric oncologists should participate in the care of such patients. Because of the high incidence of nodal metastasis and the lack of definitive data, we do lymph node dissection despite the fact that chemotherapy and radiotherapy may cure patients with positive nodes.–S.S.H.] ◄

Spermatic Cord Sarcoma in Adults. Most extratesticular scrotal tumors in the spermatic cord, epididymis or testicular tunics are derived from the cord structures. Thirty per cent of these tumors are malignant and most of these are mesenchymal sarcomas. Pramod C. Sogani, Harry Grabstald and Willet F. Whitmore, Jr.[5] (Memorial Sloan-Kettering Cancer Center) report the findings in 6 adults with spermatic cord sarcomas other than embryonal rhabdomyosarcoma. The age range was 35–62. Five tumors were intrascrotal and 1 was inguinal. There were 3 fibrosarcomas, 2 liposarcomas and 1 malignant fibrous histiocytoma. Five patients had radical orchiectomy initially and 1 had no residual tumor at orchiectomy and hemiscrotectomy 2 months after simple excision. One patient had ex-

(5) J. Urol. 120:301–305, September, 1978.

tensive local radiotherapy and 2 received chemotherapy. None had distant metastases at follow-up. Two patients were seen with locally recurrent disease after initial treatment elsewhere. Five patients have survived for up to 4 years, whereas 1 is dead at 16 years without distant metastases.

Sarcoma of the spermatic cord must be considered in the differential diagnosis of all solid tumors superior to the testis and below the internal inguinal ring. Wide excision of apparently involved adjacent soft tissues is indicated in conjunction with radical orchiectomy. Retroperitoneal node dissection, radiotherapy and chemotherapy are indicated for the treatment of embryonal rhabdomyosarcoma. The value of these measures for other sarcomas of the spermatic cord is uncertain. Node dissection is advised for children and young adults having a highly malignant sarcoma with a known tendency for lymphatic spread, such as myxosarcoma. The rate of lymphatic spread is low for liposarcoma, fibrosarcoma and leiomyosarcoma.

▶ [This report suggests that liposarcomas, fibrosarcomas and leiomyosarcomas of the spermatic cord are much less likely to exhibit distant metastasis than embryonal sarcomas and rhabdomyosarcomas. Therefore aggressive local excision may be sufficient treatment. However, Banowsky and Shultz (J. Urol. 103:628, 1970) concluded from a literature review of 101 cases, which included only 7 rhabdomyosarcomas, that 29% of patients had distant metastasis. Therefore, careful staging is clearly indicated and more aggressive therapy may be necessary.–S.S.H.] ◀

The following review articles are recommended to the reader:

Caldamone, A. A., and Cockett, A. T. K.: Infertility and genitourinary infection, Urology 12:304, 1978.

Fauer, R. B., Goldstein, A. M. B., Green, J. C., and Onofrio, R.: Clinical aspects of granulomatous orchitis, Urology 12:416, 1978

Hoppman, H. J., and Fraley, E. E.: Squamous cell carcinoma of the penis, J. Urol. 120:393, 1978.

Javadpour, N.: The National Cancer Institute experience with testicular cancer, J. Urol. 120:651, 1978.

Levitt, S. B., Kogan, S. J., Engel, R. M., Weiss, R. M., Martin, D. C., and Ehrlich, R. M.: Impalpable testis: Rational approach to management, J. Urol. 120:515, 1978.

Odell, W. D., and Swerdloff, R. S.: Abnormalities of gonadal function in men, Clin. Endocrinol. 8:149, 1978.

Savage, M. O., and Grant, D. B.: The incomplete male, Arch. Dis. Child. 53:701, 1978.

Shapiro, S. R., and Bodai, B. I.: Current concepts of the undescended testis, Surg. Gynecol. Obstet. 147:617, 1978.

Current Literature Quiz

The significant advances described in this YEAR BOOK introduce new diagnostic and therapeutic procedures useful for treating conditions seen frequently in your practice. The following questionnaire will test your familiarity with the current literature. The page references direct the reader to the articles containing the answers to the quiz.

1. What are the ingredients of the Brompton mixture that is used to manage chronic pain? (p. 74)
2. How effective is platinum in the treatment of advanced bladder cancer? (p. 228)
3. Do recurrent bladder tumors usually occur at the site of the primary tumor? (p. 224)
4. On what basis should bladder tumors in patients under age 40 be treated? (p. 220)
5. What are the presenting symptoms, signs and radiologic appearance of pediatric lower urinary tumors? (p. 219)
6. What is an alternative to the Leadbetter operation to restore continence after loss of the female urethra? (pp. 290—296)
7. What are the latest methods to predict potential invasiveness of stage A bladder cancer? (p. 222)
8. What is the latest treatment for diabetes insipidus? (p. 78)
9. What are the acute and chronic treatments of the syndrome of secretion of antidiuretic hormone? (p. 77)
10. Is there any objective evidence that varicocele repair affects the germinal epithelium? (p. 314)
11. Is the cremasteric or internal spermatic vein abnormal in patients with varicocele? (p. 315)
12. What are the most foolproof methods of doing a vasectomy? (pp. 321—323)
13. What is the latest therapy for nonspecific genital ulcers? (p. 286)
14. How should you treat a patient who requests surgery for impotency but also has significant difficulty voiding? (p. 283)
15. How can you prevent inadequate release of chordee during hypospadias repair? (p. 288)
16. How long after total occlusion of the main renal artery does the kidney remain viable? (pp. 99 and 100)

17. What is the newest treatment for renal artery stenosis? (pp. 93 and 94)
18. What is the newest treatment for intrarenal arteriovenous fistulas? (p. 105)
19. What is the incidence of renal vein valves detached during angiography? (p. 101)
20. What is the current mortality rate 1 year after renal transplantation? (p. 156)
21. What new immunosuppressive agent may represent an important advance in renal transplantation? (pp. 154 and 155)
22. What is the effect of blood transfusions on renal allograft survival? (pp. 146—152)
23. What is the value of urine cytology in detecting renal allograft rejection? (p. 141)
24. How well does flow rate during preservation correlate with postoperative function in transplanted kidneys? (p. 140)
25. What is the incidence and mechanism of nephrotoxicity due to contrast agents? (pp. 67—69)
26. What is a rapid method to detect urate nephropathy? (p. 59)
27. What is the best management of bilateral renal cell carcinomas? (pp. 109 and 115)
28. What factors predict relapse and survival in Wilm's tumor? (p. 120)
29. What is the etiology of complete (testicular feminization syndrome) and incomplete (Reifenstein syndrome) testicular feminization syndrome? (p. 327)
30. What is the etiology and management of microphallus? (p. 329)
31. What is the role of continuous ambulatory peritoneal dialysis? (p. 135)
32. What is the mechanism and treatment of impaired growth of children with renal tubular acidosis? (p. 128)
33. What is the mechanism of renal osteodystrophy? (pp. 130—133)
34. What is the etiology of the concentrating defect in pyelonephritis? (p. 19)
35. What is the etiology of acute epididymitis? (p. 26)
36. What is the major etiologic factor in nongonococcal urethritis? (p. 25)
37. What are the bacterial counts in women immediately after intercourse? (p. 12)
38. What is the incidence of residual tumor on needle biopsy after external radiation for carcinoma of the prostate? (p. 266)
39. What is the reliability of bone marrow acid phosphatase in the staging of prostatic cancer? (pp. 254—256)

40. Is the mortality of prostatic cancer the same in whites and blacks and has it changed in the past 40 years? (p. 253)
41. Does prophylactic administration of kanamycin prevent bacteriuria after transurethral prostatectomy? (p. 269)
42. What is the success rate of phosphate therapy and its mechanism of action in calcium stones? (p. 36)
43. What is the success rate and mechanisms of action of thiazide therapy in calcium stones? (p. 37)
44. What is the importance of uric acid in calcium stones? (p. 38)
45. What is the management of struvite stones with acetohydroxamic acid? (pp. 40—42)
46. What is the mechanism of secondary hyperoxaluria? (pp. 43—44)
47. What is the effect of pregnancy on nephrolithiasis? (p. 45)
48. What are the electrolyte disturbances seen with various diversions? (p. 179)
49. What is the recommended urologic management in prune belly syndrome? (pp. 201—204)
50. What is the effect of reflux on renal growth? (pp. 186—189)
51. What are the effects of pregnancy on renal failure? (p. 158)
52. What is the incidence and nature of sexual dysfunction after proctocolectomy? (p. 277)
53. How useful is computerized tomographic scanning in the localization of pheochromocytomas and adrenal adenomas? (p. 81)
54. What is the most common serious late complication of bilateral adrenalectomy for Cushing's syndrome? (p. 82)
55. Which patients with a colovesical fistula should have a two-stage repair? (pp. 239 and 241)
56. What is the psychiatric profile of women with the urethral syndrome? (p. 242)
57. What methods are in vogue to treat interstitial cystitis? (pp. 244—247)
58. How effective is low-dose cortisone therapy in the treatment of male infertility? (p. 313)
59. What happens if the peritoneum is not closed after laparotomy? (p. 71)
60. How is chyluria treated? (p. 72)
61. At what age should orchiopexy be performed in patients with prune belly syndrome? (p. 302)
62. What is the status of "sandwich" therapy for testicular tumors? (p. 309)

Subject Index

Index to Authors